Integrative Pain Management

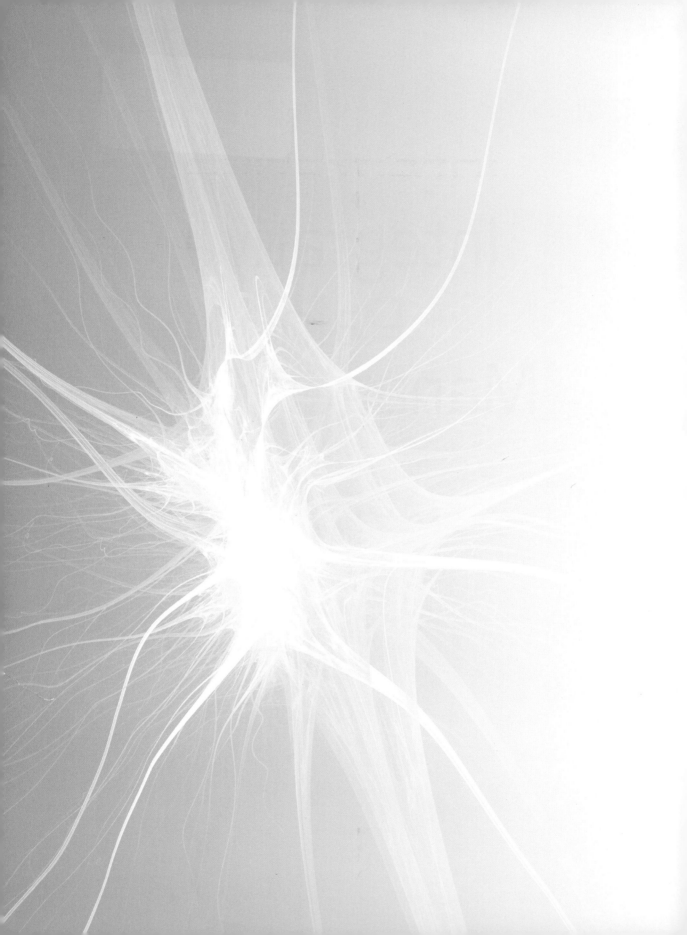

Integrative Pain Management

Massage, Movement, and Mindfulness Based Approaches

Editors

Diana L. Thompson and Marissa Brooks

Forewords by
Wayne B. Jonas - John Weeks

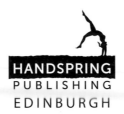

HANDSPRING
PUBLISHING
EDINBURGH

HANDSPRING PUBLISHING LIMITED
The Old Manse, Fountainhall,
Pencaitland, East Lothian
EH34 5EY, Scotland
Tel: +44 1875 341 859
Website: www.handspringpublishing.com

First published 2016 in the United Kingdom by Handspring Publishing

ISBN 978-1-909141-26-1

British Library Cataloguing in Publication Data
A catalogue record for this book is available from the British Library

Library of Congress Cataloguing in Publication Data
A catalog record for this book is available from the Library of Congress

Notice
Neither the Publisher nor the Author assumes any responsibility for any loss or injury and/or damage to persons or property arising out of or relating to any use of the material contained in this book. It is the responsibility of the treating practitioner, relying on independent expertise and knowledge of the patient, to determine the best treatment and method of application for the patient.

All reasonable efforts have been made to obtain copyright clearance for illustrations in the book for which the authors or publishers do not own the rights. If you believe that one of your illustrations has been used without such clearance, please contact the publishers and we will ensure that appropriate credit is given in the next reprint.

Commissioning Editor Sarena Wolfaard
Copy Editor Lee Bowers
Project Manager Nora Naughton
Design and illustration by Bruce Hogarth, kinesis-creative.com
Index by Annette Musker
Typeset Myriad Pro Regular, DSM Soft
Printed Pulsio, Bulgaria

The
Publisher's
policy is to use
paper manufactured
from sustainable forests

CONTENTS

Forewords   vii

Contributors   ix

Introduction   xi

Glossary   xix

1   Overview of integrative health care and pain   Bonnie B. O'Connor   1

2   Anatomy and neurobiology of pain   Ruth Werner and Geoffrey M. Bove   15

3   Pain theory and models for treatment   Bronwyn Lennox Thompson   31

4   Massage therapy: general   Susan Davis   47

5   Massage therapy: lymphatic techniques   Lisa Santoro   65

6   Massage therapy: scars and pain   Nancy Keeney Smith   79

7   Structural bodywork and fascial balancing   Lauren Christman and Richard Polishuk   95

8   Osteopathic techniques   Matthew D. Stewart   111

9   Functional taping   John Balletto   127

10   Traditional Chinese medicine bodywork: Tui Na   Benjamin Apichai   145

11   Interactive movement practices: the Feldenkrais Method®   Nancy Haller and Patricia Buchanan   159

12   Interactive movement practices: Trager   Jack Blackburn   173

13   Yoga therapy   Neil Pearson   187

14   Tai Chi/Qi Gong   Chenchen Wang and Ramel Rones   203

15   Mindfulness-based interventions   Carolyn McManus   219

16   Body awareness and pain   Cynthia J. Price and Wolf Mehling   233

17   Pathways to integrative clinical care   Marissa Brooks and Diana L. Thompson   249

Index   267

FOREWORDS

Foreword

The time for integrative pain management has arrived. The use of drugs as the main and often only approach to pain, especially the overuse of opioids, is at a tipping point. The United States President, the American Medical Association, the Institute of Medicine, the US military, the Center for Disease Control and others have all called for better management of pain and reduction in drug use – but what will be offered instead? Behavioral and integrative approaches are the logical and evidence-based alternatives. After searching for a path into mainstream care, pain is the tip of the spear for self-care, non-pharmacological and integrative approaches – perfect timing for this book.

But this is not just a book written to fill a void. *Integrative Pain Management* is a carefully and thoughtfully constructed guide on how to help patients after the drugs have been taken away. Here we have a dozen methods with pain reducing abilities. The book describes methods from massage therapy, tissue manipulation, taping, movement approaches such a yoga and Qi-Gong, and mind–body approaches such as mindfulness and body awareness. The introductory chapters provide a clear introduction to the neurobiology and theoretical models of pain. The book ends with a step-wise guide for setting up and operating an integrated team for pain management.

One of the most unique and valuable features of this book is the richness and logic of the information provided. Each chapter provides both quantitative data from the most recent research, and qualitative descriptions of patients' experiences. In addition, a history of each method is provided with the addition of recent developments in practice and a description of how the method is applied. The figures and illustrations are clear, well selected and carefully placed. Reading it provides not only information but better understanding. By the time this book is published, three large systematic reviews of massage for musculoskeletal, surgical and cancer pain will have been published showing good evidence for their use, adding to the knowledge base summarized here.

But can these approaches get into the mainstream? I see patients in an integrative pain medical clinic. Patient after patient comes in seeking rapid relief and new methods. When I speak to them about the options in this book, they are often interested, but our healthcare system cannot effectively deliver them. Reimbursement for massage and meditation therapies is thin or non-existent. Most pain centers are not trained in how to work in an integrative fashion, resulting in poorly targeted therapies. Patients often need help in engagement and lose interest in therapies that require time and new skills.

It is my hope that there will now be accelerated adoption of integrative approaches to pain in health care. As our health care system and the public awake to these methods and their growing evidence, this book should become a mainstay in that adoption.

Wayne B. Jonas, MD
President and CEO
Samueli Institute
Midville, Ohio
February, 2016

Foreword

In the United States we are witnessing a groundswell of activity that is slowly awakening policy leaders to a new strategy on the treatment of people in pain. An interprofessional group of researchers with whom I had the opportunity to work dubbed this *Never Only Opioids*. We used this title in a policy briefing published by a national organization with membership from over 40 major pain-related organizations and interests. Our subheading spoke directly to the importance of this book: "The Imperative for Early Integration of Non-Pharmacologic Approaches in the Treatment of Patients with Pain."

We suggested, but did not directly come out and name, the ultimate direction of our work. We seek to re-energize a fundamental charge that binds all health professionals. *Primum non nocere*. First do no harm. Our methods are to give practitioners more tools, and teams more players. *Integrative Pain Management* introduces the low-hanging fruit of massage, movement and mindfulness to increase options for practitioners and patients.

Health professionals in pain treatment continue to work in a context dominated by pharmaceuticals. Following the precept to choose strategies that do not bring harm to patients is at best an exercise in ambiguity. Adverse consequences of routinely prescribed agents are blasted at us *ad nauseam* via advertisements on television and in social media. The opioid epidemic in the United States, with its overwhelming rates of morbidity and mortality, is testament to how reliance on our current course will necessarily put us at odds with the Hippocratic charge.

Our ultimate mission must be nothing less than to shift the therapeutic order of the nation. From "never only opioids" to *always non-pharmacologic approaches first*. Give patients mindfulness CDs or other mind–body approaches routinely, prior to, and immediately post, surgeries. Pair non-pharmacological approaches like mindfulness and massage and acupuncture and chiropractic with pharmaceuticals. Do all we can to heal the brain to heal the pain. Create the mindset and skills in medical delivery organizations so that integrative care therapies can limit the likelihood that the reliance on pharmaceuticals will spin one into frightening downward spirals of abuse and addiction.

We are poised to make this shift. In November of 2014, the police force for most of the medical delivery organizations in the United States, the Joint Commission, finalized a two-year long review of pain-related research. This entity accredits the vast majorities of hospitals and their associated facilities. They issued a *Clarification of the Pain Management Standard*. The historic document does two things. It first highlights non-pharmacologic approaches like "acupuncture therapy, chiropractic therapy, massage therapy, osteopathic manipulative therapy" plus relaxation therapy and others. Then the Joint Commission alerts providers to the "potential risk of dependency, addiction, and abuse" from present strategies.

The depth charges in this standard are profound. End the primary reliance on pain-killers. Bring non-pharmacologic approaches toward the first line. Don't leave them as last resorts.

Integrative Pain Management offers useful how-to guidance on how massage movement and mindfulness can help bridge organizations and practices to this necessary future. This edited volume from one of the best known integrative massage leaders, Diana Thompson, LMP, and her colleague Marissa Brooks, MPH, aggregates contributions from a multidisciplinary set of well-regarded veterans. These papers are leverage tools for shifting the therapeutic order in our nation's treatment of people with pain.

John Weeks
February, 2016

CONTRIBUTORS

Benjamin Apichai, LAc, EAMP
Associate Professor, Department of Acupuncture
& East Asian Medicine, School of Traditional
WorldMedicines, Kenmore, WA, USA; Bastyr University,
Clinical Supervisor, Bastyr Center for Natural Health,
Seattle, WA, USA; private practice in Seattle, WA, USA

John Balletto, BSc, LMT, CKTP®
Licensed Massage Therapist and Certified Kinesio®
Taping Practitioner at the Center for Muscular
Therapy, Pawtucket, RI, USA

Jack Blackburn, LMP, MA (Spiritual Direction)
Certified Trager Practitioner, Certified Spiritual
Director, Founder of Trillium Institute, US and Japan,
Seattle, WA, USA

Geoffrey M. Bove, DC, PhD
Professor, Biomedical Sciences, University of New
England College of Osteopathic Medicine, Biddeford,
ME, USA

Marissa Brooks, MPH
Retired massage therapy clinician, Public Health and
healthcare professional, Seattle, WA, USA

Patricia Buchanan, PhD
Guild Certified Feldenkrais Teacher, athletic trainer,
physical therapist, and motor developmentalist,
Toledo, OH, USA

Lauren Christman, LMP, CCST, CBSI/KMI
Practitioner and teacher, specializing in structural
integration, craniosacral therapy, and visceral
manipulation, Seattle, WA, USA

Susan Davis, BHSc, MClSc (Lifestyle Medicine), RN, RMT
Member of the AAMT Research Committee Director
and Senior Therapist specializing in chronic pain at
Davis Health Centre, Sydney, Australia

Nancy Haller, MA
Guild Certified Feldenkrais Practitioner, Author,
Educator, Seattle, WA, USA

Carolyn McManus, PT, MS, MA
Physical Therapist, Swedish Medical Center,
mindfulness in health care educator and consultant,
Research Associate, VA Puget Sound, Seattle,
WA, USA

Wolf Mehling, MD
Physician, Associate Professor, University of California,
San Francisco, Family Medicine, subspecialties
Manual Medicine and Psychotherapy, Osher Center
for Integrative Medicine, USA

Bonnie B. O'Connor, PhD
Ethnographer and Emerita Faculty Member of
the Alpert Medical School of Brown University,
Providence, Rhode Island, USA

Neil Pearson, PT, MSc, BA-BPHE, CYT, ERYT500
Physical therapist, yoga therapist, Faculty Member
in yoga therapy training programs - International.
Clinical Assistant Professor, University of British
Columbia, Canada

Richard Polishuk, LMP, APP
Certified Aston-Patterning Practitioner and Teacher
with an orthopedic focus Seattle, WA, USA

Cynthia J. Price, PhD, MA, LMP
Research Associate Professor at the University of
Washington, and Director of the Center for Mindful
Body Awareness, Seattle, WA, USA

Ramel Rones
Mind–body Consultant for Dana Farber/Harvard
Cancer Center, Tufts Medical Center, Children's
Hospital, Center for Mind–Body Therapies, Boston,
MA, USA

Lisa Santoro, CMT, LLCC
Certified Lymphatic Drainage Specialist, Founder
of the Massage Program at Harvard University and
Massage Training Programs at Boston Medical Center,
Boston, USA

Contributors

Nancy Keeney Smith, LMT
Licensed Massage Therapist, Certified Manual
Lymph Drainage Therapist, author, Florida and
NCBTMB Provider of international Scar Management
Workshops, USA

Matthew D. Stewart, BAppSc, MOst, PGDipHE, LMT
(Hawaii)
Educator, education consultant, Registered
Osteopath (Australia & New Zealand), owner of North
Sydney Osteopathy, Sydney, NSW, Australia

Bronwyn Lennox Thompson, PhD, MSc (Psych),
DipOT
Senior Lecturer, Occupational Therapist, author,
University of Otago, Christchurch, New Zealand

Diana L. Thompson, LMP
Licensed Massage Therapist in private practice,
author, research consultant, educator, Past
President of the Massage Therapy Foundation,
Seattle, WA, USA

Chenchen Wang, MD, MSc
Director, Center for Integrative Medicine and Division
of Rheumatology; Professor of Medicine, Tufts
Medical Center, Tufts University, Boston, MA, USA

Ruth Werner, BCTMB
Massage therapy educator and author; Past President
of the Massage Therapy Foundation, Waldport, USA

INTRODUCTION

Diana L. THOMPSON   Marissa BROOKS

Purpose

Our understanding of the pathophysiology of chronic pain has increased substantially over the past 20 years … Pain is now considered a conscious experience

Moseley and Vlaeyen 2015

Untreated and undertreated pain is the most pervasive health problem today (Dubois, Gallagher, and Lippe 2009). Juxtaposed with the lack of adequate treatment worldwide is the dependency on prescription drug use to treat pain. There are an estimated 15 million people around the globe who suffer from opioid dependency, and an estimated 69,000 people die from opioid overdose each year (WHO 2014), many of whom are on low doses with acute and intermittent use (Fulton-Kehoe et al. 2015). Prolonged use of pain medications has been shown to worsen pain symptoms and pose substantial risk (Menard 2014; Fulton-Kehoe et al. 2015). In the USA alone, non-steroidal anti-inflammatory drugs (NSAIDs) and acetaminophen send 80,000 people to the ER annually, and NSAID use is associated with increased risk of GI bleeds, impaired renal function, and cardiovascular death (Menard 2014). The cost of pain spans economic, social, mental (Waters-Banker et al. 2014), and functional domains of human life. The economic cost of chronic pain, including lost productivity and treatment in the USA alone, is estimated at nearly $635 billion annually (Get The Facts 2014).

Failure to adequately treat pain results in an escalation of medical problems: secondary muscle changes and postural aberrations can generate additional pain (Bronfort et al. 2008). Emotional and spiritual changes affect behavior and mood. Social bonds are disrupted; inability to perform activities of daily living result in isolation, unemployment, and invalidism (IOM 2011). In addition, it is common to see depression, anger, anxiety, fear, and suicidal ideation associated with persistent pain (Goldberg and McGee 2011; Moseley and Vlaeyen 2015; European Pain Federation 2015).

Advances in understanding pain and effective treatments to address pain, coupled with inclusion of various perspectives on optimal health, are changing the landscape of what is available for individuals experiencing pain. There is an international trend towards integrative health care (IOM 2011), incorporating evidence-informed, patient-centered complementary practices that address the cadre of complications associated with pain.

Many integrative approaches to pain are non-invasive with few side effects. While the clinical safety of complementary approaches can be a concern, there is little evidence of harm in massage, movement, or mindfulness approaches (Cambron et al. 2007; Ernst 2003). Research supporting the safety and effectiveness of complementary and alternative medicine (CAM) practices is increasing. These disciplines are beneficial on many levels: approaches outlined in this book have been linked to lower healthcare utilization and costs, and better health outcomes (Martin et al. 2012; Plastaras et al. 2013).

Massage, movement, and mindfulness based approaches are most often sought by patients who have given up on, not seen improvements from, or are otherwise unsatisfied with biomedical approaches to chronic pain treatment (Clarke et al. 2015; Berman 2003). Allopathic practitioners typically have little knowledge of these less than mainstream approaches and therefore do not refer patients for care. This situation can be exacerbated by prejudice against these approaches, which is often attributed to lack of evidence. There is limited research on the effectiveness of many complementary practices, particularly an overall lack of randomized clinical trials—the gold standard in biomedical research. However, there is a wealth of clinical evidence that complementary approaches can be extremely helpful for the treatment of pain, based on patient experiences in real-life clinical practice. Research on these approaches is increasing each year, and funding for larger studies is imperative, given the positive clinical evidence for many complementary approaches. Whole systems research, based on real world practice parameters, is particularly important and this identified need has prompted a growing evidence base on the effectiveness of complementary approaches (Tick 2014).

Contents

This book was designed to provide in-depth information on safe and effective complementary approaches for pain treatment. It is our hope that biomedical providers will be encouraged to support their patients to seek and use these evidence-informed approaches in this climate of integrated care.

Audience

Our audience is twofold: the focus is on biomedical providers with the intent to ease the integration of massage, movement, and mindfulness into pain care. Complementary providers will also find this book an essential resource: an effective networking tool for participating on interdisciplinary healthcare teams. Both biomedical and complementary providers will find this text valuable for patient education, presenting research findings, providing theoretical constructs behind approaches to pain, and detailing the patient experience.

Structure

The first three chapters of the book provide an overview of integrative health care, describe the current science and understanding of pain, and detail theories to address pain. Chapters 4–16 detail massage, movement, and mindfulness-based approaches—the history of the discipline, the clinical reasoning for treating pain, the patient

encounter—demonstrating how the approach helps patients manage their pain and live fuller lives. Rather than classifying pain by diagnosis, such as fibromyalgia, the book focuses on pain symptoms and the ways in which pain is experienced by individual patients.

Included in Chapters 4–16 are Research Sidebars. These merge relevant scientific information with the clinical expertise shared by the authors. These highlight basic science research—emerging advancements in understanding mechanisms—and other sidebars summarize clinical outcomes relevant to the massage, movement, or mindfulness approach.

Interview Sidebars incorporate comments gathered from Patient and Practitioner Interview Questionnaires. Authors were asked to distribute the questionnaires to patients and referring providers. Answers illuminate the patients' experience of these complementary approaches, and offer providers insights into the value of working with complementary providers. The results are limited by small and convenient sampling; authors likely distributed these to satisfied patients and referring providers with good working relationships (see Tables 1 and 2 for results of questionnaires).

The final chapter, Pathways to Integrative Clinical Care, provides communication guidelines for building and participating on effective interdisciplinary care teams. We believe that communication is the most important tool to promote shared decision-making and implement a patient-centered approach to integrative pain management.

The Approaches

According to a 2015 report from the Centers for Disease Control (CDC), among the most commonly used complementary approaches are: yoga, Tai Chi, and Qi Gong; chiropractic or osteopathic manipulation; meditation; and massage therapy (Clarke et al. 2015). This informed our inclusion/exclusion criteria. We chose to stay within our own scope of practice

Demographics

Total respondents	25
Female	18
Male	7
Age range	22–71 years
Duration of pain	7 months – 38 years
Geographic location	Australia, Canada, Japan, USA

Table 1
Patient Interview Questionnaires: Sample questions and comments.

How did you choose this type of care?

Total respondents	25	Comment: "I met [massage therapist] through a referral from a colleague. After medical treatment and surgeries had failed to correct the root cause of my knee pain, I sought alternative therapies."
Self-referred	17	
PCP referred	3	
Ancillary referral (PT, nurse, counselor)	4	
PCP recommended/patient found provider	1	

Was your primary care provider (PCP) supportive of your decision?

Respondents (not including PCP referrals)	21	Comment: "My primary care doctor was very supportive of this decision although he admitted to me that he does not refer his patients to massage therapists primarily because he does not know many of them in the general area or what kind of therapies can be provided."
Yes	13	
No	2	
Didn't ask/Didn't tell	8	

What has changed as a result of getting this care?

a. Has your condition, symptoms, ability to function changed since receiving care?	Yes: 25	Comment: "I know I am managing my lymphedema. I can function normally or even better than most my age."
b. Do you feel differently about yourself or your pain?	Yes: 25	Comment: "Taping has changed movement habits, posture habits, and improved awareness of movement."
c. Do you do any self-care to relieve or prevent ongoing pain?	Yes: 25	Comment: "I learned a way to stretch the scar ... and self-massage."
d. What have you learned about this treatment approach or self-care that you would like other healthcare providers to know about?	Yes: 25	Comment: "Consider the mind/body/spirit connection in healing. Know that different people need different approaches ... model empathy and patience ... I only heard impatience, frustration and blame [from some providers]."

Demographics

Total respondents	8
Female	6
Male	2
Provider type	MD (3), OMD/acupuncture (2), OT, RN, counselor

Table 2
Practitioner Interview Questionnaires: Sample questions and comments.

How did you choose this type of complementary care for your patient?

Patient requested referral	2
Provider referral	6

How did you choose this complementary provider?

Personal experience of their work	8
Face-to-face meeting	4
Recommendation by colleague	4
The patient chose the practitioner	1

Why do you refer to this practitioner/discipline?

Patient satisfaction	8
Pain outcomes	8
How has it benefited your patients?	Comment: "Our clients feel stronger, more confident in their physical movement and mental approach and aware of how it benefits their overall health and pain condition. They move from a patient identity to taking charge of their own health care."

How is the communication between you and the provider? How could it be better?	Comment: "Good. More time, more in-depth discussion."
What information do you need from complementary providers to feel more confident in referring to them or the discipline?	Comments: – experience – professionalism – areas of special interest – dedication to ongoing learning – research
What are the roadblocks to referring to complementary care?	Comments: – availability – financial strain – the issue of losing patients to other practitioners when you refer them out

and focus on approaches that are commonly used by patients, have solid, emerging evidence, but are less supported by biomedical providers. In keeping with the massage, movement, and mindfulness (MMM) theme, we intentionally omitted spinal manipulation (only massage-type osteopathic techniques are included), needling (only Traditional Chinese Medicine (TCM) bodywork is included), energy work, mental health, and nutrition/supplements. Even so, there are many other modalities and disciplines within MMM, such as Alexander Technique, Shiatsu, and Watsu (water massage), that are equally effective, and we hope biomedical providers will consider these when referring patients to MMM approaches for pain management.

In particular, this book presents in-depth descriptions of a variety of massage-based disciplines (scar massage, lymphatic drainage, structural integration) and a few approaches that massage therapists integrate into practice (osteopathic techniques, functional taping, Tui Na, and Trager). Movement practices have a variety of approaches to care—active, passive, and interactive—and apply these practices in both classroom and individual settings. We included a sampling of the most common approaches: active (yoga, Tai Chi/Qi Gong), and two that incorporate passive, active, and interactive approaches (Trager and Feldenkrais Method). Mindfulness and awareness practices are interwoven into every approach, and we have a chapter dedicated to the evidence for and applications of each.

Paramount in every chapter is a focus on patient-centered care. Each author emphasizes the importance of addressing the whole person from a biopsychosocial perspective. For example, the literature states that massage is primarily biomechanical in nature yet, in practice, attention to mental, emotional, and spiritual needs are evident (Fortune and Hymel 2015).

Patient participation outside the treatment room or classroom is also emphasized. The IOM (2011) lists promoting self-management of pain as one of the critical steps to improving care. Berman asserts that complementary therapies "give people more ways to help themselves—to reduce or cope with not only pain but also other aspects of chronic conditions such as anxiety and stress, or to change to more healthy lifestyles" (2003).

Authors

The drive to expand options for care is a true expression of patient-centeredness: "There appears to be no one treatment that is best for all patients" (Maiers et al. 2012). The authors selected to contribute to this book are all experts in their disciplines, practicing in various countries around the world, treating patients with complicated health issues. We prioritized contributors that are actively practicing, in order to focus on sharing clinical expertise in treating pain. Many authors are trained in multiple modalities within their discipline, and a good number are professionals in multiple disciplines. For example, there are eleven authors practicing under massage licenses, three others with massage training but working under another license (a nurse, a medical doctor, and an osteopath). All are cross-trained in various modalities. Other authors have received biomedical academic degrees first, and later sought training in massage, movement, and mindfulness disciplines.

How to Use the Book

Because of the diversity of approaches included in this book, and the cross-disciplinary audience, definitions of some terminology will be helpful:

- Patient vs. client: these terms refer to the same individual. We allowed authors to pick the term that they use in clinical practice.

- Complementary provider: this term refers to all providers who offer the approaches described in this book. Many terms exist to describe massage, movement and mindfulness based professionals. We chose this term to illustrate the value of integration. When one approach complements another, there is good integration.

- Biomedical provider: this term includes all allopathically trained medical providers whose training is rooted in mainstream health care.

The descriptions in this book are more in-depth than the typical paragraph written in other integrative healthcare references, making this text a useful resource beyond the primary audiences mentioned above. Patients who are actively engaged in their care and are empowered to be advocates for themselves may benefit from reading these descriptions. Interdisciplinary care team members who may not have a solid understanding of the approaches included might also find this book useful.

Each of the chapters describing clinical encounters can be used as a stand-alone educational tool if a provider needs information on a particular approach. However, the front information (Chapters 1–3) and the culminating chapter (Chapter 17) are important for all providers who wish to integrate patient-centered approaches to treating people in pain.

Summary

To date, biomedical providers do not have a comprehensive tool that describes useful, substantive information about complementary care, merging research, clinical expertise, and information about current healthcare opportunities. This reference text is written by complementary providers, giving the reader inside perspectives on the clinical encounter, helping the biomedical provider understand the important role of massage, movement, and mindfulness in managing pain, and illuminating the patients' desire for human connection and interaction over pills to treat their pain.

Thus, a text that blends current mainstream understanding of pain and integrative treatment wisdom gives both biomedical and complementary providers an effective reference tool for making informed healthcare referrals for people experiencing complicated pain conditions.

Acknowledgements

We would like to thank our Foreword writers, Wayne Jonas and John Weeks.

John is an internationally-recognized organizer, writer and speaker with over 3 decades of experience working with multiple stakeholders in efforts to move the medical industry toward a system that focuses on creating health, and Wayne is the CEO and President of the Samueli Institute.

References

Berman, B. M. 2003. Integrative approaches to pain management: how to get the best of both worlds. *British Medical Journal* Jun 14; 326(7402):1320–1.

Bronfort, G., M. Haas, R. Evans, G. Kawchuk, and S. Dagenais. 2008. Evidence-informed management of chronic low back pain with spinal manipulation and mobilization. *Spine Journal* 8(1):213–25.

Cambron, J., J. Dexheimer, P. Coe, and R. Swenson. 2007. Side-effects of massage therapy: a cross-sectional study of 100 clients. *J Altern Complement Med*. Oct; 13(8):793–6.

Clarke, T. C., L. I. Black, B. J. Stussman, P. M. Barnes, and R. L. Nahin. 2015. Trends in the use of complementary health approaches among adults: United States, 2002–2012. *National Health Statistics Reports*; no 79. Hyattsville, MD: National Center for Health Statistics.

Dubois, M. Y., R. M. Gallagher, and P. M. Lippe. 2009. Pain medicine position paper. *The American Academy of Pain Medicine, Pain Medicine* 10(6). doi:10.1111/j1526-4637.2009.00696.x.

Ernst, E. 2003. The safety of massage therapy. *Rheumatology (Oxford)*. Sep; 42(9):1101–6. Epub 2003 May 30.

European Pain Federation 2015. http://www.efic.org/index.asp?sub=F8AMLHLAP9216P (accessed July 18, 2015).

Fortune, L. D., and G. M. Hymel. 2015. Creating integrative work: a qualitative study of how massage therapists work with existing clients. *J Bodyw Mov Ther* Jan; 19(1):25–34. doi: 10.1016/j.jbmt.2014.01.005. Epub 2014 Feb 7.

Fulton-Kehoe, D., M. D. Sullivan, J. A. Turner, R. K. Garg, A. M. Bauer, T. M. Wickizer, and G. M. Franklin. 2015. Opioid poisonings in Washington State Medicaid. *Medical Care* 53(8):679. doi:10.1097/MLR.0000000000000384.

Get the Facts. US Department of Health and Human Services. National Institutes of Health. National Center for Complementary and Integrative Health. 2014. https://nccih.nih.gov/sites/nccam.nih.gov/files/Get_The_Facts_Chronic_Pain_and_CHA_11-3-2014.pdf (accessed July 6, 2015).

Goldberg, D. S., and S. J. McGee. 2011. Pain as a global public health priority. *BMC Public Health* 11:770. doi:10.1186/1471-2458-11-770. http://www.biomedcentral.com/1471-2458/11/770 (accessed July 6, 2015).

Institute of Medicine (IOM). 2011. *Relieving pain in America: A blueprint for transforming prevention, care, education, and research*. Washington, DC: The National Academies Press.

Maiers, M.J., K. K. Westrom, C. G. Legendre, and G. Bronfort. 2010. Integrative care for the management of low back pain: use of a clinical care pathway. *BMC Health Serv Res* Oct 29; 10:298. doi: 10.1186/1472-6963-10-298.

Martin, B. I., M. M. Gerkovich, R. A. Deyo, K. J. Sherman, D. C. Cherkin, B. K. Lind, C. M. Goertz, and W. E. Lafferty. 2012. The Association of Complementary and Alternative Medicine Use and Health Care Expenditures for Back and Neck Problems. *Med Care* 50:1029–36.

Menard, M., A.Nielsen, H. Tick, W. Meeker, K. Wilson, and J. Weeks. 2014. Policy brief: Never only opioids: the imperative for early integration of non-pharmacological approaches and practitioners in the treatment of patients with pain. *Pains Project Transforming the Way Pain is Perceived, Judged and Treated* Fall: Issue 5.

Moseley, G. L., and J. W. Vlaeyen. 2015. Beyond nociception: the imprecision hypothesis of chronic pain. *Pain* Jan; 156(1): 35–8. doi: 10.1016/j.pain.0000000000000014.

Plastaras, C., S. Schran, N. Kim, D. Darr, and M. S. Chen. 2013. Manipulative therapy (Feldenkrais, massage, chiropractic manipulation) for neck pain. *Curr Rheumatol Rep* Jul; 15(7):339. doi: 10.1007/s11926-013-0339-x. ///C:/Users/Marissa/Downloads/Manipulative%20Therapy%20for%20Neck%20Pain.pdf (accessed July 8, 2015).

Tick, H. 2014. Integrative medicine: A holistic model of care. *IASP Pain: Clinical Updates* May; XXII: 2

Waters-Banker, C., E. E. Dupont-Versteegden, P. H. Kitzman, and T. A. Butterfield. 2014. Investigating the mechanisms of massage efficacy: The role of mechanical immunomodulation. *Journal of Athletic Training* 49(2):266–73. doi:10.4085/1062-6050-49.2.25.

World Health Organization (WHO). 2004. Media release. http://www.who.int/mediacentre/news/releases/2004/pr70/en/ (accessed July 6, 2015).

World Health Organization (WHO). 2014. Information sheet on opioid overdose. http://www.who.int/substance_abuse/information-sheet/en/ (accessed July 10, 2015).

GLOSSARY

Acupressure – a Traditional Chinese Medicine (TCM) hands-on technique based on the principles of acupuncture

Acupuncture – a key component of TCM involving the use of thin needles inserted in the body at very specific points along meridian lines to balance Qi

A-delta fibers – one of three classes of nerve fibers; fast conducting, thinly myelinated fibers that transmit information about tissue damage and pain

Afferent - the conduction of nerve impulses from the periphery of the body toward the central nervous system

Affordable Care Act (ACA) – a US healthcare reform law that expands and improves access to care and curbs spending through regulations and taxes

Allodynia – a form of central pain sensitization; pain resulting from a stimulus that would not normally provoke pain, such as light touch

Anandamide – an essential fatty acid neurotransmitter; plays an important role in the regulation of pain perception

An Mo – Chinese equivalent of the Swedish massage; to promote circulation and energy, and relieve muscular, physical and emotional stress

Anterior cingulate cortex (ACC) – part of the brain located mid frontal lobe; linked to the emotional reaction to pain rather than to the perception of pain itself

Asana – physical yoga posture or position; "to sit in ease"

Aston-Patterning – an integrated system of bodywork and movement/postural education, developed by Judith Aston, that recognizes the relationship between body and mind for well-being

Athletic taping – the application of firm, adhesive tape to the skin in order to stabilize or support muscles and joints during physical activity

Awareness Through Movement (ATM) – verbally directed movement sequences, presented primarily to groups, or individuals usually organized around a particular function, based on the Feldenkrais Method

Axon – a process of a neuron

Biomedical providers – healthcare providers that focus on biological factors for diagnosis and treatment; also called allopathic providers

Biopsychosocial – healthcare approach to diagnosis and treatment that integratates biological, psychological and social aspects of disease, human functioning, and health

Biotensegrity – a concept of musculo-skeletal relationships; tension (soft tissue) pulls on structure (bones and joints) to provide stability and efficient force transference

Body-self neuromatrix – a widely distributed neural network that includes parallel somatosensory, limbic and thalamocortical components, affective-motivational and evaluative-cognitive dimensions of pain experience

Calcitonin gene-related peptide (CGRP) – a neuropeptide with strong vasodilatory actions and released by nociceptors

Case Formulation Approach – a clinical reasoning methodology that employs biopsychosocial and patient-centered approaches to developing an individualized treatment plan

C-fibers – one of three classes of nerve fibers; slow conducting, unmyelinated fibers that transmit information related to damage to the central nervous system

Glossary

Chemoreceptors – a sensory nerve cell that detects chemical stimuli in the environment and relays the information to the central nervous system

Cicatricial scar – connective tissue that forms over a wound

Compassion meditation (CM) – a meditative practice to open one's heart to suffering and the wish for the relief of suffering in oneself and others

Complementary and alternative medicine (CAM) – healthcare practices or disciplines that have typically originated outside the realm of allopathic or biomedical health care

Conventional medicine – a system of health care that often relies on drugs, radiology, and surgery to treat symptoms and diseases; also called Western medicine, allopathic medicine, mainstream medicine, biomedicine

Counter strain (CS) – a hands-on technique using passive positional release techniques that place the body in positions of greatest comfort or ease

Craniosacral therapy (CST) – a hands-on approach using gentle manipulations of the skull in particular, and bones and fascia in general, to enhance the function of the brain and spinal fluid

Da Tui Na – "Da" means "large" and "Tui Na" is a TCM therapy hands-on approach. The treatment is performed simultaneously by more than five Tui Na practitioners while the patient is under local anesthesia after radiology lab test. Conditions suitable for Da Tui Na are herniated disc sciatica and dislocation of joints

Decompression somatics – a specific form of positional release, a hands-on technique using passive positioning of joints and soft tissue to indirectly find ease in movement, combined with client/patient somatic awareness

Deep tissue massage – massage that focuses on the deeper layers of soft tissue; often slower and deeper in pressure, and more specific in intention

Degloving injury – an injury involving a separation of the subcutaneous tissues from the deeper layers of soft tissue, severing the blood supply

Demyelinate – damage to the myelin sheath or protective covering of the nerve fibers and spinal cord

Dermatomes – an area of skin supplied by a spinal nerve root

Dharana – a yoga technique; focuses on calming the mind through concentration

Dhyana – a yoga technique; meditation; an uninterrupted state of mental concentration or higher contemplation

Dorsal root ganglion (DRG) – a cluster of sensory neuronal cell bodies, located in the vertebral foramen

Dukkha – a Sanskrit word for pain, suffering, lack of ease, sorrow

Edema – swelling; excessive fluid accumulation in body tissues and cavities

Efferent – the conduction of nerve impulses toward the periphery

Epistemology – the study or science of knowledge and ways of knowing

Evidence-based – using current research, or the best available information, to make decisions about the care of an individual patient

Evidence-informed – integrating current evidence, clinical reasoning, and patient preferences to make decisions about the care of an individual patient

Exteroception – the perception of stimuli originating from outside the body

Fascia – dense, organized connective tissue

Fear-avoidance model – a psychological model that identifies the role fear of pain plays in avoiding activities and developing disability even if physical healing has occurred

Focusing – a technique in which the therapist uses skilled listening without judgment to help fine tune the patient's internal attentiveness and become more aware of her bodily experience or "felt sense"

Functional Integration (FI) – within the Feldenkrais Method, a hands-on form of tactile, kinesthetic communication to a student about how they organize their body, and hints, through gentle touch and movement, on how to move in more expanded functional motor patterns

Functional taping – the application of stretchy, adhesive tape to the skin without binding in order to facilitate joint movement, align weak muscles, encourage circulation and proprioception, and reduce pain (see kinesiology taping)

Functional Technique (FT) – an indirect treatment approach that involves finding the dynamic balance point and one of the following: applying an indirect guiding force, holding the position or adjusting compression to exaggerate position and allow for spontaneous readjustment

Ganglion – a mass of neurons existing outside the central nervous system

Gate control theory (GCT) – a historical theory for pain modulation by Melzack and Wall in 1965, which has since been proven inaccurate, but which was influential in the investigation of pain mechanisms

Hook-up – the inner state of mind of the practitioner; presence, as coined by Milton Trager

Hyperalgesia – a form of central sensitization; an increased sensitivity to pain from a stimulus that normally provokes pain

Hypertrophic scar (HTS) – an elevated scar that stays within the boundary of the wound; excessive amounts of collagen deposited during wound healing, not to the level of a keloid scar

Hypotonia – low muscle tone and weakness

Immunomodulatory effects – modulating or regulating one or more immune functions

Integrative health care – bringing conventional and complementary approaches to health care together in a coordinated way

Integrative medicine – an approach to care, regardless of which modalities are utilized, that puts the patient at the center and addresses the full range of physical, emotional, mental, spiritual and environmental influences that affect the person's health

Inter-disciplinary care team – a collaborative group of healthcare providers from different disciplines contributing specialized skills and expertise to create an individualized treatment plan

Inter-disciplinary team – different types of healthcare providers work together with the patient to share expertise, knowledge, and skills to effect favorable patient outcomes

Interoception – the perception of sensation originating from inside the body

Keloid scar – excessive, abnormal collagen formation during wound healing; tough, irregularly shaped, grows beyond the original margins of the wound

Kinesiology taping – the application of stretchy, adhesive tape to the skin without binding in order to facilitate joint movement, align weak muscles, encourage circulation and proprioception, and reduce pain (see functional taping)

Loving kindness meditation (LKM) – a meditative practice to experience and develop friendliness, goodwill and kindness toward oneself and others

Lymphatic techniques: Lymph drainage therapy (LDT), lymphatic facilitation (LF), lymphatic pump techniques (LPT), manual

Glossary

lymph drainage (MLD) – a hands-on technique consisting of the application of gentle, rhythmic massage strokes to the skin and superficial fascia to encourage the natural drainage of the lymph fluid

Macrophage – a type of white blood cell integral in the immune response to infection and foreign particles

Mantra – a repeated word or phrase, used in mediation, prayer, or incantation

McConnell taping – a form of athletic taping developed by physical therapist Jenni McConnell for rehabilitation

Mechanoreceptor – a pressure-sensitive sensory receptor

Mentastics – a set of gentle, self-guided movements combining proprioceptive awareness and effortlessness, used for self-care, developed by Milton Trager

Meridians – twenty pathways in the body along which Qi or energy flows

Mindful awareness – the awareness that occurs through deliberately paying attention, without judgment or elaboration, to one's present moment sense experiences, thoughts and emotions

Mindful meditation – a meditative practice to cultivate present moment awareness of sense experiences, thoughts and emotions while adopting attitudes of acceptance, friendliness, and curiosity

Mindfulness-based Stress Reduction (MBSR) – an eight-session training program in mindfulness meditation and its applications to stress, illness, and daily life

Moxibustion, Moxa – the burning of dried mugwort near the skin to stimulate acupoints

Mudra – a yoga technique; a symbolic hand gesture to effect energy flow

Multidimensional Assessment of Interoceptive Awareness (MAIA) scale – a self-report instrument for experimental interoception research and for assessment of Mind–body therapies

Muscle energy technique (MET) – a hands-on technique using gentle, active muscle contractions by the patient against a practitioner-applied counter force

Myelin – a fatty sheath around a nerve to improve nerve conduction speed

Myofascia – of or relating to the fascia of muscles

Myofascial balancing, fascial balancing, fascial release, myofascial release – hands-on methods used to release restrictions in superficial, deep, muscular and visceral fascial layers

Myotome – a group of muscles that a single nerve root innervates

Neural correlates – of consciousness (NCC) constitute the minimal set of neuronal events and mechanisms sufficient to generate conscious awareness

Neuroma in continuity – a bulbous swelling in the nerve formed by sprouting axons that are intermixed with intact axons

Neuromodulation – the physiological process by which a given neuron uses one or more neurotransmitters to regulate diverse populations of neurons

Neuromodules – sub-networks that produce multiple dimensions of pain sensations, such as heightened attention to a body part, awareness of the quality of sensation, such as burning or stabbing, or 'phantom' sensations in a body part that is no longer there

Neuropathic pain – a complex, chronic pain state that usually is accompanied by tissue injury. With neuropathic pain, the nerve fibers themselves might be damaged, dysfunctional, or injured

Neuropathy – a term used to describe a problem with the nerves, usually the peripheral nerves as opposed to the central nervous system

Neuroplasticity – also known as brain plasticity—an umbrella term that encompasses both synaptic and non-synaptic plasticity—it refers to changes in neural pathways and synapses due to changes in behavior, environment, neural processes, thinking, and emotions

Neurotransmitter – endogenous chemicals that enable neurotransmission. They transmit signals across a chemical synapse, such as in a neuromuscular junction, from one neuron to another "target" neuron, muscle cell, or gland cell

Nidra – a yoga technique to induce complete physical, mental and emotional relaxation

Niyama – translates to positive duties or observances; recommended activities and habits for healthy living, spiritual enlightenment and liberated state of existence

Nociception – the encoding and processing of harmful stimuli in the nervous system, and therefore the ability of a body to sense potential harm

Nociceptor – a sensory neuron that responds to potentially damaging stimuli by sending signals to the spinal cord and brain

Opiates – analgesic alkaloid compounds found naturally in the opium poppy plant *Papaver somniferum*. The psychoactive compounds found in the opium plant include morphine, codeine, and thebaine

Opioids – artificially made rather than extracted from opium, substances that act on the nervous system by reducing the intensity of pain signals reaching the brain and affect the areas of the brain that control emotion, which diminishes the effects of a painful stimulus

Ortho-Bionomy – a gentle, non-invasive, osteopathically-based form of hands-on therapy often addressing postural and structural imbalances and associated symptoms

Osteopathy – a form of drug-free non-invasive manual medicine that focuses on total body health by treating and strengthening the musculoskeletal framework, with an aim to positively affect the body's nervous, circulatory and lymphatic systems

Pancamaya – the five aspects of the body: physical, energetic, intellect, emotion, and bliss

Patient-centered care – respectful of and responsive to individual patient preferences, needs, and values, and ensuring that patient values guide all clinical decisions

Plexopathy – a disorder affecting a network of nerves, blood vessels, or lymph vessels. The region of nerves it affects is at the brachial or lumbosacral plexus

Polyneuropathy – is damage or disease affecting peripheral nerves (peripheral neuropathy) in roughly the same areas on both sides of the body

Polyradiculopathy – damage to multiple nerve roots sufficient to produce neurologic symptoms and signs or uncommon peripheral nervous system syndromes that result from a variety of conditions. The clinical manifestations are variable but often include symmetric or asymmetric distal and proximal weakness with a variable degree of sensory loss and reduction or loss of reflexes

Practice-based research – evidence obtained from original research undertaken in order to gain new knowledge partly by means of practice and the outcomes of that practice

Pranayama – a yoga technique; gaining control of energy, typically through breath

Pratyahara – a yoga technique; drawing inward to develop a sense of self-awareness, similar but not identical to interoception

Presencing – the choice to use sensory awareness or sentience to tune into this moment, and act from one's highest potential. Presencing blends the words "presence" and "sensing" and receiving direction from our deepest source

Proprioception – the ability to sense stimuli arising within the body regarding position, motion, equilibrium and feeling awareness

Qi – an active principle forming part of any living thing. Qi literally translates as "breath," "air," or "gas," and figuratively as "material energy," "life force," or "energy flow"

Qi Gong – Chinese healthcare system that integrates physical postures, breathing techniques, and focused intention

Radiculopathy – a disease of the root of a nerve, such as from a pinched nerve or a tumor

Raja yoga – literally, royal path ("raja" means king); the path of meditation and the focus is to quiet the mind—a yoga technique to achieve control over the mind and emotions

Receptive field – of an individual sensory neuron is the particular region of the sensory space (e.g. the body surface, or the retina) in which a stimulus will trigger the firing of that neuron

Respiratory-circulatory model – one of five models used in discussion of osteopathic patient care. The goal of the respiratory–circulatory model is to improve all of the diaphragm restrictions in the body. Restriction in the diaphragms may impede the normal physiologic motion, venous and lymphatic drainage, and cerebrospinal fluid

Samadhi – a state of intense concentration achieved through meditation often described as attainment of inner peace or enlightenment

Savasana – a final posture in yoga practice, the purpose is deep relaxation, letting body and mind rest

Scale of Body Connection (SBC) – a twenty-item self-report measure, designed to assess body awareness and bodily dissociation in Mind–body intervention research

Specificity theory – a theory that the pain mechanism, like hearing and vision, is a specific modality that has its own central and peripheral apparatus

Spinal manipulative therapy (SMT) – manual therapy focusing on mobilization of joints, practiced primarily by chiropractors, but also by a small portion of osteopathic physicians and physical therapists

STarT Back questionnaire – prognostic questionnaire for clinicians to identify modifiable risk factors (biomedical, psychological and social) for back pain disability

Strain-CounterStrain (SCS) – a hands-on technique where the practitioner identifies tender points related to specific strain patterns and positions the body to alleviate or reduce the tenderness

Structural Integration (SI) – a hands-on technique that focuses on realigning structure, increasing awareness and educating the person regarding posture, body usage, and ease of movement; based on the work of Ida P. Rolf

Structural relief therapy – a hands-on technique in which the practitioner positions the body and identifies tender points, utilizing osteopathic principles of muscle energy technique and strain, counter strain, to address unwanted symptoms

Summation theory – a pain theory from the 1800s; excessive or intense stimulation of nerves will eventually produce a disagreeable or unwanted sensation

Tai Chi (includes Chen, Wu, Hao, Sun and Yang styles) – a martial art originating in China; utilizes breathing, visualizations and movements to work on the entire body, integrating physical, psychosocial, spiritual, and behavioral elements; currently used as a mind–body approach/practice for self-management of chronic conditions

Tellington Touch – a hands-on technique applied to animals; additional training and licensure may be needed

Traditional Chinese medicine (TCM) – holistic system of health and healing, based on the notion of harmony and balance; employs the ideas of moderation and prevention

Tui Na – a form of Chinese therapeutic massage. "Tui" meaning to push and "Na" to grasp

Ujjayi breathing – a diaphragmatic breath, which first fills the lower belly, rises to the lower rib cage and moves into the upper chest and throat. It is sometimes called "the ocean breath." The ujjayi breath is typically done in association with yogic asana practices

Viscerotomes – the visceral area innervated by the spinal segment

Yamas – in yoga, one's ethical standards and sense of integrity, focusing on our behavior and how we conduct ourselves in life

Yang – the male principle of the universe that is considered light and active and is associated with heaven

Yin – the female principle of the universe that is considered dark and passive and is associated with earth

Yoga – a discipline involving controlled breathing, prescribed body positions, and meditation, with the goal of decreasing suffering and attaining a state of spiritual insight and tranquility

Yoga therapy – a process in which an individual, trained and experienced in the entire spectrum of yoga modalities and philosophy, guides individuals through yoga techniques and practices specific to the client's therapeutic needs

Zangfu – traditional Chinese medicine recognizes five yin organs (zang) and six yang organs (fu) in nature. The zang and fu organs are not simply anatomical substances; the term represents the generalization of physiology and pathology of certain systems of the human body

Zero balancing – a body–mind therapy that focuses primarily on key joints that conduct and balance forces of gravity, posture, and movement to address the relationship between energy and structures of the body

Overview of integrative health care and pain

Introduction

Pain is a universal human experience. It is also a singular motivator for people to seek attention and care: to help determine its origins and meanings, as well as to help alleviate its ravages. The longer pain persists, the more disabling or frightening it is, the greater the suffering it causes, the greater the range of possible treatment and coping resources people are likely to seek as they pursue relief. Throughout the developed world, conventional medical care has in recent decades been supplemented—and sometimes even replaced—by other diagnostic and therapeutic choices for treating and managing pain; and the more refractory an individual's pain is to medical treatment, the likelier it is that the sufferer will explore and multiply other avenues of aid.

There is presently a large-scale, international movement toward integration of conventional medical approaches to pain treatment and management with other modalities originating outside the medical domain. Each country has its variants of social and political responses to this growing phenomenon known as **Integrative Medicine** or **Integrative Health Care,** but many of the general issues that arise are common to all. To illustrate, this chapter takes the United States as an example of the potential benefits, tensions, and vigorous debate that characterize the rise of integrative approaches to pain.

Integrative Health Care in the United States

Chronic pain is the primary reason that patients in the United States seek treatment from integrative healthcare clinics (Abrams et al. 2013). To fully understand and critically assess the current state of the field of integrative pain management and to strategize for its immediate and longer-term future, it is important to get a sense of the short

(30–40 years), epistemologically complex, and politically fraught history of complementary—and subsequently, integrative—approaches to health care in the USA.

Alongside the "official," conventional, biomedical system, people have always had recourse to numerous other modalities for maintaining and restoring health (Hufford 1995; O'Connor 1995). Irrespective of recognition from the conventional system we have, from the perspective of popular usage (i.e. what people *actually do* to take care of health concerns), long had *de facto* healthcare pluralism. This has been true of minor ailments, life-threatening illnesses, and chronic or debilitating conditions such as severe or persistent pain. Until very recently—since about the mid-1990s—the response of **conventional medicine** to other healthcare modalities has typically been one of alarm that proponents and users of nonbiomedical healing modalities might be causing themselves harm, either directly, as a primary consequence of the practice in question, or indirectly, by delaying their presentation for conventional care while sampling other approaches.

In part, this medical concern was predicated on the unexamined assumption that people selected *either* the conventional healthcare pathway, *or* some alternative(s) to that pathway, in a pattern of serial usage. We now know that is rarely the case; rather, the pattern is virtually always one of simultaneous use of healthcare resources from various pathways (Eisenberg et al. 1993; Hufford 1995; O'Connor 1995; Astin 1998). The alternative pathways, about which relatively little was known in the conventional medical setting, were presumed, by comparison to "officially" accepted practice, to be inferior at best and dangerous or even deadly at worst, irrespective of the conditions they were being used to treat. The long-held general assumption in professional and academic thought was that use of such therapies was largely found among socially "marginal" populations: people who for reasons of poor education, recency of immigration to the USA (implicit: particularly from non-anglophone countries), lack of acculturation to the USA "mainstream," poverty or other lack of access to the conventional system, either didn't *know* any better or couldn't *do* any better (Hufford 1995). We also now know this is incorrect: rather, the majority of complementary and alternative medicine (CAM) use is found among the college-educated middle class (Cassileth et al. 1984; Eisenberg et al. 1993; O'Connor 1995; Astin 1998; Barnes, Bloom, and Nahin et al. 2008.)

Among the general public, a lively interest in all manner of popular healthcare movements, modalities, and practitioners continued to grow exuberantly from about the 1960s onward, and information about these resources abounded in the popular press, then as now. Large numbers of ordinary folks were confident in using their own experiences or those of trusted others to decide what modalities to try and to assess whether the things they tried produced any apparent benefit. People used a basic problem-solving approach to health disruptions (Hufford 1995), particularly those that presented impediments to functioning, ability to work, or enjoyment of everyday life.

Chronic conditions including pain and debilitating diseases were particular candidates, partly because they were often refractory to conventional treatment, partly because their seriousness called for "trying anything," and partly because many people seemed to find benefit from the nonbiomedical interventions they tried. Most were using alternative options alongside conventional medicine, hoping to derive from each what it did best. At the same time, popular movements in health foods and nutrition became part of a growing grass-roots interest in prevention, health promotion, and wellness—a holistic state of health and

well-being encompassing body, mind, emotions, and (for many) spirit, much further-reaching than the mere absence of disease. This kind of "high-level wellness" was not addressed in conventional medicine, so its support structures and services at the time were almost entirely to be found along alternative pathways, even well after the late-1970s introduction into conventional medical education and practice of the then-revolutionary **biopsychosocial** model (Engel 1978).

Defining a New Area of National Research Interest

By the early 1990s, governmental assessments of "unorthodox" or "unconventional" therapies began to be carried out in earnest. The Congressional Office of Technology Assessment examined unconventional cancer therapies in 1990 (US Congress 1990). In 1992, under the sponsorship of Senator Tom Harkin (D, Iowa, himself a proponent of certain nonbiomedical therapies), Congressional legislation appropriated $2 million, a very modest sum, for the establishment within the National Institutes of Health (NIH) of an Office for the Study of Unconventional Medical Practices (Marwick 1992a, 1992b). Proponents and practitioners of nonbiomedical therapies, included as members of an ad hoc advisory committee assembled to plan the research agenda for this new entity, unsurprisingly objected to this name.

There has been considerable tussling over terminology and definitions since the early use of objectionable identifiers. "Every definition reflects a particular worldview and is formulated as part of a specific agenda (consciously or unconsciously)" (Boon et al. 2004, 50). "Many constituencies participate in [this] discourse … and each has viewpoints and interests to advance, often for disparate – and sometimes mutually exclusive – ends" (Committee on Definition and Description 2007). The new NIH office opened formally in 1992 as the Office of Alternative Medicine (OAM). The term "alternative medicine/therapies" was fairly rapidly amended to "complementary and alternative medicine," as being a more accurate descriptor (although arguments about it still persist). This usage also suited a particularly American propensity for pronounceable acronyms (CAM), and this shorthand form quickly became the common collective term for the many pathways and resources for health care "with origins outside of mainstream medicine" (Briggs 2014). The OAM was reconfigured as the National Center for Complementary and Alternative Medicine (NCCAM) in 1998; and in December 2014, it announced a new name change, to the National Center for Complementary and Integrative Health (NCCIH), stating "[t]he intent of an integrative approach is to enhance overall health …, prevent disease, and alleviate debilitating symptoms such as pain and chemotherapy-induced nausea, among others" (nccam/nih.gov/news/press/12172014; accessed December 17, 2014).

Wake-up Call

In 1993, a group of academic medical researchers published in the *New England Journal of Medicine* the results of a survey, begun in 1991, to seek the patterns and prevalence of use of "unconventional medical therapies" in the United States (Eisenberg et al. 1993). Their findings indicated that roughly one-third of the American public used CAM therapies, a much higher percentage than had been anticipated, and that the majority of CAM users were "nonblack" (*sic*), more educated, and had higher incomes. The profile of all CAM users neatly corresponded with that of Cassileth and colleagues' 1984 profile of users of CAM therapies for cancer, completely contradicting the "marginality" theory. Eisenberg and colleagues (1993) found that the "vast majority" of CAM users used CAM therapies together with conventional medicine to treat the same conditions, and, of those, the substantial majority did not discuss their CAM usage with their medical doctors.

In my own ethnographic research in the early to mid-1990s, CAM users reported that they did not discuss this with their MDs for one or more of three main reasons: (1) they did not expect their MDs to be knowledgeable about CAM therapies or to be able to offer advice within that realm; (2) they expected their MDs to be hostile to or dismissive of CAM therapies, and perhaps even to speak disapprovingly to them or laugh them off; or (3) they respected their MDs and did not wish to offend them by implying, through their use of additional therapeutic modalities, that there was anything "wrong" with their medical treatment; they were simply seeking the rest of what they needed from other sources (O'Connor 1995).

What most galvanized the medical establishment about that 1993 report, however, were two particular findings: (1) the enormous number of annual visits to CAM providers (425 million in 1990, outnumbering all visits to primary care providers in that year by 37 million); and (2) total expenditures on CAM therapies of approximately $13.7 billion, of which some $10.3 billion came from out-of-pocket, non-insurance-covered costs (Weil 2000). This single article, published at a time when biomedical and governmental interest was already piqued, provided a stunning wake-up call that something very important was going on in "the patient population," and that this popular groundswell had very real significance for the health of the public, for conventional medicine, and for healthcare economics and policy. This realization quickly stimulated interest in learning more about what was available within the great diversity of CAM disciplines, and whether/how it might be possible to invite these modalities and practitioners (or at least selected ones) into a new conversation with a biomedical profession that had heretofore largely shut them out.

Enter Integrative Medicine

When differing worldviews meet and attempt to establish, as it were, diplomatic relations, one option is *accommodation*, in which each paradigm becomes modified and expanded by taking on some new characteristics or qualities introduced by the other (Hufford 1984). In an accommodative model, conventional medicine and those CAM disciplines working with it would function as partners, each with its own recognized and respected contributions to make, each purposively learning from the other and broadening its former horizons incrementally. A second option is *pluralism*—in which the broad domains of conventional medicine and CAM approaches "relate to each other as separate but cooperative medical systems [… or as] a coalition of allies, characterized by honest agreement and disagreement" (Kaptchuk and Miller 2005, 286). In its strongest form, pluralism is egalitarian: two or more paradigms maintain autonomous standing while engaging cooperatively in a shared effort or working toward a common goal. Another option is *assimilation*, in which a dominant paradigm incorporates characteristics or qualities of another, but changes these to conform with its own epistemological rules, without substantially altering itself (Hufford 1996; Coulter 2004; Boon and Kachan 2008; Hollenberg and Muzzin 2010). In this model, there is an inherent status inequality, and the minority view is subsumed as secondary or subordinate (Hufford 1996; Coulter 2004; Hollenberg and Muzzin 2010). In the case of conventional and CAM disciplines, the specific *techniques* of CAM modalities might be accepted and put to use, but the underlying theories and sometimes even the "indigenous" practitioners (as, for example, with **acupuncture**, commonly) discarded or replaced (Bell et al. 2002; Coulter 2004; Hollenberg and Muzzin 2010). Hollenberg and Muzzin (2010) consider this type of assimilation a form of colonialism and refer to this practice as "paradigm appropriation."

Almost from the moment that CAM therapies began to be recognized outside their own borders as serious subjects for study, the notion of integration of conventional and CAM modalities also emerged. At the time of the first NIH ad hoc advisory committee meeting for what became the OAM, one physician member was already pursuing a five-year funded project to investigate possible models for integrating conventional medicine with "other forms of care" (Marwick 1992a, 957). A PubMed search undertaken in September 2014 found a single article using the term "integrative medicine" or "integrative health care" in the decade from 1980 to 1989; that paper referred to integration among specialty disciplines within conventional medicine ("integrative care" does continue to be used in this sense.) From 1990 to 1999, there were thirty indexed papers, twenty-seven of which were clearly about integrative medicine/integrative health care as we recognize the terms today. The accumulation of such papers now numbers in the thousands.

From the conventional medical perspective, the impetus for and excitement about research on CAM therapies arose from a desire to discover "what works" and thereby expand the conventional medical therapeutic armamentarium (Hufford 1996). Although early physician advisors had stressed as "essential" (Marwick 1994) the inclusion of knowledgeable CAM figures into design of the OAM research program, the goal of the research was primarily assimilationist, as revealed by various language usages in the medical literature. For example, use of terms like "incorporate *into*" or "integrate *into*" as opposed to, say, "integrate *with*" reveals a medicocentric focus in which the tacit—and sometimes explicit—assumption is that any practice discovered to be of "actual" therapeutic value would be incorporated into what conventional medicine would offer (US Congress 1990; Hufford 1996; Coulter 2004; Horrigan 2007).

In its strongest form, this perspective is reflected in statements asserting that, if a therapy has been proven efficacious for a particular indication through rigorous scientific testing, "it no longer matters whether it was considered alternative at the outset" (Angell and Kassirer 1998); or that the ultimate, desirable goal is not to have conventional medicine and CAM (or even Integrative Medicine), but "just good medicine" (Snyderman and Weil

2002; Rayner, Willis, and Pirotta 2011; Rakel and Weil 2012; Holmberg, Brinkhaus, and Witt 2012), the arbiters of which would be conventional physicians, trained to a broadened medical worldview. Underlying statements of this type is the unspoken assumption that what truly matters in the CAM disciplines are their techniques and particular skills, and that these are readily transferrable to conventional medical settings if proven useful. This perspective is not always appreciated or accepted by CAM practitioners, who value their own disciplinary perspectives and training and typically feel that a crucial part of what their disciplines have to offer is precisely the lenses through which they see and interpret patients' problems, together with their philosophies of care (Boon et al. 2009; Holmberg et al. 2012). They tend to see disassociated skill and technical transfer as "co-optation" by biomedicine (Coulter 2004; Hsiao et al. 2006).

Defining Integrative Medicine/Integrative Health Care

If the struggle for defining and naming what we have settled on, despite its drawbacks, as "CAM" was politically charged, hotly contested, context dependent, and deeply confusing (Caspi et al. 2003; Hufford 1995; Committee on Definition and Description 2007), then identifying and defining terms for Integrative Medicine (IM) or Integrative Health Care (IHC) is a virtual battleground beset with complexity and conflict, as many different stakeholders attempt to claim their territories and influence or control the public discourse (Clouser, Hufford, and Morrison 1995; O'Connor 1995; Boon et al. 2004; Holmberg et al. 2012). Shaping the public discourse, especially in a newly emerging and promising field of endeavor, has important political and practical ramifications (Hufford 1995; Committee on Definition and Description 2007; Holmberg et al. 2012).

The inclusion/exclusion of terminology and conceptual models will affect statuses, relationships, policy, practice, education of multiple stakeholders (Porcino and MacDougall 2009), regulation, and the direction, designs, and funding of research (Clouser et al. 1995; Porcino et al. 2013), along with fundamental and far-reaching consequences such as who qualifies as a healthcare professional and for what purposes. For example, the National Center for Health Workforce Analysis presently includes massage therapists in its Allied Health category, and the Bureau of Labor Statistics recognizes massage therapists in tracking healthcare workforce statistics. But it remains to be seen how the various states will interpret "essential health benefits" and their providers under the terms of the 2010 Patient Protection and **Affordable Care Act (ACA)**.

There is currently an enormous range of definitions of IM/IHC, including particular requirements, and there are at least as many proposed models of implementation. Some definitions *include* specification of a practice model, a more overt placement of a stake in this contested ground. Here is a sampling of some published definitions:

- "[IM] shifts the orientation of medicine to one of healing rather than disease, engaging the mind, spirit, and community as well as the body. The integrative approach is based on a partnership of patient and practitioner within which conventional and alternative modalities are used to stimulate the body's innate healing potential" (Gaudet 1998).

- "An 'integrative' model of care is interdisciplinary whereby biomedical and other therapies outside its boundaries work together in non-hierarchical ways for the good of the patient" (Schroeder and Likkel 1999, cited in Boon et al. 2004).

- "The care, while multi-disciplinary, is physician directed. [...] Conventionally degreed physicians oversee the care and personally deliver conventional medical services, mind–body interventions, nutritional counseling, and in some cases acupuncture." (Horrigan 2007, 13).

- [IM] means "… combining CAM and conventional medical therapies in an **evidence-based** approach to providing patient care" (Boon and Kachan 2008).

- "… [IM] is healing-oriented and emphasizes the centrality of the physician *(sic)*–patient relationship. It focuses on the least invasive, least toxic, and least costly methods to help facilitate health by integrating both allopathic and complementary therapies. These therapies are recommended based on an understanding of the physical, emotional, psychological and spiritual aspects of the individual" (Rakel and Weil 2012, 6).

The wide range of elements and qualifiers stipulated in this small sample gives an idea of who is trying to ensure what perspectives and operating conditions are incorporated into a definition of IM/IHC. Clearly, not all of the stakeholders will agree to particular qualifiers, for example: the body's having an innate healing potential; that the pattern of working together will be non-hierarchical; that care delivery will be physician-directed; that conventional physicians should deliver certain CAM-originating treatment modalities; that the *physician* (vs. "practitioner")–patient relationship is central; or that either community or spirit (in the religious or metaphysical sense of the term) is necessarily entailed. The common denominator in all of the definitions is some kind of incorporation into patient care of both conventional and CAM therapeutic approaches (see also Institute of Medicine, 2009); about this much, there appears to be universal agreement.

Separating "Integrative Medicine" from "Integrative Health Care"

As early as the mid-1990s, proposals began to be put forward suggesting modifications to medical school curricula to teach IM. IM Fellowships opened in some academic medical centers, with the purpose of training "integrative physicians" (Gaudet 1998). Warnings were forthcoming that the public

were "voting with their feet" in huge numbers by choosing to add CAM to their healthcare resources, essentially making a public announcement that conventional medicine was missing the mark in meeting patient needs (Weil 2000). This view provided additional impetus to a growing movement within biomedicine to create educational guidelines, competencies, and programs for educating new generations of physicians to be integrative thinkers and practitioners. The Consortium of Academic Health Centers for Integrative Medicine (CAHCIM) had its inaugural planning meeting in 1999, coalesced under its current name the following year, and has grown in membership continually since. This consortium is composed only of medical schools/academic health centers (MD and DO). Its purpose is to promote scientific research and (specifically) *medical* education in IM. In 2004, members of the CAHCIM Education Working Group published a proposed set of "core competencies in integrative medicine for medical school curricula" (Kligler et al. 2004).

That same year, the Academic Consortium for Complementary and Alternative Health Care (ACCAHC) was founded "as a project of the Integrated Healthcare Policy Consortium (IHPC), an organization dedicated to promoting policies and action to advance integrated health care" (http://accahc.org/brief-history; accessed October 6, 2014). This consortium primarily represents educational and accrediting organizations in the five "licensed complementary and alternative healthcare professions [in Canada]" (acupuncture and oriental medicine, chiropractic, direct-entry midwifery, naturopathic medicine, and massage therapy) (Cambron and Schwartz 2012). ACCAHC initiated collaboration with CAHCIM in 2004 in an effort to include the voices and perspectives of CAM professions in CAHCIM's process of developing definitions, educational goals, and standards for IM in medical curricula. Milestones in this collaboration are listed on the ACCAHC website (http://accahc.org), and include publication of a peer-reviewed paper

(Benjamin et al. 2007) in response to the CAHCIM "core competencies" paper (Kligler et al. 2004). The ACCAHC response "underscored the importance of integrating disciplines and practitioners, not just therapies, in 'integrative medicine'" (http://accahc.org; accessed October 6, 2014). Among the responding authors' five key concerns with the CAHCIM proposal were "the definition of IM as presented in the paper; … omission of competencies related to collaboration between MDs and CAM professionals in patient care; and … omission of potential areas of partnership in IM education." (Benjamin et al. 2007, 1021).

Vigorous debate continues about the respective roles of conventional physicians and CAM professionals in integrative care. Some authors use the terms essentially interchangeably: "Integrative Medicine or Integrative Health Care [is] any approach that uses a partnering of both biomedicine … and complementary and alternative medicine" (Porcino and MacDougall 2009, 21). For others, the choice of the term *health care* instead of *medicine* "may reflect an author's views on the centrality of physicians in health care delivery systems" (Boon et al. 2009, 717). Some favor separating the terms as having genuinely differing referents. IM might be retained for what goes on in the integrative education, training, and practice of conventional physicians, to whom the term "medicine" has long referred (or some might say "belonged") (Boon et al. 2004). This may be especially apt as IM develops into an officially sanctioned medical specialty, as indicated by the creation in mid-2013 of the American Board of Integrative Medicine (a member of the American Board of Medical Specialties), which offered its first board-certification examinations to MDs/DOs in November 2014 (http://www.abpsus.org/integrative-medicine-board-january-2014-update; accessed November 18, 2014).

Boon and colleagues (2009) found that their interviewees across many healthcare disciplines considered IM to imply physician dominance, as exemplified both by the membership of CAHCIM and by that organization's definition of IM as: "a new approach to *medicine* that embraces the concerns of the public and *medical profession* for more effective, compassionate, *patient-centered medicine*" (CAHCIM website; as accessed February 27, 2009; emphasis added by Boon et al. 2009, 719). It is noteworthy that his definition was edited in both May and November 2009 (partly as a result of the ACCAHC critique), and now reads: "[IM] is the practice of *medicine* that reaffirms the importance of the relationship between practitioner and patient, focuses on the whole person, is informed by evidence, and makes use of all appropriate therapeutic approaches, healthcare professionals and disciplines to achieve optimal health and healing" (http://www.imconsortium.org/about/home.html; accessed October 7, 2014; emphasis added).

By contrast, Integrative Health Care or IHC would refer to the entire spectrum of healthcare delivery, in recognition of the facts that "medical care is but one of the many factors that contribute to … health" (Boon et al. 2004); that there are many disciplines and providers involved in this still-developing approach to patient care; and that this terminology reflects actual patterns of use of multiple healthcare resources by the public. In this usage the term "integrative" implies some form of conscientious coordination among multiple providers involved in particular patients' care.

Multiple Models of Integrative Care

There are as many models of what integrative care should look like as there are definitions of the key terms. These range from organizational integration of a team of conventional and CAM providers conjointly trained and working as clinical partners in the same outpatient clinical setting with shared electronic record-keeping (O'Connor, Levy, and Eisenberg 2013); to an in-hospital, inpatient integrative pain management service with full access to patient information and documentation in the electronic record (Dusek et al. 2010); to creation of several compositions of **interdisciplinary/ multidisciplinary teams** with active cross-referrals; to various forms of collaboration across/ among disciplines; to varied patterns of patient co-management with "informed referral" (Ben-Arye et al. 2008, 395). When Boon and colleagues (2009) interviewed key informants working in multiprofessional healthcare teams, they found "differences in stakeholder perceptions of the terms *collaboration* and *integration*." In discussions of care delivery models "any model that resulted in perceived loss of autonomy by any participant was generally considered less desirable" (Boon et al. 2009, 719).

A majority of the definitions and models of integrative care delivery describe ideal goals and may not accurately portray programs that are in operation as they actually function (Boon et al. 2004). Several authors have noted that, even in the idealized program model of all providers working as clinical partners in a single organization or clinical entity, conventional and CAM providers may in actuality occupy separate office spaces, on separate floors, buildings, or campuses; use separate patient records and case conferences; or "collaborate" in name only while communicating very little and actively maintaining the boundaries of their own professions (Shuval and Mizrachi 2004; Shuval Mizrachi, and Smetannikov 2002; Hollenberg 2006; Hsiao et al. 2006). In some settings, MDs decline to associate with their nominal CAM "partners," or to include them in patient case conferences (Shuval, et al. 2002); establish themselves as the primary providers for, and initial assessors of, patients, who see the "in-house" CAM providers only by MD referral (Boon and Kachan 2008); or assert dominance by creating situations in which the only commonly accepted language of interdisciplinary communication is the language of biomedicine (Anderson 1999; Hollenberg 2006). Boon and colleagues found that many of their [CAM] interviewees felt that multidisciplinary collaboration, rather than actual integration, was their ideal goal for patient care, perhaps because "collaboration involves structures and

processes that … preserve the uniqueness of philosophy and values of the players" (2009, 720). This preference leans toward the cooperative model of pluralism suggested by Kaptchuk and Miller (2005).

Most likely, many different models of collaboration will continue to emerge under the umbrella of integrative care, and the range of concept implementation will provide a living laboratory for discovering and testing what sorts of disciplinary arrangements work best to meet the needs of both patients and providers. There are already inpatient and outpatient specialty models such as Integrative Oncology, Integrative Pediatrics, Integrative Women's Health; and outcome-driven models such as Integrative Pain Management that cross many disciplinary and specialty boundaries and are adaptable to clinical settings from clinic or hospital to rehab to continuing patient self-care. The term "integrative" in the sense of incorporating both biomedical and CAM approaches can also be applied to particular patient-centered actions, such as formulating and implementing an integrative care plan.

Evidence-based vs. Evidence-informed Care

Among the many conceptual disputes with which the field of IM/IHC is fraught is the determination (by whom?) of how much of what kind(s) of evidence is required (by whom?) for a given modality/therapy to be considered "accepted" (by whom?) and brought into a formalized integrative care practice structure. Indeed, the very question of what *counts* as evidence remains open in this discussion. Since the inception of conventional medicine's interest in exploring therapies arising outside of its own borders, entities aligned with conventional medical research and practice have insisted that CAM therapies be subjected to the identical standards of scientific inquiry as biomedical therapies, and meet the exact same standards of proof of efficacy. Debates about this proposition have repeatedly noted two significant incongruities.

First, the reductionist approach of conventional scientific research (study the parts to understand the whole) is incongruent with exploration of systems that are inherently holistic, synergistic, context-dependent, or individualized in character and that claim their effects on the basis of precisely these qualities (Bell et al. 2002; Porcino et al. 2011, 2013; Abrams et al. 2013). In these cases, reductionist approaches lack construct validity within the framework of the systems/modalities under study, and thus are fundamentally altering at the outset what they claim to be studying.

Second, the conventional "gold standard," the double-blind, randomized, controlled clinical trial (RCT) is not a research design well suited to *any* therapies (e.g. involving touch, needles, or instruments which are impossible to blind to providers and very challenging (at best) to blind to patients). (This is an extremely simplified representation of a *very* complex and heated argument that involves many stakeholders [including the pharmaceutical industry, which also has vested interests here]; touches upon many elements, questions, subtleties, and subdebates; and is far too vast to be summarized in detail here.)

These challenges call for methodological innovation (much more easily said than done) that realistically reflects actual definitional criteria and parameters of practice of nonbiomedical therapies (Institute of Medicine 2005; Verhoef and Vanderhayden 2007; Bennell et al. 2011; Porcino et al. 2013), by realistically expanding the range of acceptable research designs, and by a measure of pragmatism. Research monies are limited, and time is short. It is as monstrously expensive—and time-consuming—to thoroughly study a nonbiomedical therapy as it is to study a biomedical one. One important contribution to a more rapid and less costly approach is outcomes or comparative outcomes research: how do patients actually *do* with this therapeutic approach? This is a widely accepted approach in both conventional and integrative healthcare research (Bell et al. 2002), and it is now supported

fiscally by a clause in the ACA that established the Patient-Centered Outcomes Research Institute (PCORI) in 2010. Outcomes research and other forms of pragmatic research/pragmatic trials are preferentially used by corporate entities (Kimbrough et al. 2010) and the military services (Pain Management Task Force 2010) to select which kinds of therapeutic approaches to approve for health insurance coverage based on their discoverable "track records" in returning employees to work or personnel to their posts of active duty or lives free of crippling pain. These entities have a primary interest in practical, workable solutions to the problem of loss of service by their constituents/employees, the largest cause of which by far is acute and chronic pain (Pain Management Task Force 2010). Mechanisms of action (*how* it works) are of less practical relevance than positive outcomes (*that* it works). Outcome measures that matter are success of treatment in terms of quality of life and return to work. The same can be said from the perspective of patients.

The rise of the evidence-based medicine (EBM) movement in conventional medicine is coincident with the growth of interest in CAM and IM (e.g. Guyatt et al. 1992). The ideal standard for EBM is rarely attained in actual biomedical practice. "Anyone strictly practicing evidence-based medicine bases his or her practice decisions on guidelines backed by the highest-quality evidence derived from multiple, [well-designed], congruent RCTs with perhaps a confirmatory meta-analysis or systematic review. The reality is that when a discipline looks closely at the evidence behind current practice guidelines, it is the minority of recommendations that attain this standard" (Donald B. Levy, MD, Medical Director, Osher Clinical Center for Integrative Medicine, Brigham and Women's Hospital, Brookline, MA, personal email, October 5, 2014; see also Tricoci et al. 2009). It is more factually accurate to refer to "**evidence-informed** practice" (Levy, personal communication 10/5/14, emphasis in original; Werner 2013), even within conventional medicine. Evidence-informed practice is generally defined as a practice or care plan formulation that combines the best available evidence, the clinician's experience, and the patient's preference for a particular therapeutic approach (Maiers et al. 2010). Given that real access to research funding for most CAM modalities has been possible in the USA for less than 20 years, and given the very large number and variety of researchable modalities, interventions, and combinations and the time it takes to accumulate a substantial research base, evidence-informed practice is a realistic, practical, and honest goal for CAM and for integrative models of health care.

Evidence Supporting Integrative Treatment of Pain

Chronic pain is the primary reason that patients in the US seek treatment from **integrative healthcare** clinics (Abrams et al. 2013). A substantial majority of integrative health centers associated with hospitals or medical schools report chronic pain as being among the five conditions most effectively treated by integrative methods or CAM providers (Horrigan et al. 2012). The two modalities to which pain patients are most commonly referred in these settings are **yoga** and massage (Cambron and Schwartz 2012; Horrigan et al. 2012). The majority of existing research on integrative pain management has focused on low back pain (LBP), and particularly on chronic low back pain (cLBP), an enormous public health problem in the USA. A research review by Chou and Huffman (2007) found "good evidence that cognitive-behavioral therapy, exercise, spinal manipulation, and interdisciplinary rehabilitation [not further specified] are all moderately effective for chronic or subacute (>4 weeks' duration) [LBP]" and "fair" evidence that massage and yoga are also effective for cLBP (p. 492). The most recent available update of the Cochrane Back Group's review of CAM therapies for LBP (Furlan et al. 2008) found that "massage might be beneficial for patients with subacute and chronic [>12 weeks] non-specific low-back pain, especially when combined with exercises and education" (http://onlinelibrary.wiley.com/

doi/10.1002/14651858. CD001929. pub2/abstract; accessed October 10, 2014). Maiers and colleagues, in a study of treatment models for cLBP, also report that "massage therapy reviews, combining evidence from higher-quality recent trials, [demonstrate] evidence of overall benefit and some pain relief lasting up to a year" (2010, 301).

In other causes of pain, a 2000 nationwide survey of rheumatologists regarding efficacy of CAM treatments for osteoarthritis and joint pain yielded a total of 345 respondents (of 600 surveyed); of these, 70% indicated that body work (defined only as "practices such as massage") was "either 'very beneficial' or 'moderately beneficial;' the modality with the next highest perceived benefit was meditation at 63%. … Rheumatologists were 'very' or 'somewhat likely' to recommend bodywork (65%), followed closely by meditation (64%)" to their patients experiencing joint pain (Manek et al. 2010, 7). Perlman and Njike conducted a prospective randomized controlled trial finding that Swedish massage was "safe and effective for reducing pain and improving function in patients with symptomatic [osteoarthritis] of the knee" (2006, 2536). Other studies have shown benefit for juvenile rheumatoid arthritis (Field et al. 1997), for pain relief in fibromyalgia (Sunshine et al. 1996; Brattberg 1999) and pain associated with cancer and its treatment (Cassileth and Vickers 2004), although systematic reviews of clinical trials of massage for cancer pain (e.g. Ernst 2009) have found that, while evidence is encouraging, the small size of trials and poor quality of study designs prevents this conclusion from being definitive at present.

Reporting on experiences with an inpatient integrative pain management (IPM) service, Dusek and colleagues found that across six hospital services (cardiovascular, medicine/surgery, orthopedics/spine, acute care rehabilitation, oncology, and women's health) and pain of all causes "[p]rovision of integrative services had immediate and beneficial effects … reducing self-reported pain by more than 50%" (2010, 45). Practitioners are hired by the hospital, and services are offered to patients without charge. IPM services include a range of mind–body therapies (including acupuncture and **acupressure**). In addition to significant pain reduction, IPM services enhanced patient safety by substituting for modalities including medications with higher risks of adverse side effects, and reduced length of stay by an average of half a day (Dusek et al. 2010).

An encouraging research direction with potential to elucidate and test mechanisms of action in pain control through bodywork is application of the **Multidimensional Assessment of Interoceptive Awareness (MAIA)** to pain patients. Mehling and colleagues, using this instrument, suggest that "[a]ttention regulation … appears to be a major element of **interoception** with potential applications for pain management" (2013, 404). These authors find that "[c]linical trials of mind–body therapies such as mindfulness meditation, yoga, **Tai Chi**, and Feldenkrais, for patients with pain, including [LBP], have provided encouraging results for these approaches that claim to improve body awareness as one potential mechanism of action" (Mehling et al. 2013, 404). Avenues for further research in this area include testing whether patient "training in mind–body approaches may lead to a different coping style with pain, possibly based on a different style of interoceptive attention regulation" (p. 415). This is an extremely promising line of inquiry.

The current research base for pain management incorporating manual and mind–body therapies is small but encouraging. For most therapeutic massage and bodywork disciplines (as for nursing, physical therapy, and occupational therapy) "case reports provide the foundations of practice-based evidence" (Munk and Boulanger 2014, 32); research sources are still relatively scarce. The large number of specific techniques and approaches (Sherman et al. 2006) and wide variability in training and personal practice styles (Porcino et al. 2011) make practice assessment and study design challenging.

Nevertheless, innovative designs have succeeded in obtaining meaningful results using mixed qualitative and quantitative methods (Porcino et al. 2011). One study created a clinical pathway for pain management incorporating individualization of therapeutic plans and coordinated use of multiple therapies, while providing for "consistent application of evidence-based care for [LBP] in the context of an integrative setting" (Maiers et al. 2010).

These are felicitous developments. Such innovations are likely to become more widespread in view of the Institute of Medicine's (IOM) 2011 report, *Relieving Pain in America*, which decries our current, inadequate state of pain treatment; calls for multidisciplinary approaches to pain management (occasionally mentioning "complementary and alternative medical providers" [e.g. IOM 2011, 10]); and strongly recommends "tailoring pain care to each person's experience" (IOM 2011, 8, Finding 3-1). Tailoring treatment plans to individual patients has always been an integral part of bodywork and mind–body therapies, and it appears now to be an approach whose promise and whose skilled practitioners are overdue for recognition in pain management.

References

Abrams, D. I., R. Dolor, R. Roberts, C. Pechura, J. Dusek, S. Amoils, S. Amoils, K. Barrows, J. S. Edman, J. Frye, et al. 2013. The BraveNet prospective observational study on integrative medicine treatment approaches for pain. *BMC Complementary and Alternative Medicine* 13:146–54.

Anderson, R. 1999. A case study in integrative medicine: alternative theories and the language of biomedicine. *Journal of Alternative and Complementary Medicine* 5(2):165–73.

Angell, M., and J. Kassirer. 1998. Alternative medicine: The risks of untested and unregulated remedies. *New England Journal of Medicine* 339(12):839–41.

Astin, J. 1998. Why patients use alternative medicine: Results of a national study. *Journal of the American Medical Association* 279 (19):1548–1553.

Barnes P. M, B. Bloom, and R. L. Nahin. 2008. Complementary and alternative medicine use among adults and children: United States, 2007. *National Health Statistics Reports*; no 12. Hyattsville, MD: National Center for Health Statistics.

Bell, I. R., O. Caspi, G. R. E. Schwartz, K. L. Grant, T. W. Gaudet, D. Rychener, V. Maizes, and A. Weil. 2002. Integrative medicine and systematic outcomes research: Issues in the emergence of a new model for primary health care. *Archives of Internal Medicine* 162:133–40.

Ben-Arye, E., M. Frenkel, A. Klein, and M. Scharf. 2008. Attitudes toward integration of complementary and alternative medicine in primary care: Perspectives of patients, physicians and complementary practitioners. *Patient Education and Counseling* 70(3): 395–402.

Benjamin, P. J., R. Phillips, D. Warren, C. Salveson, R. Hammerschlag, P. Snider, M. Haas, R. Barrett, T. Chapman, R. Kaneko, et al. 2007. Response to a proposal for an Integrative Medicine Curriculum. *Journal of Alternative and Complementary Medicine* 13(9):1021–34.

Bennell, K. L., T. Egerton, Y. H. Pua, J. H. Abbott, K. Sims, and R. Buchbinder. 2011. Building the rationale and structure for a complex physical therapy intervention within the context of a clinical trial: A multimodal individualized treatment for patients with hip osteoarthritis. *Physical Therapy* 91(10):1525–41.

Boon, H. S., and N. Kachan. 2008. Integrative medicine: A tale of two clinics. *BMC Complemenatry and Alternative Medicine* 8:32–51.

Boon, H. S., S. A. Mior, J. Barnsley, F. D. Ashbury, and R. Haig. 2009. The difference between integration and collaboration in patient care: Results from key informant interviews working in multiprofessional health care teams. *Journal of Manipulative and Physiological Therapies* 32(9):715–22.

Boon, H., M. Verhoef, D. O'Hara, B. Findlay, and N. Majid. 2004. Integrative health care: Arriving at a working definition. *Alternative Therapies in Health and Medicine* 10(5):48–56.

Brattberg, G. 1999. Connective tissue massage in the treatment of fibromyalgia. *European Journal of Pain* 3:235–44.

Briggs, J. P. 2014. NCCAM proposed name change (video). http://search.usa.gov/search/news/videos?affiliate=nccam&query=proposed+name+change, posted May 16, 2014 (accessed September 16, 2014).

Cambron, J., and J. Schwartz. 2012. What is the Academic Consortium for Complementary and Alternative Health Care (ACCAHC)? *International Journal of Massage Therapy and Bodywork* 5(2): 9–11.

Caspi, O., L. Sechrest, H. Pitluk, C. L. Marshall, I. R. Bell, and M. Nichter. 2003. On the definition of complementary, alternative, and integrative medicine: Societal mega-stereotypes vs the patients' perspectives. *Alternative Therapies in Health and Medicine* 9(6):58–62.

Cassileth, B. R., and A. J. Vickers. 2004. Massage therapy for symptom control: outcome study at a major cancer center. *Journal of Pain and Symptom Management* 28(3):244–9.

Cassileth, B. R., and E. J. Lusk, T. B. Strouse, and B. J. Bodenheimer. 1984. Contemporary unorthodox treatments in cancer medicine: A study of patients, treatments, and practitioners. *Annals of Internal Medicine* 101:105–12.

Chou, R., and L. H. Huffman. 2007. Nonpharmacologic therapies for acute and chronic low back pain: A review of the evidence for an American Pain Society/American College of Physicians clinical practice guideline. *Annals of Internal Medicine* 147:492–504.

Clouser, K. D., D. J. Hufford, and C. J. Morrison. 1995. What's in a word? *Alternative Therapies in Health and Medicine* 1(3):78–9.

Committee on Definition and Description, Office of Alternative Medicine, CAM Methodology Conference, 2005. 2007. Defining and describing complementary and alternative medicine. *Alternative Therapies in Health and Medicine* 3(2):49–57.

Coulter, I. 2004. Integration and paradigm clash. In *The Mainstreaming of Complementary and Alternative Medicine: Studies in Social Context*, eds. P. Tovey, G. Easthope, and J. Adams 103–22. London: Routledge.

Dusek, J. A., M. Finch, G. Plotnikoff, and L. Knutson. 2010. The impact of integrative medicine on pain management in a tertiary care hospital. *Journal of Patient Safety* 6(1): 48–51.

Eisenberg, D., R. Kessler, C. Foster, F. E. Norlock, D. R. Calkins, and T. L. Delbanco. 1993. Unconventional medicine in the United States: Prevalence, costs, and patterns of use. *New England Journal of Medicine* 328:246–52.

Engel, G. 1978. The Biopsychosocial Model and the education of health professionals. *Annals of the New York Academy of Sciences* 310:169–81.

Ernst, E. 2009. Massage therapy for cancer palliation and supportive care: A systematic review of randomized clinical trials. *Supportive Care in Cancer* 17:333–7.

Field, T., M. Hernandez-Reif, S. Seligman, J. Krasnegor, W. Sunshine, R. Rivas-Chacon, S. Schanberg, and C. Kuhn. 1997. Juvenile rheumatoid arthritis: Benefits from massage therapy. *Journal of Pediatric Psychology* 22:607–17.

Furlan, A. D., M. Imamura, T. Dryden, and E. Irvin. 2008. Massage for low-back pain. Cochrane Database of Systematic Reviews 2008, Issue 4. Art. No.: CD001929. DOI: 10.1002/14651858. CD001929.pub2.

Gaudet, T. W. 1998. Integrative medicine: The evolution of a new approach to medicine and to medical education. *Integrative Medicine* 1(2):67–73.

Guyatt, G., J. Cairns, D. Churchill, D. Cook, B. Haynes, J. Hirsh, J. Irvine, Mark Levine, Mitchell Levine, J. Nishikawa, et al. (Evidence-Based Medicine Working Group). 1992. Evidence-based medicine: A new approach to teaching the practice of medicine. *Journal of the American Medical Association* 268(17):2420–5.

Hollenberg, D. 2006. Uncharted ground: Patterns of professional interaction among complementary/alternative and biomedical practitioners in integrative health care settings. *Social Science and Medicine* 62:731–44.

Hollenberg, D., and L. Muzzin. 2010. Integrative medicine: An anti-colonial perspective on the combination of complementary/alternative medicine with biomedicine. *Health Sociology Review* 19(1):34–56.

Holmberg, C., B. Brinkhaus, and C. Witt. 2012. Experts' opinions on terminology for complementary and integrative medicine – a qualitative study with leading experts. *BMC Complementary and Alternative Medicine* 12:218–24.

Horrigan, B. (in collaboration with other Bravewell representatives). 2007. Integrative medicine best practices: Introduction and summary. Minneapolis, MN: The Bravewell Collaborative, 2007.

Horrigan, B., S. Lewis, D. Abrams, and C. Pechura. 2012. Integrative medicine in America: How integrative medicine is being practiced in clinical centers across the United States. Minneapolis, MN: The Bravewell Collaborative.

Hsiao, A.-F., G. W. Ryan, R. D. Hays, I. D. Coulter, R. M. Andersen, and N. S. Wenger. 2006. Variations in provider conceptions of integrative medicine. *Social Science and Medicine* 62:2973–87.

Hufford, D. J. 1984. *American healing systems: An introduction and exploration.* (Medical Ethnography Collection, George T. Harrell Library.) Hershey, PA: Milton S. Hershey Medical Center, Pennsylvania State University Medical School.

Hufford, D. J. 1995. Cultural and social perspectives on alternative medicine: Background and assumptions. *Alternative Therapies in Health and Medicine* 1(1):53–61.

Hufford, D. J.1996. Culturally grounded review of research assumptions. *Alternative Therapies in Health and Medicine* 2(4):47–53.

Institute of Medicine. 2005. *Complementary and Alternative Medicine in the United States.* Washington, DC: National Academies Press.

Institute of Medicine. 2009. *Integrative Medicine and the Health of the Public: A Summary of the February 2009 Summit.* Washington, DC: National Academies Press.

Institute of Medicine. 2011. *Relieving Pain in America: A Blueprint for Ttransforming Prevention, Care, Education, and Research.* Washington, DC: National Academies Press.

Kaptchuk, T. J., and F. G. Miller. 2005. What is the best and most ethical model for the relationship between mainstream and alternative medicine: Opposition, integration, or pluralism? *Academic Medicine* 80(3):286–90.

Kimbrough, E., L. Lao, B. Berman, K. R. Pelletier, and W. J. Talamonti. 2010. An integrative medicine intervention in a Ford Motor Company assembly plant. *Journal of Occupational and Environmental Medicine* 52(3):256–7.

Kligler, B., V. Maizes, S. Schachter, C. M. Park, T. Gaudet, R. Benn, R. Lee, and R. N. Remen. 2004. Core competencies in integrative medicine for medical school curricula: A proposal. *Academic Medicine* 79(6):521–31.

Maiers, M. J., K. K. Westrom, C. G. Legendre, and G. Bronfort. 2010. Integrative care for the management of low back pain: Use of a clinical pathway. *BMC Health Services Research* 10: 298–307.

Manek, N. J., C. S. Crowson, A. L. Ottenberg, F. A. Curlin, T. J. Kaptchuk, and J. C. Tilburt. 2010. What rheumatologists in the Unites States think of complementary and alternative medicine: Results of a national survey. *BMC Complementary and Alternative Medicine* 10:5–12.

Marwick, C. 1992a. Congress wants alternative therapies studied; NIH responds with programs. *Journal of the American Medical Association* 268(8):957–8.

Marwick, C. 1992b. Alternative therapies study moves into new phase. *Journal of the American Medical Association* 268(21):3040.

Marwick, C. 1994. Advisory group insists on 'alternative' voice. *Journal of the American Medical Association* 272(16):1239–40.

Mehling, W. E., J. Daubenmier, C. J. Price, M. Acree, E. Bartmess, and A. L. Stewart. 2013. Self-reported interoceptive awareness in primary care patients with past or current low back pain. *Journal of Pain Research* 6:403–18.

Munk, N., and K. Boulanger. 2014. Adaptation of the CARE guidelines for therapeutic massage and bodywork publications: Efforts to improve the impact of case reports. *International Journal of Therapeutic Massage and Bodywork* 7(3):32–40.

O'Connor, B. 1995. *Healing Traditions: Alternative Medicine and the Health Professions.* Philadelphia: University of Pennsylvania Press.

O'Connor, B., D. B. Levy, and D. M. Eisenberg. 2013. Case study: Osher Clinical Center for Complementary and Integrative Medical Therapies. In *Beyond The Checklist: What Else Healthcare Can Learn From Aviation Safety and Teamwork*, ed. S. Gordon, P. Mendenhall, and B. O'Connor, 102–16. Ithaca, NY: Cornell University Press.

Pain Management Task Force. 2010. Providing a standardized DoD and VHA vision and approach to pain management to optimize the care for warriors and their families. Washington, DC: Office of the Army Surgeon General.

Perlman, A. I., and V. Y. Njike. 2006. Massage therapy for osteoarthritis of the knee: A randomized controlled trial. *Archives of Internal Medicine* 166:2533–8.

Porcino, A. J., and C. MacDougall. 2009. The integrated taxonomy of health care: Classifying both complementary and biomedical practices using a uniform classification protocol. *International Journal of Therapeutic Massage and Bodywork* 2(3):18–30.

Porcino, A. J., H. S. Boon, S. A. Page, and M. J. Verhoef. 2011. Meaning and challenges in the practice of multiple therapeutic massage modalities: A combined methods study. *BMC Complementary and Alternative Medicine* 11:75–85.

Porcino, A. J., H. S. Boon, S. A. Page, and M. J. Verhoef. 2013. Exploring the nature of therapeutic massage bodywork practice. *International Journal of Therapeutic Massage and Bodywork* 6(1):15–24.

Rakel, D., and A. Weil. 2012. Philosophy of integrative medicine. In *Integrative Medicine*, ed. D. Rakel, 3rd edn, 2–11. Philadephia: Elsevier/Saunders.

Rayner, J., K. Willis, and M. Pirotta. 2011. What's in a name? Integrative medicine or simply good medical practice? *Family Practice* 28:655–60.

Schroeder, C. A., and J. Likkel. 1999. Integrative health care: The revolution is upon us. *Public Health Nursing* 16(4):233–34.

Sherman, K. J., M. W. Dixon, D. Thompson, and D. C. Cherkin. 2006. Development of taxonomy to describe massage treatments for musculoskeletal pain. *BMC Complementary and Alternative Medicine* 6:24–30.

Shuval, J., and N. Mizrachi. 2004. Changing boundaries: Modes of coexistence of alternative and biomedicine. *Qualitative Health Research* 14:675–90.

Shuval, J. T., N. Mizrachi, and E. Smetannikov. 2002. Entering the well-guarded fortress: Alternative practitioners in hospital settings. *Social Science and Medicine* 55:1745–55.

Snyderman, R., and A. T. Weil. 2002. Integrative medicine: Bringing medicine back to its roots. *Archives of Internal Medicine* 162:395–7.

Sunshine, W., T. Field, O. Quintino, K. Fierro, C. Kuhn, I. Burman, and S. Schanberg. 1996. Fibromyalgia benefits from massage therapy and transcutaneous electrical stimulation. *Journal of Clinical Rheumatology* 2:18–22.

Tricoci, P., J. M. Allen, J. M. Kramer, R. M. Califf, and S. C. Smith. 2009. Scientific evidence underlying the ACC/AHA clinical practice guidelines. *Journal of the American Medical Association* 301(8):831–41.

US Congress, Office of Technology Assessment. 1990. Unconventional Cancer Treatments (OTA-H-405). Washington, DC: US Government Printing Office.

Verhoef, M., and L. Vanderhayden. 2007. Combining qualitative methods and RCTs in CAM intervention research. In *Researching Complementary and Alternative Medicine*, ed. J. Adams, 72–86. Milton Park, Oxon: Routledge.

Weil, A. 2000. The significance of integrative medicine for the future of medical education. *American Journal of Medicine* 108:441–3.

Werner, R. 2013. We should do a journal: A brief history of the IJTMB. *International Journal of Massage Therapy and Bodywork* 6(2):1–2. (Open access, electronic-only journal at http://www.ijtmb.org; accessed October 3, 2014.)

Champagne for my real friends, and real pain for my sham friends.

Tom Waits

Introduction

This chapter examines some of the basic human anatomy and neurobiology related to the perception of pain. In this context we will discuss how the nervous, endocrine, and musculoskeletal/**fascial** systems all contribute to our experience of this important sensation. We will look at some of the pathologic changes that occur when short-term pain becomes a long-term problem, and how stress can exacerbate pain perception. Finally, we will discuss how manual therapies may access peripheral nervous system structures in order to address some of the factors that can contribute to chronic pain patterns.

What is Pain?

The concept of pain has many definitions, but for the purposes of this chapter, this one is a good fit:

> *Pain is an unpleasant sensory and emotional experience associated with actual or potential tissue damage, or described in terms of such damage.*
>
> (Merskey and Bogduk 2012)

This description introduces several important points. First is the term "unpleasant": who decides if an experience is unpleasant? Only the person experiencing it can make this judgment. Pain is a completely subjective phenomenon (Coghill 2010). While we can empathize with another person's pain, it is not possible to feel or interpret it in comparison to any other person's experience.

Also, according to this definition, pain has both sensory and emotional components. The interconnectedness of our emotional state to our physical state cannot be overemphasized. For many people whose pain is long-lasting, these two aspects of experience become inextricably entangled, to the extent that physical pain often cannot be successfully treated without addressing emotional pain, and vice versa (Deligianni, Vikelis, and Mitsikostas 2012).

Finally, pain may occur in association with actual or potential damage. The perception of pain may occur with anticipation alone, separate from that caused by tissue damage. All of these ideas figure prominently in this chapter, but we will start with pain that begins from an environmental, rather than an emotional trigger.

Pain as Part of the Sensory System

The great art in life is sensation, to feel that we exist, even in pain.

Lord Byron

Pain serves a vital function to healthy people: it lets us know when we are at risk for injury. If we lose this function, then ordinary normal interactions with our environment can quickly lead to tissue damage. Imagine not knowing that the oven rack is hot, that you have a blister on your toe, or that you broke a bone. The threat of invading infection and challenging complications is significant, which is why we need an effective reaction to this type of stimulus (see Sidebar 2.1).

Sidebar 2.1 Numbness is Dangerous

Leprosy, nowadays known as Hansen's disease, is a collection of bacterial infections of nerve endings in the skin and mucous membranes where the temperature is relatively low. Unlike other nerve infections, Hansen's disease leads to dangerous numbness rather than pain. The result is a gradual atrophy of healthy skin and small muscles, accrual of minor injuries, and tissue-destroying secondary infections coupled with poor healing. These accumulate to the point that extremities such as fingers, toes, ears, and the nose appear to simply "fall off."

At its most elemental, pain is simply a signal of real or potential damage. It is often classified by the source of that damage. Examples include mechanical injury (caused by impact, pressure, or swelling), temperature-related injury (for instance, frostbite or burns that can range from a mild sunburn to extreme of third-degree charring), or chemical injuries (various toxins, infection, or ischemia).

Pain is often multifactorial: it is rarely only one type of damage that creates this perception.

Many of us learned in elementary school that we have five senses: seeing, hearing, smelling, tasting, and touch. Vision, hearing, taste, and smell are called special senses because their receptors are located in isolated, specialized areas. But the sensation of touch is called a general sense because our touch receptors are located all over the body, in our skin, connective tissue, and internal organs. For more on the general senses of heat and cold, see Sidebar 2.2.

In fact, the term "touch" covers several distinct senses, including light and deep pressure, texture, hot, cold, and pain. Each of these sensations has a dedicated type of receptor neuron.

> **Sidebar 2.2 Fun Facts about Food and Sensation**
> Imagine eating a minty breath freshener. Now imagine taking a sip of water—even warm water. Feels colder than usual, right? The reason for this is that menthol in mint hypersensitizes our receptors to cold, so everything feels colder.
>
> The opposite is true of capsaicin, the substance that puts the "heat" in hot peppers: it hypersensitizes our receptors to heat, so that everything, even the cold beer that you gulped after your five-alarm chili verde, feels hot.

It is critically important to understand the definitions of the language used in the study of pain. These definitions are regularly updated by groups of scientists and clinicians and published by the International Association for the Study of Pain. For our discussion, the most important definitions are those of pain and nociception:

- *Pain*, a sensation that integrates multiple pathways of nerve transmission, has been defined above.

- *Nociception* describes the neural processes of encoding and managing noxious, or potentially painful stimuli.

Not all pain requires nociception, and not all nociception leads to pain. **Nociceptors** are sensory neurons in the peripheral or central nervous system (PNS, CNS) that carry signals. Nociceptors convert, or transduce, various stimuli (energy forms), such as might occur from a cut or other injury, into electrical impulses that communicate with the CNS, where we interpret the information. No single chain of neurons leads to the perception of pain; it takes many neurons in multiple pathways to create this awareness.

By contrast, nociceptor discharge, or nociception, happens regardless of whether we interpret pain as the outcome of the nerve transmission. It can be measured directly by recording from the neuron, even if the neuron is disconnected from the body.

Once a noxious stimulus begins, the signals travel through complex pathways within the CNS. Signals can be amplified or suppressed in several places along the way. The details of these pathways and interactions are far beyond the scope of this chapter. We will focus on the part of the system with which we most often directly interact: the nociceptors of the peripheral nervous system.

Pain Pathways: From Outside to Inside

The process of turning an environmental trigger into pain perception takes several discrete steps.

Transduction

The first step, transduction, occurs when nociceptors are activated by a trigger, such as pressure, high or low temperature, or chemical irritation. The stimulus is converted into an action potential by specialized receptor channels in the cell membrane. It is important to remember that activated nociceptors also simultaneously secrete proinflammatory chemicals, which contribute to the inflammatory response at the site of injury.

Transmission

After transduction, the **axon** transmits the message from the body to the spinal cord's dorsal horn through the dorsal root. Here the axon branches to multiple segments and to multiple levels. If the input is sufficient to propagate at this level, it crosses to the contralateral side of the spinal cord and travels to the thalamus (see Figure 2.1).

Perception

The thalamus, which functions somewhat like an old-fashioned switchboard, transmits incoming signals to the appropriate cerebral cortical centers for consciousness and interpretation. Unlike our other senses, we have no specific area in the brain to receive information about pain or tissue damage. Instead, the thalamus sends these messages toward the reticular center for autonomic motor responses; the somatosensory cortex for interpretation, evaluation and memory; and the limbic system: the source of our emotional and behavioral responses.

Modulation

While the major part of messages in sensation travel from the peripheral nervous system up to

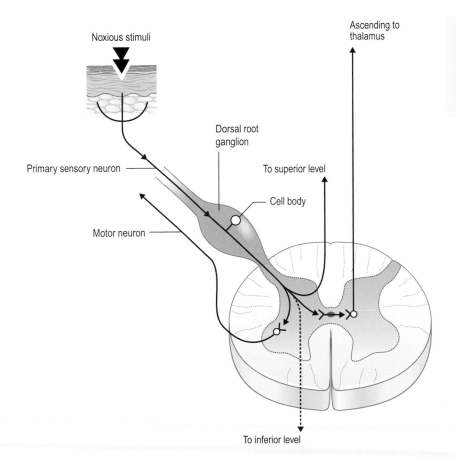

Noxious stimuli

Ascending to thalamus

Dorsal root ganglion

Primary sensory neuron

To superior level

Cell body

Motor neuron

To inferior level

Figure 2.1
From stimulus to perception of pain, nociception is a complicated pathway.

the brain, at each step of the way the transmission can be either amplified or depressed, by activity in descending pathways. These interactions are all neurochemical; excitatory neurotransmitters make our pain sensation more intense, while inhibitory neurotransmitters act as organic analgesia, subduing our perception of pain. (For more on organic analgesics, see Sidebar 2.3.) All of this happens below levels of consciousness, even before we may become conscious of ongoing pain signals.

Sidebar 2.3 Fun Facts about Neuromodulation
It is no surprise that opium and marijuana are such popular drugs. Our bodies produce very powerful versions of both, and both can have profound suppressing influences on pain.

Opium poppies secrete morphine in their "milk," the base for heroin, morphine, and codeine. Oxycodone and similar drugs are synthesized versions of the same chemicals. Endorphins are endogenous **opiates**, and they all inhibit critical pain pathways.

The active ingredient in marijuana is a *cannabinoid*. We produce **anandamide** (based on a Sanskrit word for bliss), and many other cannabinoids. While these affect many systems, in relation to pain, these chemicals are powerful pain suppressants. Acetaminophen works in the cannabinoid pathways as well.

Understanding the steps in the transmission of signals that are eventually interpreted and consciously perceived as pain provides important treatment strategies, because different types of analgesics act at different sites in the transmission process. Over-the-counter anti-inflammatories, for instance, act at the tissue level by working to reduce the mechanical pressure and chemical irritation that may trigger pain signals at the site of an injury. Antiseizure drugs, by contrast, are powerful pain modulators because they suppress the secretion of excitatory **neurotransmitters** in the central nervous system. Antidepressants are sometimes used as pain treatments because they do exactly the opposite: they promote the secretion and uptake of inhibitory neurotransmitters, which leads to the same result: the reduced perception of pain.

Pain is sometimes called the "fifth vital sign" because a patient's report of pain must inform the priorities for his or her treatment. This is a complicated issue, however, because when a patient reports acute or severe pain, treatment is often limited to opioid drugs, which are fraught with problematic side effects and undesired consequences (Morone and Weiner 2013) and have little effect on the primary afferent nociceptor. That said, the experience of being in pain gives rise to several stress-related reactions that can increase the risk of serious health problems. Increased potential for blood clots, hypertension, depression, and insomnia (which deprives us of sleep, our best opportunity for tissue repair) comprise a short list of the consequences of long-term pain. All of this points to a need to develop more and better strategies for dealing with pain in acute and chronic settings.

Nociceptors: Pain Signal Initiators

Nociceptors are the first sensors in the pathways to pain. The neuronal cell bodies are located in the dorsal root ganglia, which lie in the intervertebral foramina. The cell bodies extend one axon, which splits into two branches before leaving the **ganglion**. One branch goes to the spinal cord through the dorsal root, and the other one extends to the peripheral structures through the spinal nerve. Nociceptors innervate almost every structure and tissue type in the body (exceptions include the nucleus pulposis of intervertebral discs and hyaline cartilage).

When nociceptors reach their target, they branch into numerous very fine processes, and are called "nerve endings." Unlike other sensory neurons, nociceptor processes have no obvious capsule or structure around them, so they are often referred to as "free" nerve endings. However, nociceptors are not nerves; they are single neurons. Further, functionally these are not endings; they are beginnings, in that the impulses begin here. Nociceptor processes are sensitive specifically to the types of stimuli that lead to the brain's interpretation of pain. In the skin, these include mechanical, thermal, and chemical triggers. In the deeper structures, the nociceptors respond to these stimuli as well, but thermal stimuli may be less important, as the body keeps internal temperature relatively constant.

Nociceptors that supply the skin look like a spray of flowers; these define the "**receptive field**" for the individual neuron. Receptive fields are usually relatively small, but they can be discontinuous and may or may not overlap with other neurons' receptive fields. In fact, the skin has some areas that are not innervated at all, where a needle can pierce without pain.

The receptive fields of the skin are relatively well established, but we know less about the receptive fields of muscle and other deep nociceptors. It is clear that they can be larger and involve multiple tissue types (Bove and Light 1995). This means that a nociceptor innervating a muscle might also innervate the tendon associated with that muscle, and also the nerve sheath in which it is encased (see Figure 2.2). This may explain the generally poor spatial localization of pain from deep structures compared to that of skin.

Types of Nociceptors

The nomenclature that scientists currently use to describe nociceptors is a bit clumsy. The distinctions between types of nociceptor are described here for completeness but are by no means critical to the understanding of pain anatomy. However, these terms frequently appear in the literature, so it can be helpful to have a basic idea of their characteristics.

- C-fibers
  Afferent or sensory axons within a peripheral nerve are various sizes (see Figure 2.3). The smallest diameter axons, **C-fibers,** are about 1–2 µ diameter, they are unmyelinated, and they conduct action potentials very slowly (under 2.5 m/sec). These are typically associated with nociceptor function, although

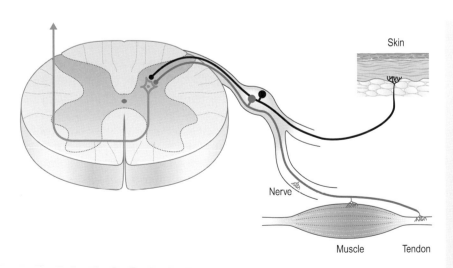

Skin

Nerve

Muscle   Tendon

Figure 2.2
Individual nociceptors to skin and deep structurs have fundamental differences. Among these, skin nociceptors innervate discrete areas of skin, while deep nociceptors may innervate several tissue types. This may explain why sometimes it is more difficult to identify where the initial signals in the deep pain pathways arise.

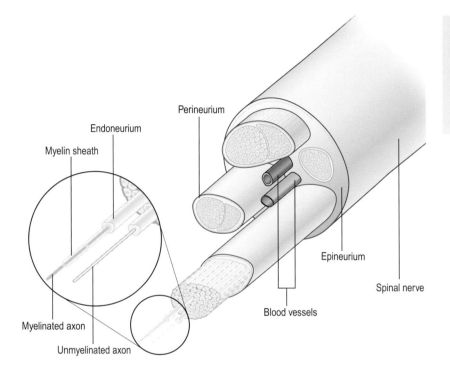

Figure 2.3
Peripheral nerve anatomy showing C-fibers (unmyelinated) and A-delta fibers (myelinated) within their fascia.

Perineurium

Endoneurium

Myelin sheath

Epineurium

Spinal nerve

Blood vessels

Myelinated axon

Unmyelinated axon

not all C-fiber axons are nociceptive. In skin, nociceptors with C-fiber axons are called C-nociceptors. In muscle and other deep structures, nociceptors with C-fiber axons are called Group IV nociceptors.

- A-delta nociceptors
  A-delta axons are slightly larger than C-fibers. These axons have a thin myelin sheath, and conduct action potentials at 2.5–10 m/sec. In skin, nociceptors with A-delta axons are called A-delta nociceptors, while in muscle and other tissues they are called Group III nociceptors.

The sensations associated with **A-delta fiber** stimuli are highly localized, and often described as "sharp," "stinging," or "pricking." C-fibers, by contrast, are slow conductors, and several different types of stimuli can trigger them. Mechanical distortion, thermal injury, and chemical irritations can all activate C-fibers, hence the common term "polymodal nociceptor." Descriptors of C-fiber related pain

include "diffuse," "dull," and "aching;" these also reflect the slower nature of C-fiber stimulation.

Nociceptor Activation

When an event such as pressure, thermal injury, or chemical imbalance causes tissue damage, a flood of proinflammatory substance is released into the local tissues (see Figure 2.4). Prostaglandin behaves like a localized hormone, promoting pain sensitivity and vasodilation; bradykinin, serotonin, potassium, and histamine all prolong and reinforce the inflammatory response. When these chemicals activate nociceptors, they release two substances that are key to inflammation. **Calcitonin gene-related peptide (CGRP)** causes blood vessels to dilate, and Substance P (SP) causes the fenestrations in the blood vessels to open. This allows immune cells to cross from the blood to the extracellular matrix to do their job of cleaning up the damage. This essential endocrine function of nociceptors is referred to as neurogenic inflammation, and it occurs whenever nociceptors are activated.

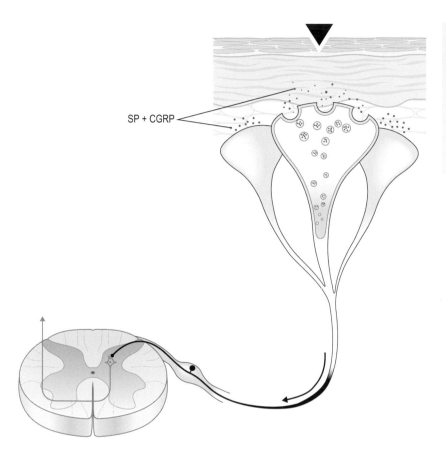

SP + CGRP

Figure 2.4
Nociceptors release pro-inflammatory chemicals at the site of tissue damage, at the same time as carrying nociceptive signals to the CNS.

The need for nociceptors in acute pain is not controversial, but their involvement in chronic pain is hotly debated. All pain scientists recognize that pain can exist without any peripheral input. However, data are accumulating that indicate that even in the most reticent chronic pain cases a source of peripheral nociception often maintains the centrally mediated pain processes (Gracely, Lynch, and Bennett 1992; Staud 2011). This means that a client who has long-term pain related to central nervous system hypersensitivity probably also has a source of nociception, from peripheral tissues, that contributes to the problem. This is good news, because if a manual therapist can identify and help to resolve those irritants, then at least some contributors to the pain cycle can be interrupted.

Good Pain, Bad Pain

While the experience of pain is not something we generally look forward to, pain processes can be highly useful, or dangerously dysfunctional.

Nociceptive Pain

The most highly functional form of pain is sometimes called *nociceptive pain*, referring to the perception of something noxious. This is a normal, healthy process: a signal of tissue damage is modulated by inflammatory responses, including the secretion of proinflammatory chemicals at the site of injury. These chemicals tend to reinforce and prolong the pain messages. Pain helps us make appropriate accommodations to limit further damage: we limp, taking pressure off our sprained ankle, or we avoid re-injuring our hurt finger by using other fingers instead. As the tissue heals, inflammatory chemicals subside, and pain sensation diminishes.

Ectopic Nociceptive Pain

Under normal circumstances, axons are not sensitive to normally encountered stimuli along the length of the fiber; they only pick up messages at their "flower spray" end points. This is good, because it provides spatial specificity for the sensation: we need to be able to tell exactly where a signal comes from. This is easily demonstrated. If you pinch your little finger on the palmar side, you will feel the nociception as coming from the pinched spot. However, if you press moderately hard on the ulnar nerve as it passes behind your ulnar medial epicondyle, you should not feel any sensation into your fingers, even though you are pressing on the axons that were carrying the previous message of

"pinch." That said, we have all banged our "funny bone" and felt pain and tingling in our fingers, through mid-axonal activation of the ulnar nerve. Although the axons are being activated in their middle, the impulses going to the CNS are perceived as coming from the fingers (see Figure 2.5). This activation of the axons is *ectopic*, meaning that our interpretation of the source of pain is in the wrong place, like an ectopic pregnancy, which may occur in a uterine tube rather than in the uterus.

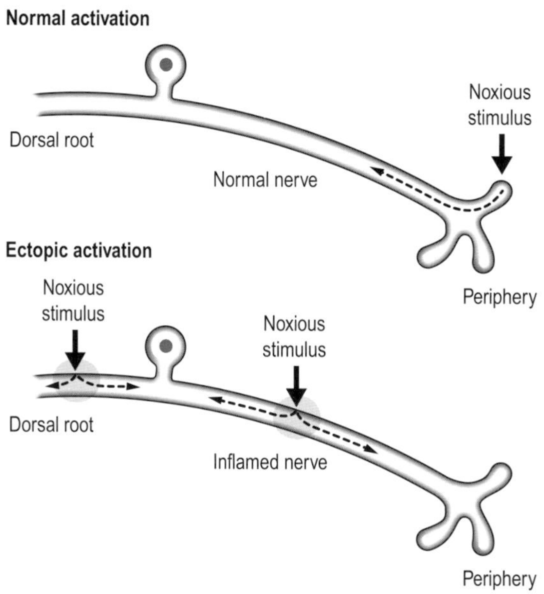

Ectopic nociceptive pain is a term coined by Geoffrey Bove and David Seaman (Bove and Seaman 2010), based on observations of the effects of inflammation of nociceptor axons. As axons wind through nerves and between various structures, they can be exposed to inflammation when they pass through an injured or damaged area. For instance, a deep bruise of the posterior thigh can affect the sciatic nerve and create symptoms that seem to come from the leg, or a constricted carpal tunnel may compress the median nerve, causing pain that appears to come from the hand. The nerve, which might be otherwise normal, then becomes an "innocent bystander" of the local inflammation (see Sidebar 2.4).

Figure 2.5
Ectopic axonal activation: No matter where a particular axon is activated, the sensation will be perceived in the innervated structure, not at the site of activation.

> ### Sidebar 2.4 Inflamed Axons and Cutaneous vs. Deep Pain
>
> Inflammation alone does not damage axons. Inflammation has been found to evoke sensitivity only from nociceptor axons that go to deep structures (Bove et al. 2003). When inflamed, deep nociceptor axons display sensitivity to mechanical and chemical stimuli. Nociceptors to the skin do not show these sensitivities. This is a critical difference between the innervation of the skin and that of other structures. Think about it. How many of our clients in pain describe that pain as being just in their skin? Patients with radiculopathy (radiating or distal pain that is due to dorsal and/or ventral root pathology, including inflammation) do not usually report cutaneous pain (Bove, Zaheen, and Bajwa 2005).

Using our previous example, if the ulnar nerve was inflamed, pressing on it could cause pain to be felt into the hand. This radiating pain would be appropriately called ectopic nociceptive pain. Likewise, leg pain from the sciatic nerve or hand pain from the median nerve is ectopic nociceptive pain. This phenomenon is the basis of positive nerve provocation tests, where the nerve is stressed along its length but the symptoms are reported distal to the stimulus.

Inflamed axons can also generate action potentials without any other stimulus (Bove 2009). This is called "ongoing activity," and it results in the sensation of pain at rest or with no identified trigger. But again, the site of action potential generation is not the site of symptom perception, so the whole situation can be very confusing. In this situation, a thorough knowledge of nociception patterns allows manual therapists to untangle some of these confusing symptoms, and to get at the root of their clients' problems.

Nerve Trunk Pain

The term "nerve trunk" describes any large section of a peripheral nerve. When you palpated your ulnar nerve (a nerve trunk) at the medial elbow, you may have felt pain at that site. To feel something and be able to localize it, a receptor must be tuned to the stimulus and located appropriately. For nerve trunks, these receptors are called the nervi nervorum, or the "nerves on the nerves." Like other structures, nerves have their own sensory innervation, which includes nociceptors (Bove and Light 1997). These nociceptors run within the connective tissue of the nerves and neurovascular bundle, and—at least in rats—branch and innervate relatively long stretches of the nerve. Clinical examination often identifies sections of nerves that are locally tender: this sensation is mediated by the nervi nervorum, and is appropriately called nerve trunk pain.

Peripheral Nerve Damage

The word **neuropathy** refers to a lesion of part of the nervous system. In the peripheral nervous system (PNS), neuropathy refers to damage to the sensory cell bodies found in the **dorsal root ganglion (DRG)**, and to sensory and motor axons within a peripheral nerve, including cranial nerves. The dorsal and ventral roots are usually considered parts of the PNS as well. In the CNS, neuropathy is used to describe damage to CNS structures such as the spinal cord and brain. We need to remember that the autonomic nervous system, consisting of the sympathetic and parasympathetic divisions, also sends axons to peripheral and cranial nerves, and contributes to pain under certain circumstances. To remain in the scope of this chapter, we will limit our discussion to effects of damage to peripheral nerves.

Peripheral nerves can be damaged in numerous ways, including by trauma, infection, chemotherapy, radiation therapy, fascial entrapment, and pathologies such as degenerative disc disease. It is important to remember that not all nerve injuries are painful, and most heal with no lasting pain. Nerve injury symptoms indicate what types of axons have been damaged. That is, if motor axons are damaged in isolation, the denervated muscle will be paralyzed, but not painful. If the sensory axons are damaged in isolation, the denervated territory will be numb, but moveable. If the sympathetic axons within a peripheral nerve are damaged, symptoms can include decreased blood flow, goose bumps, and/or sweating in the denervated area.

When nociceptor axons within a peripheral nerve are damaged, they develop spurious activity, which can be perceived as pain. They regenerate rapidly, but while most peripheral nerve injuries heal well, in some cases the healing fails and the endings form a neuroma: a tangled mass of axons growing in a ball, or a sort of tumor, with no well-defined receptive field. If the injury was diffuse, and axons were damaged along a length of nerve, the result is often called a **"neuroma in continuity."** Injuries in which nerves are stretched, like brachial plexus injuries, often lead to neuroma in continuity, which can be devastating. Neuromas can develop and then remain hypersensitive to all kinds of stimuli, becoming a source of strong afferent discharge that causes a more intense, severe experience than most other sources of pain. The signals from damaged nociceptors seem particularly efficient at evoking central sensitization, a potentially serious phenomenon that contributes to neuropathic pain.

Neuropathic pain: a description, not a diagnosis

Neuropathic pain is an abnormal sensation, usually caused by a lesion or disease of the somatosensory nervous system; that is, it is often caused by a type of neuropathy, as described above. It is critical to understand that "neuropathic pain" is a *clinical description* rather than a *diagnosis*. It is equally critical to understand that neuropathies do not necessarily cause neuropathic pain, and that neuropathic pain can exist in the absence of neuropathy. The effects of persistent nociceptive pain and ectopic nociceptive pain can include symptoms that qualify as neuropathic pain, but with no true neuropathy. This is why the definition has recently been amended to a clinical description and is under constant revision as our knowledge base grows.

The complex of symptoms that we call neuropathic pain usually includes the presence of a peripheral generator or initiating trigger, though one cannot always be found. The term peripheral generator describes a source of nociceptor discharge. As has been pointed out, neuropathies are often a source of this discharge, but they are not requisite.

Even a single bout of intense niciceptor discharge can induce and maintain changes in the CNS, most of which have been studied in the dorsal horn of the spinal cord. These changes are currently referred to as central sensitization. It is the combination of the persistent **afferent** discharge and the effects of central sensitization that comprise neuropathic pain. The qualities of neuropathic pain can be different from other pain sensations. While the perception of typical tissue damage might be described as "dull," "sharp," "achy," or "throbbing," in the context of directly damaged nerve tissue patients often use adjectives like "burning," "electric," and "tingling."

Neuropathic pain has several possible causes. For a list of common diagnoses associated with neuropathic pain, see Sidebar 2.5.

Sidebar 2.5 Common Descriptors and Diagnoses for Neuropathic Pain

- Diabetic neuropathy
- Postherpetic neuropathy
- Entrapment neuropathies (carpal tunnel syndrome, thoracic outlet syndrome, etc.)
- Nerve compression or infiltration by tumor
- Chemotherapy-induced peripheral neuropathy
- Post-radiation plexopathy
- Phantom limb pain
- Acute and chronic dymelinating **polyradiculopathy** (e.g. Guillain-Barre syndrome)
- Alcoholic **polyneuropathy**
- **Radiculopathy**
- Complex regional pain syndrome
- HIV sensory neuropathy
- Nutritional deficiency neuropathies
- Toxic exposure neuropathies
- Tic douloureux (trigeminal neuralgia)

Altered Neural Processing, aka Central Sensitization

Central sensitization (CS) refers to a complex change in the CNS induced by abnormal peripheral activation. When painful, CS can be devastating. A perfect example is the too-frequent complication of adult herpes zoster infections (aka "shingles"), called postherpetic neuralgia. The first appearance of the infection for most people is as a childhood bout with chickenpox, but the virus then goes into dormancy, usually residing in a dorsal root or trigeminal ganglion. Later in adulthood it may reactivate: after a prodromal period usually described as a tingling sensation, painful blisters form on the skin all along the dermatome of the affected nerve. It is thought that the infection causes the degeneration of the nociceptor terminals, causing spurious activation and pain. If the symptoms persist after the visible lesions heal, the condition is called postherpetic neuralgia. The skin becomes hypersensitive to light touch, and even a slight breeze will cause excruciating pain. Patients often cannot wear clothes or have bedsheets covering the affected area. These symptoms are not likely to be mediated by nociceptors; sensors that normally carry the sensation of light touch and temperature mediate them. So why do these neurons suddenly relay pain messages? And why can the changes persist, often for the lifetime of the patient?

Hyperalgesia

Hyperalgesia is increased pain from a stimulus that normally provokes pain, and is a clinical term that does not imply a mechanism (Merskey and Bogduk 2012). When damaged, nociceptors demonstrate increased sensitivity at their peripheral processes, and this effect can occur in the spinal cord as well. The nociceptors can secrete more neurotransmitter per action potential, and the corresponding spinal cord neuron can also become more responsive. Therefore, less nociceptor input will lead to stronger relaying of the information. Moreover, with persistent stimulation, nociceptors can grow more branches. This has the effect of extending the signal to more neurons. These changes serve to "turn up the volume" of pain.

Allodynia

More problematic even than increased reactivity to nociceptor activity is the strengthening of a pathway from the low threshold non-nociceptive receptors to the same dorsal horn neurons. This means that normally nonpainful or innocuous stimuli such as warmth or light touch can lead to a sensation of pain, in a situation called **allodynia**. In other words, even very minor, subtle sensory signals create a perception of pain. These light touch neurons are capable of very high frequency discharge, which may account for the very intense nature of pain once this pathway had been established (see Figure 2.6).

Neuroplasticity

When peripheral nociceptors enter the spinal cord, they branch to span multiple spinal segments, and they also reach multiple levels of the spinal cord. In response to injury, this branching pattern becomes more extensive. If the new branches reach more nociceptive-specific cells, the expected phenomenon would be an increased pain perception, or hyperalgesia. If the new branches reach more wide dynamic range cells, which respond to many types of input, the expected phenomena include the perception of pain when there was no noxious stimulus, or allodynia. These phenomena, combined with new CNS receptor sites, may account for the perception of an increased "volume" of pain following nerve injury.

Loss of pain filters

The problems carry on within the brain as well as in the spinal cord: in the presence of central sensitization, descending pain-modulating pathways in the brain—those innate processes that act as organic analgesia by inhibiting our responses— may become dysfunctional. In other words, we cannot filter out the pain sensation. The peripheral neurons become sensitized; the ascending tract becomes sensitized; the brain perceives pain out of proportion to the nature of the damage, and finally our

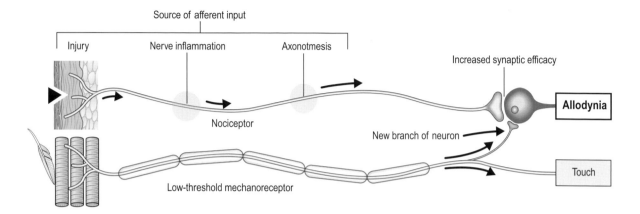

Figure 2.6

Peripheral sensory sensitization. Normally, nociceptor activation (top) and low threshold stimulation of the skin (bottom) contribute to pain and light touch, respectively. However, when primary afferent nociceptors are injured by damageto any part of the axon (axonotmesis), by degeneration, or pass through a region of inflammation, persistent afferent activity is possible. Over time, this persistent activity may lead to a strengthening of the synaptic efficiency of the synapses between the nociceptor and the low threshold mechanoreceptor on the wide dynamic range neurons (WDRN). Additionally, such input can cause tonic depolarization of the WDRNs. Under these conditions, light touch may be perceived as painful, a symptom called allodynia.

ability to control our perception of pain with internal neurotransmitters is lost as well: we hurt more, because we hurt more.

The good news is that these changes may not be permanent in most people. Theoretically, if the peripheral generators are located and effectively treated, the changes in the CNS leading to neuropathic pain should, and do, revert. If interventions were never successful, all those who have had these injuries and hypersensitivities—which includes most people to some extent—would have chronic pain forever. After all, these phenomena occur without CNS damage; some would even state that in central sensitization the CNS is behaving exactly as designed. But instead of facing a lifetime of debilitating pain, many people get better, and manual therapies are often listed among the most effective interventions for this population (Nijs, Van Houdenhove, and Oostendorp 2010; Courtney et al. 2011).

As with many other facets of pain, this topic is vigorously debated, and viewpoints continue to change with the publication of new research findings.

The diagnosis of *chronic regional pain syndrome* (CRPS) is given to individuals who have experienced some sort of nerve injury, but who develop a perplexing myriad painful symptoms that endure long after the tissue seems healed. These vexing disorders were originally identified in gunshot wound patients from the American Civil War, in what may be the first documented cases of central sensitization. In that era, it was called "causalgia," from the Greek "*kausis*," which means burning. This descriptor was derived from patients who talked about how even the gentlest of touch felt like "red hot file, rasping the skin." Since then, the name has changed to reflex sympathetic dystrophy and now to CRPS. Pain in CRPS seems completely out of proportion to the severity of any injury, and it impacts the well-being of the patients so that eventually their general health seriously declines (American RSDHope 2014). While CRPS begins with a neuropathy, it evolves to include painful central sensitization and autonomic changes, including **edema**, and/ or abnormal trophic findings, such as abnormal fingernail or toenail growth, and keratinization of the skin. The etiology of these symptoms is largely unknown.

Responses to Pain

We cannot be more sensitive to pleasure without being more sensitive to pain.

Alan Watts

Regardless of what the trigger might be, when we encounter a stimulus that causes pain, a limited number of things can happen. The fastest response to pain is a reflex action: a stimulus (a hot iron) encounters some skin. Rather than waiting for the scent of burning flesh to reach our nose, we are wired to withdraw from this dangerous and painful trigger. The stimulus activates nerve endings in the skin (transduction); the message is transmitted via sensory neurons to the dorsal root ganglia, and in the spinal cord neurons synapse with both the ascending tract, and with motor neurons at the same level. These transmit the instructions to contract the appropriate muscles in our hand and arm, and we pull away from the iron before much damage can accrue. This is an example of a relatively simple withdrawal reflex. Others can be much more complex, with sensory input and motor responses occurring at multiple levels, but all below our consciousness; we become aware of the stimulus and our responses after they have already taken place.

Pain sensations do not always create a withdrawal reflex. Tissue damage can develop without an initially dangerous trigger (think of a sunburn, for example, or overworking our muscles so that we're sore the next day), and in the best of these circumstances we experience functional nociceptive pain, which is simply the first step of going through a healthy healing process.

When the situation is long-term and frequently repeated, we may become vulnerable to more serious dysfunction and ultimately to painful central sensitization. Conditions ranging from fibromyalgia

syndrome to migraine headaches to chronic pelvic pain syndrome for men and women have been described using this model.

What we have described here is a worst-case scenario by which an injury causes changes to nervous system structures, and because of those changes, the sensation of pain becomes self-perpetuating and chronic. The chronification of pain is a leading challenge in healthcare delivery, as our ability to intervene in these processes is limited at best.

The Body and the Mind are NOT Separate Entities

Fear is pain arising from the anticipation of evil

Aristotle

In our culture we place great value on the power of human cognition, sometimes at the expense of how we view the more primitive experience of sensation. Eighteenth-century philosopher Rene Descartes suggested that our ability to doubt our own existence is, in fact, proof that we exist; this is the origin of the "I think, therefore I am" philosophical argument (see Sidebar 2.6). Notice that our existence is demonstrated by thinking, not by our perception of feeling. The saying is not, "I *sense*, therefore I am." This foundation for Western philosophy and identification of consciousness (which has roots far deeper than Descartes) has given rise to an assumption that what happens in our brain is both separate from and superior to what happens in our body.

> **Sidebar 2.6**
> One wet, stormy day in Paris a hungry Rene Descartes visited his favorite restaurant and very much enjoyed a bowl of cassoulet. He ate it to the very dregs. When his server asked him if he would like some more, he paused for a moment and considered. "I think not," he replied. And he disappeared.

This is a false paradigm.

Our physical experiences of pleasure and pain, of hunger and satiety, of energy and fatigue, all have influence on our mood, our cognition, and our ability to function intellectually. Likewise, our emotional state drives many of our motor behaviors. Our posture is a reflection of our habits, and these are influenced by many emotional responses. To suggest that our body and our brains can somehow function separately or be valued differently is a mistake. One of the most important connectors in the loops between the brain and the body is the limbic system.

The Limbic System

The limbic system is a collection of structures deep in the brain that includes the hypothalamus, the hippocampus, and the amygdala. The hypothalamus, readers may recall, is essentially the mediator of many of our homeostatic processes. It does this in an immediate way through the autonomic nervous system, and in a slower, longer-lasting way through the endocrine system. The hippocampus is a structure mainly understood to assist in the formation of memories, and the amygdala is a center for the interpretation of emotion (Weinberg and Krebs ND).

When the limbic system is activated, a response is translated through the motor fibers of the autonomic nervous system. When that reaction is triggered by a perceived threat, our stress response system is recruited.

Stress Response Systems: Hormonal Reactions

Through the limbic system we delineate between the need for two connected-but-distinct stress response loops. The SAM (sympathetic adrenal medulla) axis refers to the activation of the adrenal medulla and the secretion of catecholamines, epinephrine, and norepinephrine: the hormones that regulate immediate, short-term, high-grade, *WE'RE ALL GONNA DIE NOW* stress. It has special

impact on heart rate and respiratory rate, two mechanisms that help to determine our ability to fight or to run away. The HPA axis, by contrast, refers to the hypothalamus–pituitary–adrenal connection that leads to the secretion of cortisol from the adrenal cortex. This hormone helps us to mobilize our resources to respond to long-term, low-grade, *hold-on-grit-your-teeth-here-it-comes* stress.

Stress Response Systems: Motor Reactions

The limbic system also connects to the basal ganglia and cerebellum for the translation of a stress response into a behavioral response (see Sidebar 2.7). This can impact our breathing, our muscle tone, our posture, and the efficiency of movement (which, ironically, can influence our risk for injury and more pain). In the context of pain, therefore, the limbic system determines our emotional and behavioral responses to a threatening situation. Through electrical and chemical messages it influences our mood, our attention and cognitive function, and our ability to take action— or not—on our own behalf.

Sidebar 2.7 Emotional Body Language

Our state of mind and emotion influences every nuance of our motor behavior, even if we don't pay attention. Emotional body language (EBL) refers to the motor expression of emotions, through posture, gestures, and facial expression. Humans innately respond to the EBL of others.

Much of this motor function relies on basal ganglia and the secretion of dopaminergic neurotransmitters. One of the distinguishing features of Parkinson's disease, in which parts of the basal ganglia fail and dopamine is not adequately available, is the "Parkinson's mask": a phenomenon in which a person's facial muscles become rigid and unable to convey expression or EBL (Weinberg and Krebs ND).

Many of us live in an ongoing state of perceived threat, and this leads to pain-promoting behaviors such as collapsed shoulders, teeth grinding, shallow breathing, and increased general muscle tension. In turn, the physical experience of being in this state can reinforce and prolong the long-term sense of threat or stress. In this way, we can enter a particularly vicious circle of pain, stress, motor responses that cause pain, ad infinitum. Add the other stress-related responses that influence blood pressure, heart rate, and immune system function, and it is not a stretch to track the relationship between pain, stress, and generalized disease.

Manual Therapies and Pain

To truly laugh, you must be able to take your pain, and play with it!

Charlie Chaplin

What can a manual therapist do in the context of pain? If this sensation is related to triggers that are mostly transmitted via the skin, don't we, even with the best intentions, simply risk exacerbating an already bad situation? Fortunately, usually not.

One way to think about debilitating pain is that it is cumulative: enough small things must be wrong to add up to one large, complicated thing. But if that is true, then some of those small things (peripheral generators) can possibly be undone. If some of the contributors to pain can be addressed, then the partnership between a manual therapist and a hurting client yields a virtuous circle: reduced pain leading to improved mood and function, leading to reduced pain-promoting behaviors, and even better function, ad nauseam. The finding that massage has a generally positive effect in the context of many pain-experiencing populations (Abdulla et al. 2013; Gelinas et al. 2013; Somani, Merchant, and Lalani 2013) supports this hypothesis.

The challenge then becomes finding how to unlock the altered patterns.

> *Pain is not just a stimulus or a response, but both together. Hence successful pain practitioners need, oddly, to have a willingness to play in their work. We must guess at the primary drivers of pain … This approach is greatly aided by a three-dimensional visualization of fascial planes as they relate to nerve trunks and interwoven branches as they transverse throughout the tissues of the body. At the same time, it's important to consider the manifold influence of the central nervous system, often conditioned by years of input. The brainstem, thalamus, limbic system must constantly question the therapist's friendliness, trying to ascertain how much protective stasis is warranted. The more we can convince central and peripheral nervous systems of our essential benevolence, the more the client becomes our ally in the hard-but-rewarding work of creating a pathway toward pain relief.*
> *(Michael Hamm, massage therapist)*

Manual therapists have a unique role to play with our clients who live in pain: what other healthcare provider is in a position to offer such prolonged, undivided attention?

> *Pain can be terribly lonely and isolating. Most interventions, however sympathetic, just check in and check out: "Here's a pill, here's an exercise, here's a suggestion, maybe this will help?" But we manual therapists really want to know: exactly how does it hurt, exactly where? Does this touch "reach" it, or that touch?*
>
> *It's rare for a massage therapist to be able to fix pain altogether, which can be frustrating, but we can always, always at least recognize it: lay hands on it and be with it. Nobody else in the healthcare world really does that. When the pain alters mood, as it so often does, the fact that we are willing to be there and stay there with a patient can be profoundly moving and important.*
> *(Dale Favier, massage therapist).*

The most important take-away ideas about central sensitization and chronic pain are these:

- The pain is common, real, and not imaginary.
- The pain was triggered by some event outside the CNS.

- The pain can be reversible—and manual therapy may help.

Chronic pain and central sensitization take an enormous toll on every affected individual, and on society as a whole, with lost productivity and increased disability. Many conventional interventions are extremely expensive, risky (with highly addictive drugs) or invasive (with surgically implanted equipment to alter pain sensation), and many patients report being dissatisfied with these options (Anderson, Wang, and Zlateva 2012; Jouini et al. 2014). Unlike many conventional practitioners, manual therapists have the time and space to patiently and safely approach the body-and-brain as a unified whole, looking for ways to undo some of the contributing factors, and to create an oasis of safety in the midst of the perception of unrelenting threat. We may not be able to unpin every tethered neuron, or to reset every hypersensitive synapse, but our contribution to solving the pain puzzle can be valuable and effective.

References

Abdulla, A., N. Adams, M. Bone, A. Elliott, J. Gaffin, D. Jones, R. Knaggs, D. Martin, L. Sampson, and P. Schofield, British Geriatric Society. 2013. Guidance on the management of pain in older people. *Age Ageing* 42 Suppl 1:i1–57.

American RSDHope. 2014. CRPS origins. http://www.rsdhope.org/crps-or-rsds.html.

Anderson, D., S. Wang, and I. Zlateva. 2012. Comprehensive assessment of chronic pain management in primary care: a first phase of a quality improvement initiative at a multisite Community Health Center. *Qual Prim Care* 20:421–33.

Bove, G. M. 2009. Focal nerve inflammation induces neuronal signs consistent with symptoms of early complex regional pain syndromes. *Exp Neurol* 219:223–7.

Bove, G. M., and A. R. Light. 1995. Unmyelinated nociceptors of rat paraspinal tissues. *J Neurophysiol* 73:1752–62.

Bove, G. M., and A. R. Light. 1997. The nervinervorum: missing link for neuropathic pain? *Pain Forum* 6:181–90.

Bove, G. M., B. J. Ransil, H. C. Lin, and J. G. Leem. 2003. Inflammation induces ectopic mechanical sensitivity in axons of nociceptors innervating deep tissues. *J Neurophysiol* 90:1949–55.

Bove, G. M., and D. R. Seaman. 2010. Subclassification of radicular pain using neurophysiology and embryology. In *7th Interdicsciplinary World Congress on Low Back and Pelvic Pain, 2010 Los Angeles*, ed. A. Vleeming, 155–9. San Diego: University of California at San Diego.

Bove, G. M., A. Zaheen, and Z. H. Bajwa. 2005. Subjective nature of lower limb radicular pain. *J Manipulative Physiol Ther* 28(1):12–14.

Coghill, R. C. 2010. Individual differences in the subjective experience of pain: new insights into mechanisms and models. *Headache* 50:1531–5.

Courtney, C. A., J. D. Clark, A. M. Duncombe, and M. A. O'Hearn. 2011. Clinical presentation and manual therapy for lower quadrant musculoskeletal conditions. *J Man Ther* 19(4):212–22.

Deligianni, C. I., M. Vikelis, and D. D. Mitsikostas. 2012. Depression in headaches: chronification. *Curr Opin Neurol* 25:277–83.

Gelinas, C., C. Arbour, C. Michaud, L. Robar, and J. Cote. 2013. Patients and ICU nurses' perspectives of non-pharmacological interventions for pain management. *Nurs Crit Care* 18:6, 307–18.

Gracely, R. H., S. A. Lynch, and G. J. Bennett. 1992. Painful neuropathy: altered central processing maintained dynamically by peripheral input. *Pain* 51:175–94.

Jouini, G., M. Choiniere, E. Martin, S. Perreault, D. Berbiche, D. Lussier, E. Hudon, and L. Lalonde. 2014. Pharmacotherapeutic management of chronic noncancer pain in primary care: lessons for pharmacists. *J Pain Res* 7:163–73.

Merskey, H., and N. Bogduk. 2012. *IASP Taxonomy* [Online]. International Association for the Study of Pain.: https://www.iasp-pain.org/Education/Content.aspx?ItemNumber=1698.

Morone, N. E., and D. K. Weiner. 2013. Pain as the fifth vital sign: exposing the vital need for pain education. *Clin Ther* 35:1728–32.

Nijs, J., B. Van Houdenhove, and R. A. Oostendorp. 2010. Recognition of central sensitization in patients with musculoskeletal pain: Application of pain neurophysiology in manual therapy practice. *Man Ther* 15(2):135–41.

Somani, S., S. Merchant, and S. Lalani. 2013. A literature review about effectiveness of massage therapy for cancer pain. *J Pak Med Assoc* 63(11):1418–21.

Staud, R. 2011. Peripheral pain mechanisms in chronic widespread pain. *Best Pract Res Clin Rheumatol* 25:155–64.

Weinberg, J., and C. Krebs. ND. *Neuroanatomy tutorial*. University of British Columbia.

Bronwyn Lennox THOMPSON

Chapter 3

Pain theory and models for treatment

Introduction

We are all familiar with what it feels like to experience our own pain and we usually understand our pain and why we have it. We learn as youngsters that pain helps us to protect our bodies when we are threatened and keep us safe when our body must rest to repair. We need pain to stay healthy. Without pain, we risk living short and disabled lives (Emad et al. 2007).

> Let's think about Mark. He is experiencing pain in his shoulder. It's been there for 2 weeks now. It bothers him at night. It nags at him when he brushes his hair and cleans his teeth. He remembers the last time he had pain like this, when he had back pain that dragged on for months. He thinks about his busy day ahead in his job as a builder and wonders how he will get through the day. He makes a mental note to do something about it when he gets a chance during the day. In the meantime, he reaches for an anti-inflammatory tablet and swallows it with water.

This is an unremarkable story of a person-in-pain that many people will recognize.

When we think about a person-in-pain, understanding what it means and what to do about it reflects the time and culture in which the pain is experienced. Mark's pain has, at various times in history, been interpreted as Mark being punished by wicked spirits or tormented by unhappy tribe members (Karenberg and Leitz 2001). Mark's pain has also been viewed as a revelation from God, or a way for him to achieve spiritual cleansing. It has been a way for Mark to demonstrate moral character, and an opportunity for others to care for him (Bourke 2014). It has been considered random bad luck or bad genes, or both (Griffiths et al. 2000). His pain has been seen as a result of repressed desires

(Elfant, Burns, and Zeichner 2008), mental health problems (Reid et al. 2001) or a sign he doesn't want to work (Pearce 2002).

Mark could have sought help from spiritual advisors, elder tribe members, or healers depending on the practices of the time. He may have chanted, danced, prayed, taken herbal concoctions, rubbed ashes or fat or blood on his shoulder. He might have made offerings to deities, performed rituals including cutting himself or fasting or having heat applied to his shoulder or his feet. He may possibly have held a magnetized piece of metal while soaking his feet in a water bath. He could have applied electric shocks to his body or reclined on a couch and be asked to "free associate." More recently his grimaces and occasional groans may have been ignored in favor of praise whenever he uses his arm in daily activity or he may have been given an injection into the joint, or mobilization, exercises, medication, or surgery.

The way we, people-in-pain and those looking on (including treatment providers), conceptualize pain varies considerably depending on prevailing models of the human body, psyche, and spirit, as well as social rules and practices.

Today, pain is usually thought of as indicating the presence of a threat to the tissues (Moseley 2007). Nociceptors, or sensory neurons that respond to potentially damaging stimuli, have been activated and have transmitted information from the periphery to the spinal cord. Neurotransmitters released as part of this process have activated secondary transmissions. Eventually, the information has reached Mark's brain where various centers of his brain attend to, and judge the meaning of the information in terms of its threat value compared with his current goals. At every point in the journey from the peripheral tissues to the cortex, this information has been subject to modifying influences. These descend from cortical structures and vary depending on past experiences, anticipated futures, and beliefs drawn from the community, as well as biological variability.

Alongside the biological mechanisms involved in Mark's pain, Mark also makes decisions to do something about his shoulder pain based on broader social factors such as service availability, cost, social acceptability, and his personal preferences. Health professionals, however, see only Mark as he presents himself, the person-in-pain, how he describes his experience, and what he does. They may see their task as primarily to diagnose the cause of tissue damage, provide a treatment to remove the cause, and reduce or abolish the pain (Hanchard, Goodchild, and Kottam 2014). If they proceed on this understanding alone, without considering why Mark does what he does, there is an opportunity for misunderstanding and dissatisfaction for both parties.

Many contemporary textbooks consider only the biological mechanisms involved in nociceptive information transmission between the periphery and the central nervous system. This account fails to recognize that no matter how pain arises, its primary characteristic is its negative emotional valence, while the decision to become a patient and seek treatment reflects a very broad range of factors.

Pain is not simply a product of neural activity; it is an event we recognize, having experienced it before. It is an event that is personal and holds meaning for an individual in the context of his or her life. Pain is not the tissue damage or noxious stimulus, but is the way we *evaluate* tissue damage or noxious stimuli (Bourke 2014). Pain is influenced by where it occurs, when it occurs, and how long it is present. Some people greet noxious stimuli with reverence (body suspension practitioners, worshippers of the Hindu god Murugan); some fear and interpret the stimulus with horror (torture, children attending a dental clinic). The relationship between stimuli and experience is not straightforward, and people-in-pain judge their experience in light of their history and with an eye to their possible future.

Healthcare providers attending only to tissue damage must wrestle with difficult questions.

> Why do some people fail to act on their tissue damage? Why does the boxer, reeling from a powerful blow to the head remain in the ring rather than turning away to leave? Why do some people describe excruciating pain when tissue damage is invisible or no one can find any damage? Why is one person comforted by hands being laid on her head, while another gets angry when strong medications leave him with even the tiniest ache? Why do some return to activities quickly despite considerable pain, while others remain disabled and distressed even though their pain is mild?

Can we ever know what it is like to have someone else's pain? Unlike taste or color, we cannot point to an external object to compare experiences about that "thing." Pain is not a "thing" although we may talk about our experience as if it is separate from "us." It is a personal experience.

This chapter introduces selected models of pain, both historical and contemporary. It will show how views of pain and the way it is managed are fluid, shifting over time on the basis of context and ideas. Knowledge and beliefs about pain from past theories do not entirely disappear; we are all influenced by the legacy of what was previously "truth."

Defining Pain

The current internationally accepted definition of pain is: "Pain: An unpleasant sensory and emotional experience associated with actual or potential tissue damage, or described in terms of such damage" (International Association for the Study of Pain, IASP 2014).

This definition distinguishes between what we experience and what occurs in body tissues. It is not necessary to have tissue damage to have pain. Not only can we experience pain *before* tissue damage occurs, but we can also experience pain long after tissue healing is complete. Pain is also subjective; there is no way to determine whether another person has or does not have pain. Neither can we share the peculiar, particular quality of a pain that another person experiences. Instead, we interpret, on the basis of language and behavior, that someone is experiencing what it is like to have pain.

Mark, like all of us, learned about pain and how it relates to injury as part of his childhood development. This learning occurs within a social environment. We all develop an association between our *internal* experience of pain, and *external* events, so that we can recognize and avoid actual or potential harm, and learn about normal behavior associated with these events. This process begins at birth and continues as we mature. We develop greater voluntary control over the ways we express our pain at the same time as we develop greater emotional regulation and cognitive sophistication (Noel, Petter, and Chambers 2012). We also learn about pain and what to do about it by interacting with family and community. Mark's attitudes and typical behaviors regarding pain are more similar between him and his family members than between his neighbours, and among communities in his country of origin than communities from another country (Rollman 2004; Throop 2008; Ness 2009; Goubert et al. 2011; Hsieh, Tripp, and Ji 2011). Differences in what one person considers "typical" responses can create problems when people from another culture try to interpret language and gesture associated with pain, and as a result pain may not be recognized and treated appropriately.

The word *pain* is derived from the Latin word *poen*, meaning "punishment" or "penalty," while the word *poena* comes from the Latin word *patior*, which means "to endure suffering or pain." It is easy to see how *pain* and *suffering* have come to be used together to describe the emotional impact of unrelieved pain.

Healthcare providers enter health as a profession because, by and large, they care. Clinicians can hold strong beliefs that it is wrong to have to experience pain and that by alleviating pain they are restoring individual dignity—even though the process of treatment may temporarily increase pain. For example, Mark may undergo surgery to remove a bone spur from his painful shoulder. The process of recovery is painful for at least several weeks. This pain is usually acceptable because people expect long-term improvement in pain and reduced disability.

Not all pain is bad. Without pain alerting people to change position, blink, or avoid contact with hot objects, humans may not have survived. People who have inherited insensitivity to pain often die young from complications arising from undetected tissue damage (Cox et al. 2006; Emad et al. 2007; Young 2008), while one of the most important habits a person with spinal cord injury develops is to check their skin integrity, because tissue breakdown can occur without the usual warning indication from pain (Henzel et al. 2011).

While most people try to avoid pain, there are many occasions where people accept pain as integral to what they are doing. If Mark was an Army recruit, he could learn "pain is weakness leaving the body," and he has probably watched boxers "pushing through the pain barrier." Mark's partner may choose to have no pain relief while giving birth. His friends may voluntarily experience pain when getting a tattoo (see Figure 3.1) (particularly those getting an authentic Samoan tatau or Maori tattoo), having body modifications, and participating in body suspension.

Understanding pain and why people seek help for their pain is complex. Pain research is growing at an exponential rate. Through technological advances such as imaging techniques and neurophysiological

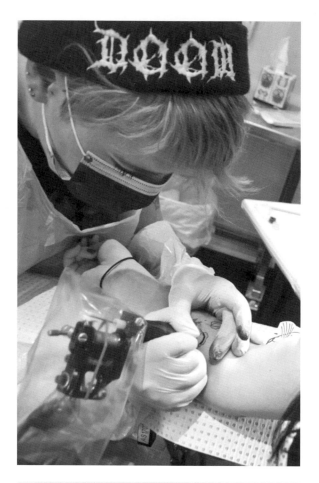

Figure 3.1
People around the world have endured painful body modification as part of rites of passage, to conform to cultural norms of beauty, or to express themselves.

In response to the question, "What information helped you decide to go to complementary treatment sessions or classes?", a 62-year-old female, living with pain for 15 years, replied: "I was not getting help to deal with the pain levels that were out of proportion to my physical problems and their unrelenting nature. So, my physical therapist suggested I meet with Neil to begin to work to understand my pain, how pain works, and on calming my wound-up central nervous system. I was just blessed that while my GP was in the way of my recovery for her lack of understanding about pain, and how it is different with people like myself, my physiotherapist knew of Neil and his work and that there was much more to my pain than what I was being taught or treated for."

Historical Theories of Pain

Humans develop explanations to make sense of what has happened to them. Sociohistorical contexts shape these explanations and they belong to and emerge from a place and time. It seems natural today to use images of the brain to illustrate pain processes, but earlier in history Hippocrates thought pain was an imbalance of the humors, while Galen and Aristotle believed it was a passion of the soul, and for many years pain was attributed to hysteria, or "the wandering womb" (Sir Thomas Sydenham in 1681) (Bonica and Loeser 2001).

Pain has not always been a clinician's domain. Pain relief, with the exception of opiates or alcohol, has only been widely available since the mid-1800s (Thernstrom 2010), and even now is not widely available in developing countries. Many people in earlier times would have experienced not only acute pain from injury or illness, but also

testing, the various biological processes involved in pain are being uncovered. Despite these advances, however, if we want to know about Mark's pain, we must communicate with him, and he with us. There is still no way to share what it feels like to have my pain, your pain, or their pain. Perhaps this is why pain is such an enigma, and why understanding it is so important in health care.

ongoing or persistent pain from the ailments we live with today (Rogers, Watt, and Dieppe 1981; Meng et al. 2011). In many pre-European cultures, pain not directly associated with visible injury was believed to involve "magic fluids, evil spirits, or pain demons" intruding into the body (Bonica and Loeser 2001). Pain could be the result of spiritual inattention, deliberately committing sins, or evil-doers attacking the individual on both a physical and spiritual plane. People, therefore, looked for spiritual help. If injury and pain could be the result of mischievous spirits, malevolent ancestors, or act as punishment for transgressions by the person in pain, the person-in-pain and family could at least appease the spirits (Bonica & Loeser 2001; Valadas 2011; Bourke 2014). Even today, spiritual approaches help some individuals to make meaning from the internal experience of pain (Ashby and Lenhart 1994; Dunn and Horgas 2004; Rippentrop 2005; Andersson 2008; Bussing et al. 2009).

Pain has not always been seen in spiritual terms, however, and explanations for pain have varied widely over the course of history. In the following sections, I explore what is known about historical practices and beliefs about pain to provide a context from which the current models of pain have developed.

Ancient Models: Early Egyptian

Records from ancient Egypt show that Egyptians believed demons caused pain. Then in Egyptian history, partially digested food was supposed to generate "pain-matter" that went through the body and caused painful ailments (Karenberg and Leitz 2001). In the Fifth Dynasty (2450 BC), Egyptians understood that body mixtures such as fluids and gases needed to be in the correct state of "continuity." Ill health was due to "loss of continuity;" therefore, treatments such as blood-letting, administering enemas, lancing pus, or coughing sputum were aimed to rid the body of substances interfering with the free flow of fluids and gases. Prayers or spells were also administered (Ansary, Steigerwald,

and Esser 2003). Natural analgesics were also used including opium, *Salix alba* (willow bark), and a mix of calcium carbonate with acetic acid which, when heated, generates CO_2 and was used to cool the painful area (Ansary et al. 2003).

Ancient Models: Greek

Aristotle (348–322 BC) believed the heart to be the seat of feelings, and classified pain as an emotion or "passion of the soul." At the time, health was thought to depend on "balancing the four humors" (blood, phlegm, yellow bile, and black bile). Hippocrates proposed that pain arose because of deficiencies or excesses in these substances. Galen (AD 129–c. 200/c. 216) was a Greek surgeon, physician, and philosopher who studied in Alexandria. He introduced the idea that the brain was the organ of feeling and identified the anatomy of the major spinal and cranial nerves. Galen classified pain as a sensation, and in terms of its sensory qualities, such as stabbing, shooting, and burning (Ansary et al. 2003).

Galen was undoubtedly influenced by Hippocrates and also considered "balancing the humors" to be an important part of health. He drew upon ancient Egyptian treatments such as applying heat and using enemas, as well as analgesic agents to manage pain. Blood-letting was also a common practice for many painful conditions, and this continued even until the 1800s. In 1833, Dr. D. Davis describes a theory proposed by Dr. Gooch, that the "exquisitely painful disease" of hysteralgia was caused by "a painful over-plenitude of a part at least of the internal iliac and pubic systems of bloodvessels (sic)" (Davis 1833), for which the treatment was to apply leeches. Some decades later, the explanation given by Dr. Lombe Atthill, in a lecture published in the *British Medical Journal*, explains that the treatment of "chronic endometritis" is to "ensure the free escape of the contents of the uterus" (1878, 779). While he suggests applying nitric acid to the "whole of the cavity of the uterus," along with "dividing the cervical canal," his recommendation is for the doctor to first apply "local blood-letting." The basis for this practice was Dr. Atthill's belief that impeded blood flow from the uterus meant the retained blood was "virtually a foreign body" (Atthill 1878).

Atthill and Davis were both influenced by the ideas developed by the philosopher and anatomist, Rene Descartes, and his contributions are discussed next.

Descartes and the "Mind–body" Divide

It was not until the Middle Ages in Europe that the idea of the brain as the center of sensation began to emerge. Descartes (1596–1650) tried to show that people were made of two parts: the "earthly machine," or the body; and the "soul," which was rational and governed the body. At least part of his rationale for this argument was to satisfy the requirements of the Church. By successfully claiming that the *body* and *soul* were separate, Descartes paved the way for researchers to study anatomy, opening up a world of discovery (Engel 1977, 131).

When Descartes won this argument, he also completed the move separating *physical* pain from *spiritual* or *emotional* pain, at least in Western civilizations (Bonica and Loeser 2001). This perspective lasted until the **Gate Control Theory** was introduced in 1965.

The main legacies of a Cartesian model of pain are the ideas that there is a one-to-one relationship between tissue damage and what we experience; therefore, a small paper cut should hurt very little, while a large leg fracture should hurt a great deal. In addition, the body and body parts became separate entities housing the soul or spirit. Pain became viewed as a by-product of the body, with rather less attention to the entirety of the way it is experienced by a person in his or her daily context. It also led to the long-lasting belief that pain experienced in the absence of tissue damage must therefore be "of the mind" (Cohen et al. 2011).

For our patient Mark, with his painful shoulder, the Cartesian influence means that his shoulder should not be painful if there is no evidence of tissue derangement, while his pain (and actions associated with his pain such as grimacing, guarding, and seeking treatment) should be in proportion to the degree of visible tissue damage. Any distress Mark experiences should be managed by priests or ameliorated by his devotion to God (Bourke 2014; Thernstrom 2010).

Post-Cartesian Models

During the nineteenth and twentieth centuries, scientific experimentation meant researchers proposed new models of pain. Progress in physiological research led to developments in understanding sensation and pain, with Johannes Müller (July 14, 1801–April 28, 1858), a physiologist and anatomist, proposing that the brain played a primary role in receiving information via sensory nerves; Müller also identified the five senses, although he believed that sensations were transmitted, without alteration, from the body to the part of the brain responsible for sensation (Bonica and Loeser 2001, 7; Wade 2009).

Three schools of thought emerged during the mid- to late-1800s regarding pain:

- *specificity theory* in which specialized nerve fibers were thought to transmit pain, independent of other senses

- *summation theory* in which any stimulus could produce pain given sufficient intensity

- the *traditional* view held since Aristotle, that pain was an affective, or emotional quality (Raj 2010).

Philosophers and psychologists primarily held this latter belief, believing that pain contributed to motivation (Bonica and Loeser 2001, 8). In 1895, these competing views were brought together by Strong, the president of the American Psychological Association at the time. He proposed that pain consisted of two parts: the *physical sensation* and the *psychic reaction* to this sensation (Strong 1895).

Researchers maintained this view until the 1940s, believing that pain could be separated into the *perception* of pain, and the *reaction* to pain. In this model, pain *perception* was a neurophysiologic process involving relatively simple and primitive neural mechanisms while the pain *reaction* involved complex psychophysiological processes including cognition, learned experiences, cultural, and other psychological factors (Bonica and Loeser 2001). While psychosocial factors were incorporated into the model, neurophysiological processes involved in transmitting "pain signals" or nociception were believed to be the primary mechanisms. More importantly, the pathways identified during this period were thought to transmit *unmodified* information from the periphery to an as-yet unidentified pain center in the brain. Health professionals and researchers could not conceive of a situation in which a person-in-pain might fail to show evidence of a visible pathology; therefore, these individuals were demonstrating "functional" or psychiatric pathology.

The impact of this view of pain lingers. As a result of the idea that the physical sensation of pain was governed by biological mechanisms, while pain perception and expression by a person-in-pain was governed by "psychological" factors, clinicians could judge patients' moral worthiness. Those that "suffered in silence" were, if they were from the same culture and gender as the clinician, considered heroic, while if they were of a different culture and gender they could simply be "less sensitive" (Bourke 2014, 192–230). Today, judgments are often made to determine whether someone like Mark with his sore shoulder is truly incapacitated for his work. In compensation environments, clinicians are often asked to determine if an individual's pain "does not correlate with objective findings or body part dysfunction" (Ekstrom 2012; US Department of Labor 2013). This approach fails to account for the many factors that influence Mark as he seeks to carry on with life despite his painful shoulder.

While the idea that pain occurs within the tissues and that the person-in-pain simply responds to this continues, the concept as a whole began to be overturned in the mid-1960s. Ronald Melzack and Patrick Wall proposed that, while information from the periphery to the central nervous system was important, transmitting this information was not as simple as connecting to a telephone exchange. The Gate Control Theory (GCT) has now been superseded with new research, but it heralded one of the most profound shifts towards a contemporary understanding of pain, and it is to this model I now turn.

The Gate Control Theory

Strong's model of pain perception and response held sway until the mid-1960s when Melzack and Wall published their work, *Gate Control Theory* (GCT) of pain. The GCT proposed that neural impulses are transmitted to the dorsal horn of the spinal cord, then *modulated* via descending inhibitory fibers to influence the amount of information transmitted to the brain (Melzack and Wall 1967). There have been significant revisions to the model since then, but the key contributions of this theory led to re-evaluating the importance of psychological and social factors in an individual's experiences of pain. Rather than passively processing information arriving from the peripheral nervous system, the brain was seen to be actively involved in selecting and modifying neural input from the periphery. Melzack put it this way:

> *Pain processes do not begin with the stimulation of receptors. Rather, injury or disease produces neural signals that enter an active nervous system that (in the adult organism) is the substrate of past experience, culture, and a host of other environmental and personal factors. These brain processes actively participate in the selection, abstraction, and synthesis of information from the total sensory input. Pain is not simply the end product of a linear sensory transmission system; it is a dynamic process that involves continuous interactions among complex ascending and descending systems.*
>
> (Melzack and Katz 2013, 1)

At every level of the spinal cord, Melzack and Wall identified interactions between ascending and descending neurons. These functioned to either amplify or reduce the action potential moving across the synapse and transmitted to the next neuron. This they called the *gate control system*. The interactions were triggered by what Melzack and Wall called the *central control system* which descended from various parts of the brain. They also challenged the idea of a central pain center where pain sensation and response were coordinated in the brain, identifying that the thalamus, limbic system, hypothalamus, reticular formation, parietal cortex, and the frontal cortex were all implicated in pain perception (Melzack and Wall 1965, 976). Pain biology suddenly became a great deal more complex, but several major conundrums were also settled as a result of their hypotheses, such as why there is no one-to-one relationship between stimulus and pain; why rubbing a painful area results in less pain; why nociceptive stimuli can sometimes not be perceived at all; and why pain can be experienced in a phantom limb.

Research into psychosocial aspects of pain has flourished since the 1965 GCT as neurologists and psychologists began to examine the contributions of cortical processes on the experience of pain. For our patient Mark, this would have meant that attention, memory, emotions, and planning began to be acknowledged as not just psychological responses to what was going on in his tissues, but were integral to the experience of his pain. The new relevance of psychological processes on pain led to psychological theories and treatments based on them. As a result, in the late 1960s and 1970s, Mark could begin to have treatment based on cognitive and behavioral principles along with his medical treatment (Fordyce 1981; Main and Williams 2002). This may have included relaxation training, cognitive therapy for his unhelpful beliefs about his pain, and reinforcement schedules to encourage "well" behavior, with any illness behavior ignored by clinicians.

The legacy of the GCT continues today, although specific hypotheses proposed within the GCT have been superseded. Pain is now broadly acknowledged as an individual's experience that is shaped by past events, present interpretations, and future predictions as well as biological events. More recently, Melzack has proposed the neuromatrix model. The neuromatrix model is an integrated model in which pain is identified as an *output* of the brain produced by characteristic "neurosignature" patterns of nerve impulses generated by a widely distributed neural network called the *body-self neuromatrix*. Melzack proposes that the body-self neuromatrix activates perceptual, homeostatic, and behavioral "programs" or outputs when information received by the neuromatrix from the periphery indicates tissue injury, pathology, or chronic stress. These patterns form sensory, affective, and cognitive **neuromodules** or programs that produce the multiple dimensions of pain such as heightened attention to the relevant body part, awareness of the quality of sensation (burning, aching, stabbing, intermittent, or ongoing), and emotional responses that generate action to respond to the threat to the self. Melzack suggests that these responses indicate loss of homeostasis, with the neuromatrix then activating mechanisms to shift the organism towards homeostatic balance. This hypothesis may explain why some individuals develop phantom limb pain. In the absence of normal input to the neuromatrix from the missing limb, homeostatic balance is disturbed. The neuromatrix activates sensory, affective, and cognitive neuromodules that are experienced by the individual as pain arising from a body part that is no longer there. Mirror therapy treatment based on this model attempts to provide visual evidence to show that there is no threat to tissue integrity of the missing limb by essentially fooling the neuromatrix through visual illusion (Foell et al. 2014).

Modern neuroscientific studies support the premises of the neuromatrix and show the widely activated pathways associated with our experience of pain (Tracey and Bushnell 2009). Studies (mainly conducted using functional MRI) still cannot determine who is and is not experiencing pain, however, and neither can they indicate the quality of "what it is like" to experience pain. The reasons one person looks for treatment while another carries on cannot be explained by biology alone, and for this reason I now discuss the relevance of the biopsychosocial model proposed by George Engel.

Biopsychosocial Model

George Engel (December 10, 1913–November 26, 1999) was an American psychiatrist with a particular interest in psychosomatic medicine and most renowned for introducing the general health model known as the biopsychosocial model. The fundamental assumption of this model is that health and illness are consequences of an *interplay* of biological, psychological, and social factors (Engel 1977). As a framework for understanding how and why an individual experiences and expresses ill health, the model has provided considerable understanding.

Engel's work emerged from his fascination with psychosomatic health problems, and his appreciation of General System Theory (Von Bertalanffy 1956). At the time he wrote his paper "The need for a new medical model: A challenge for biomedicine" (Engel 1977), the field of psychiatry was being challenged by the emergence of:

> A hodgepodge of unscientific opinions, assorted philosophies and "schools of thought," mixed metaphors, role diffusion, propaganda, and politicking for "mental health" and other esoteric goals.
>
> (Ludwig 1975)

Engel believed that psychiatry had to either withdraw from medicine as a whole, or "adhere strictly to the 'medical model' and limit psychiatry's field to behavioral disorders consequent to brain dysfunction" (1977, 129). He accused followers of the medical model of conforming to a caricature of the model in which disease, both physical and mental, emerged purely from "natural causes" defined as "biological," while disorders such as problems of living, social adjustment, dependence, depression, and social deviancy were not considered illnesses because they were produced by psychosocial variables. With no evidence of biological pathology, mental illnesses such as depression and addiction could not be a concern for psychiatrists under this interpretation and would instead be managed by nonmedical clinicians.

Engel did not find this palatable, and he argued instead that the medical model itself was flawed. The basis for this was his argument that, although the reductionist approach in which various parts of a condition were examined in isolation had merit, it had become a dogmatic position in which health problems that could not readily be reduced to component parts were at risk of not being considered disease despite their apparent effects on health (Engel 1977, 196). He was acutely aware that social factors influenced what was defined as ill health and what should be done about it, arguing that medical practice had come about because of the decision by the Church in Descartes' time to allow the physical body to be examined, while leaving the spirit and emotions to spiritual advisors.

Engel's model was controversial, but it rapidly gained recognition. Pain clinicians and researchers, already considering psychological approaches for managing chronic pain, began to reconceptualize pain in biopsychosocial terms. Two clinicians, psychologist John Loeser from the USA, and orthopedic surgeon Gordon Waddell from the UK, recognized the relevance of psychosocial factors, particularly in those individuals experiencing chronic pain (Loeser 1982; Waddell 1987). Waddell pointed out that the majority of individuals will experience low back pain, while only a small percentage of those people will seek treatment for their pain. He identified that in countries where orthopedic or Western medicine had been only recently introduced, while people experienced low back pain, they did not become disabled by it, and remained actively engaged in daily life. This was in contrast to Western societies in which the disability associated with low back pain, and the costs of treatment, had rapidly escalated between the 1950s and 1970s. Back pain was, he argued, a problem of extended disability created by psychosocial contexts including clinician's beliefs and behavior, rather than exclusively a biological phenomenon.

Loeser developed a model of pain based on the biopsychosocial model in which he depicted concentric circles with nociception in the centre, and ending with the social environment as the final ring in what has become known as the "onion ring" model (Loeser 1982). In it, he depicted the experience of pain as being distinct from what people do when they experience pain, otherwise known as pain behavior. Pain behaviour, according to psychologists such as Loeser (1982), Main and Williams (2002), and Wilbert E. Fordyce (1988), was subject to the mechanisms influencing all behavior including conditioned learning, observational learning, and beliefs, and was developed from reflexes but shaped by learning and social interaction.

If this model is applied to Mark's situation, he may have nociceptive input from bone spurs in his shoulder (inner circle), but this is only experienced as pain (second ring) in the context of influences from all the remaining rings.

For example, he may identify what is going on in his shoulder as highly distressing and a sign that he is aging more quickly than he wants and an indication he will need to change his job (third ring). He believes, because he lives in a modern, Western country, that he should not have to tolerate this pain (fifth ring), so he visits his primary health provider or general practitioner, and grimaces and cradles his arm while he is examined (fourth ring). His mother Julie and coworker encourage him to seek treatment (fifth ring), and he remembers the last time he had shoulder trouble (third ring) (see Figure 3.2).

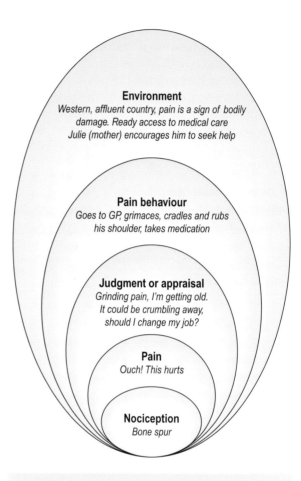

Figure 3.2
This diagram illustrates the relationships between various influences on the human pain experience. The only aspect able to be shared between two people is pain behaviour—what a person does when he or she experiences pain.
(Drawn from Loeser 1982.)

Clinical Reasoning within the Biopsychosocial Framework

Throughout this chapter I have pointed out that pain is an experience we cannot share directly with anyone else. This means we rely on what people say and do to indicate that they have pain, and we interpret this behavior in light of our own experiences and learning. There is much room for misinterpretation because each one of us has followed a unique pathway to reach where we are today. The biopsychosocial model provides a useful framework for beginning to understand an individual's experience, and to disentangle the various factors that explain how and why an individual is presenting in a particular way, at any point in time. This is important when we hope to help a person with their pain, because if we only attend to the biological, we may forget that someone like Mark continues to interpret what has happened to him, is currently happening in treatment, and may happen in the future, and he does so in the context of his family, community, and wider society.

The Case Formulation Approach

Clinicians identify patients' needs on the basis of the model of pain they have adopted. Hence, a clinician employing a strongly biomedical model in the clinical encounter and treatment application will tend not to incorporate psychological or social factors, while a clinician with a strong psychological model will tend to focus primarily on psychological factors. The biopsychosocial model is intended to integrate all three recognized elements in the experience of pain. The challenge, however, is that each patient has followed a unique pathway towards the point at which they seek attention.

While diagnoses are useful to collect signs and symptoms that co-occur, they fail to explain how and why an individual presents with a particular set of problems. Diagnoses often fail to incorporate the necessary information to identify the individual's illness experience, illness being the experience of what it is like to have a disease, and includes understanding role disruptions, social sanctions, and the threat to identity that these changes bring about (Eisenberg 1977; Armstrong 2011; Jutel 2011). Clinicians working with people who have pain may use a diagnosis to classify the proposed mechanisms underpinning an individual's presentation, but unless they incorporate the unique psychosocial factors, they may well fail to address the illness experience. This can give rise to extended disability, where an individual does not return to "normal" or regain function.

When considering how to help Mark with his painful shoulder, there are good reasons for using a **case formulation approach** as a clinical reasoning methodology:

1. Pain is complex, as are both illness and disability. There are many factors to consider, and the weighting of these factors will be different for Mark and for his mother Julie.

2. The biomedical diagnosis he receives tells us little about his experience of pain and how it has affected his life. While his clinician might give him a diagnosis of "a bone spur on the clavicle," confirming for Mark that he does indeed have a problem that is understood as a disease, this diagnosis does not allow his treatment providers to identify or address what this means to Mark in his daily life.

3. Mark has had a shoulder impingement problem before, and this has influenced the way he uses his shoulder, and his expectations for treatment. He also has intermittent low back pain which has limited his ability to carry out his job over the past 2 years. Both of these problems influence how he manages his current shoulder pain and need to be considered.

4. Finally, because Mark's primary care clinician wants to ensure the interventions offered to Mark hold to the principles of patient-centered health care, case formulation allows for shared decision-making when making referrals.

The Case Formulation Process

Case formulations can be developed in many different ways, but a useful step-by-step approach is described below. Engel originally considered the biopsychosocial model to be a way for two people to collaborate on the many factors leading to the person seeking help, so it is also helpful to think of developing a case formulation as a dialogue between two experts: one is an expert on his or her own experience, while the other is an expert on the various processes and causal relationships that can influence health.

Case formulations can be developed using the following steps:

1. Identify the person's problems from their perspective.

2. Detect the underlying patterns and identify those that conform to known diagnoses, but include those that appear consistently but are not recognized as disease entities.

3. Infer causal mechanisms based on recognized processes from the research literature.

4. Draw a causal model showing the relationships between the various factors and their mechanisms.

5. Evaluate the causal model by monitoring the outcome of interventions provided.

6. Confirm the case formulation.

Identifying the person's problems may seem straightforward: they have pain; it is "caused" by some mechanism which requires treatment for cure. It is important to extend the range of potential problems and contributory factors to include biological, psychological, and social factors that can explain the person's presentation because pain is a multidimensional experience. Bodywork practitioners from a range of approaches address the multiple dimensions of Mark's experience in similar ways: by hearing Mark, not only his words, but the story his body tells, acknowledging his pain experience through touch, reflection, and compassion, and using gentle movement to discover pain-free ways to function.

In practice, this means listening to Mark's story, considering two primary questions that guide assessment: (1) Why is Mark presenting in this way at this time? (2) What can be done to reduce his distress and disability?

Perhaps Mark's main reason for seeing his treatment provider is so he can be reassured that he doesn't have cancer or need surgery; perhaps he wants to reassure his employer and his mother Julie that he genuinely has a problem. He may be working very hard at work but failing to rest when he returns home, leading to fatigue and greater attention to his aches and pains when he collapses into bed. When he tries to sleep, he may find he rolls on to his sore shoulder and his sleep has consequently been fragmented and compounding his tiredness. He may have limited awareness of ways he can relax effectively and need to learn to move with more mindfulness. Mark may be worrying about the viability of his building business, which has led him to be more anxious than usual and activating his sympathetic nervous system. He may also be fearful and worry that, if he moves his arm normally, he may be doing damage to an already worn-out joint.

All of these different concerns will respond to different treatment approaches, and, while simply abolishing his pain by using medication could address some of his immediate problems, this strategy will fail to address Mark's underlying concerns. This is how long-standing disability can arise from what appears to be a very simple physical problem. The diagram below provides an indication of the influences on Mark's presentation, and some suggestions for referrals to help reduce both his distress and his disability (see Figure 3.3).

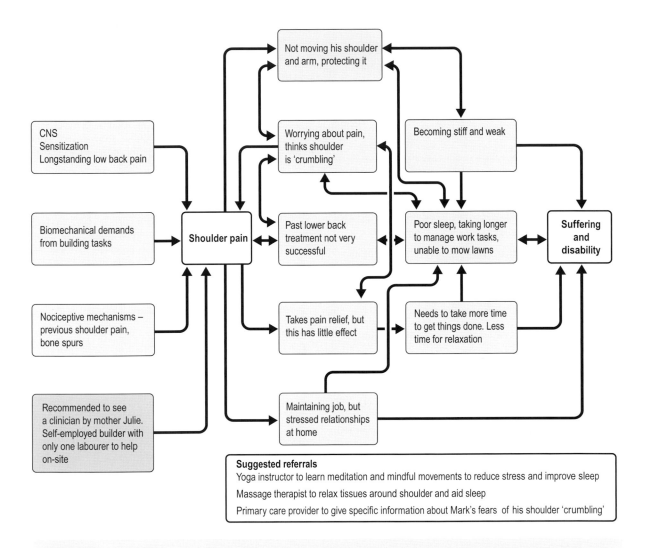

Figure 3.3
Example of case formulation showing the relationships between biological, psychological, and social factors as they influence suffering and disability.

Conclusion

Pain is complex and many different factors can influence how people experience it. While neurobiological mechanisms are certainly a major part of the experience, psychological and social aspects are equally important contributors to the illness associated with pain.

The models clinicians and patients bring with them when thinking about pain influence the factors that are considered and addressed during treatment. By exploring a broad range of biopsychosocial factors, clinicians can move beyond simply addressing a "diagnosis" which fails to explain how and why this person is presenting in this way at this time, and begin to unravel the many different factors that can influence the individual's experience of pain and maintain their disability.

References

Andersson, G. 2008. Chronic pain and praying to a higher power: Useful or useless? *Journal of Religion and Health* 47(2):176–87. doi: http://dx.doi.org/10.1007/s10943-007-9148–8.

Ansary, M. E., I. Steigerwald, and S. Esser. 2003. Egypt: Over 5000 years of pain management—cultural and historic aspects. *Pain Practice* 3(1), 84–7. doi: 10.1046/j.1533-2500.2003.00010.x.

Armstrong, D. 2011. Diagnosis and nosology in primary care. Social Science & Medicine, 73(6):801–7. doi: http://dx.doi.org/10.1016/j.socscimed.2011.05.017.

Ashby, J. S., and R. Lenhart. 1994. Prayer as a coping strategy for chronic pain patients. *Rehabilitation Psychology,* 39(3): 205–9.

Atthill, L. 1878. *Clinical lecture on the treatment of chronic endometritis* (Vol. 1).

Bonica, J. J., and J. D. Loeser. 2001. History of pain concepts and therapies. In *Bonica's Management of Pain* ed., 3rd ed., J. D. Loeser, (Vol. 1, 3–16). Philadelphia: Lippincott, Williams & Wilkins.

Bourke, J. 2014. *The story of pain: From prayer to painkillers.* Oxford: Oxford University Press.

Bussing, A., A. Michalsen, H. J. Balzat, R. A. Grunther, T. Ostermann, E. A. Neugebauer, and P. F. Matthiessen. 2009. Are spirituality and religiosity resources for patients with chronic pain conditions? *Pain Medicine* 10(2):327–39. doi: http://dx.doi.org/10.1111/j.1526-4637.2009.00572.x.

Cohen, M., J. Quintner, D. Buchanan, M. Nielsen, and L. Guy. 2011. Stigmatization of patients with chronic pain: The extinction of empathy. *Pain Medicine* 12(11):1637–43.

Cox, J. J., F. Reimann, A. K. Nicholas, G. Thornton, E. Roberts, K. Springell, Y. Raashid, et al. 2006. An scn9a channelopathy causes congenital inability to experience pain. *Natur,* 444(7121):894–8.

Davis, D. 1833. On hysteralgia, or irritable uterus. *The Boston Medical and Surgical Journal* (11): 165–9. doi:10.1056/NEJM183310230091101.

Dunn, K. S., and A. L. Horgas. 2004. Religious and nonreligious coping in older adults experiencing chronic pain. *Pain Management Nursing* 5(1):19–28.

Eisenberg, L. 1977. Disease and illness distinctions between professional and popular ideas of sickness. *Culture, medicine and psychiatry* 1(1):9–23.

Ekstrom, L. W. 2012. Liars, medicine, and compassion. *Journal of Medicine & Philosophy* 37(2):159–80.

Elfant, E., J. W. Burns, and A. Zeichner. 2008. Repressive coping style and suppression of pain-related thoughts: Effects on responses to acute pain induction. *Cognition and Emotion* 22(4): 671–96. doi: http://dx.doi.org/10.1080/02699930701483927.

Emad, Y., A. El Yasaki, A., Y. Ragab, M. Khalifa, O. Moawayh, and M. Salama. 2007. Arthritis in a child secondary to congenital insensitivity to pain and self-aggression. Why and when pain is good? *Clinical Rheumatology* 26(7):1164–6.

Engel, G. L. 1977. The need for a new medical model: A challenge for biomedicine. *Science* 196(4286):129–36. doi: http://dx.doi.org/10.1126/science.847460.

Foell, J., R. Bekrater-Bodmann, M. Diers, and H. Flor. 2014. Mirror therapy for phantom limb pain: Brain changes and the role of body representation. *European Journal of Pain* 18(5):729–39. doi: 10.1002/j.1532-2149.2013.00433.x.

Fordyce, W. E. 1981. Behavioral methods in medical rehabilitation. *Neuroscience & Biobehavioral Reviews* 5(3):391–6.

Fordyce, W. E. 1988. Pain and suffering: A reappraisal. *American Psychologist* 43(4):276–83.

Goubert, L., J. W. S. Vlaeyen, G. Crombez, G., and K. D. Craig. 2011. Learning about pain from others: An observational learning account. *Journal of Pain* 12(2):167–74.

Griffiths, B., R. D. Situnayake, B. Clark, A. Tennant, M. Salmon, and P. Emery. 2000. Racial origin and its effect on disease expression and hla-drb1 types in patients with rheumatoid arthritis: A matched cross-sectional study. *Rheumatology* 39(8):857–64.

Hanchard, C. A. N., L. M. Goodchild, and L. Kottam. 2014. Conservative management following closed reduction of traumatic anterior dislocation of the shoulder. *Cochrane Database of Systematic Reviews* (4).

Henzel, M. K., K. M. Bogie, M. Guihan, and C. H. Ho. 2011. Pressure ulcer management and research priorities for patients with spinal cord injury: Consensus opinion from sci queri expert panel on pressure ulcer research implementation. *J Rehabil Res Dev* 48(3):xi–xxxii.

Hsieh, A. Y., D. A. Tripp, and L. J. Ji. 2011. The influence of ethnic concordance and discordance on verbal reports and nonverbal behaviours of pain. *Pain* 152(9):2016–22.

Jutel, A. 2011. Classification, disease, and diagnosis. *Perspectives in Biology & Medicine* 54(2):189–205.

IASP http://www.iasp-pain.org/Taxonomy. 2014. 1510 H Street NW, Suite 600, Washington, DC 20005-1020, USA © 2015 International Association for the Study of Pain.

Karenberg, A., and C. Leitz. 2001. Headache in magical and medical papyri of ancient Egypt. *Cephalalgia* 21(9):911–916. doi: 10.1046/j.1468–2982.2001.00274.x.

Loeser, J. 1982. Concepts of pain. In *Chronic low back* pain, ed. M. Stanton-Hicks and R. Boas, 145–8. New York: Raven Press.

Ludwig, A. M. 1975. The psychiatrist as physician. *JAMA*, 234(6): 603–4. doi: 10.1001/jama.1975.03260190031016.

Main, C. J., and A. C. d. C. Williams 2002. Abc of psychological medicine: Musculoskeletal pain. *BMJ: British Medical Journal* 325(7363):534–42.

Melzack, R., and J. Katz. 2013. Pain. *Wiley Interdisciplinary Reviews: Cognitive Science* 4(1):1–15. doi: 10.1002/wcs.1201.

Melzack, R., and P. D. Wall. 1965. Pain mechanisms: A new theory. *Science* 150(3699):971–9.

Melzack, R., and P. D. Wall 1967. Pain mechanisms: A new theory. *Survey of Anesthesiology* 11(2):89.

Meng, Y., H. Q. Zhang, F. Pan, Z. D. He, J. L. Shao, and Y. Ding. 2011. Prevalence of dental caries and tooth wear in a neolithic population (6700–5600 years bp) from northern China. *Archives of Oral Biology* 56(11):1424–435.

Moseley, G. L. 2007. Reconceptualising pain according to modern pain science. *Physical Therapy Reviews* 12(3):169–78.

Ness, S. M. 2009. Pain expression in the perioperative period: Insights from a focus group of Somali women. *Pain Management Nursing* 10(2): 65–75. doi: http://dx.doi.org/10.1016/j.pmn.2008.05.001.

Noel, M., M. Petter, and C. T. P. Chambers. 2012. Cognitive behavioral therapy for pediatric chronic pain: The problem, research, and practice. *Journal of Cognitive Psychotherapy* 26(2): 143–56. doi: 10.1016/j.pain.2005.10.027.

Pearce, J. M. 2002. Psychosocial factors in chronic disability. *Medical Science Monitor* 8:12.

Raj, P. P. 2010. The 2009 John J. Bonica award lecture: The impact of managing pain in the practice of medicine through the ages. *Regional Anesthesia & Pain Medicine* 35(4):377, 378–85.

Reid, S., D. Whooley, T. Crayford, and M. Hotopf. 2001. Medically unexplained symptoms: GPs' attitudes towards their cause and management. *Family Practice* 18(5):519–23.

Rippentrop, A. 2005. A review of the role of religion and spirituality in chronic pain populations. *Rehabilitation Psychology* 50(3):278–84.

Rogers, J., I. Watt, and P. Dieppe. 1981. Arthritis in Saxon and mediaeval skeletons. *Br Med J (Clin Res Ed)* 283(6307): 1668–70.

Rollman, G. B. 2004. Ethnocultural variations in the experience of pain. *In Pain: Psychological perspectives,* ed. T. Hadjistavropoulos and K. D. Craig, 155–78. Mahwah, NJ: Lawrence Erlbaum.

Strong, C. A. 1895. The psychology of pain. *Psychological Review* 2(4):329–47.

Thernstrom, M. 2010. *The pain chronicles: Cures, myths, mysteries, prayers, diaries, brain scans, healing, and the science of suffering.* New York: Farrar, Straus and Giraux.

Throop, C. J. 2008. From pain to virtue: Dysphoric sensations and moral sensibilities in Yap (Waqab), Federated States of Micronesia. *Transcultural Psychiatry* 45(2):253–86.

Tracey, I., and M. C. Bushnell. 2009. How neuroimaging studies have challenged us to rethink: Is chronic pain a disease? *Journal of Pain* 10(11):1113–20.

US Department of Labor. 2013. *Division of Federal Employees' Compensation (DFEC).* Washington, DC: US Department of Labor. http://www.dol.gov/owcp/dfec/regs/compliance/DFEC-folio/FECA-PT2/group2.htm.

Valadas, M. A. 2011. A short history of pain and its treatment. In *Maldynia: Multidisciplinary perspectives on the illness of chronic pain,* ed. J. Giordano, 7. Boca Raton, FL: CRC Press.

Von Bertalanffy, L. 1956. General system theory. *General systems* 1(1):11–17.

Waddell, G. 1987. Volvo award in clinical sciences: A new clinical model for the treatment of low-back pain. *Spine* 12(7):632–44.

Wade, N. J. 2009. Beyond body experiences: Phantom limbs, pain and the locus of sensation. *Cortex* 45(2):243–55. doi: http://dx.doi.org/10.1016/j.cortex.2007.06.006.

Young, F. B. 2008. A life without pain? Hedonists take note. *Clinical Genetics* 73(1):31–3.

Introduction

Massage is a global and ancient practice used by many cultures as a remedy for pain and muscular discomfort (Calvert 2002). Evidence of massage has been found as far back as 15,000 BC in European cave paintings (Krieger 1979) and in nearly every known culture on our planet. There is a healing effect in human touch that modern science is still researching to adequately explain. We instinctively press our hands to our head if it is aching, rub our leg if we bang it, or tap an area that is numb. This "hands to soothe" reflexive response to pain is arguably the prototype for the development of massage as a deliberate treatment.

Massage is a therapy that utilizes touch, pressure, and movement to improve the physical state of the recipient over a broad range of responses, from simple relaxation to complex remedial and therapeutic benefits. Massage can enhance awareness in the recipient on an explicit level, such that they have a greater sense of what is happening in their body, and also on an implicit level, where the body becomes "aware" of its condition, activating natural processes that may initiate a healing response. Cherkin et al. (2011) demonstrated that benefits continued implicitly for some 6 months following treatment with both relaxation and structural massage for chronic lower back pain.

Around 1945, a group of nurses was chosen to participate in a program using a controversial polio treatment developed and taught by Sister Elizabeth Kenny. The treatment included a form of massage, heat application, and passive exercise to affected limbs. One of those nurses was my mother, Sister Cynthia Davis, and so began the use of massage for the treatment of chronic pain in Australia.

Research shows massage is a complementary modality commonly chosen by both the general public and a diverse range of healthcare practitioners. Massage therapy is sought out to minimize or eliminate pain, increase relaxation, assist in their capacity to deal with activities of daily life, and as prevention to further injury (Barnes et al. 2004; French et al. 2010; Armstrong, Thiebaut, and Brown 2011). It is practiced as a stand-alone treatment, as part of an integrative treatment for rehabilitation, a preventive treatment for musculoskeletal activity, and as part of a person's healthy lifestyle program.

Unfortunately, the term "massage" has become a colloquial umbrella for almost anything to do with touch. It is even used to describe general softening or manipulating, such as "massaging the company figures" or "massaging your ego." In health practices, "massage" can simplistically be used to describe any rubbing of the skin to soothe and/or to make it feel better. There are medical descriptions such as "external heart massage" or "carotid artery massage" that add to the confusion. It has, therefore, become necessary to clarify definitions of massage and massage therapy for professional practice.

The term "massage therapy" has been professionally accepted as: an individual treatment, by a trained practitioner who utilizes established techniques (Rich 2010). The action of massage has been defined as: "certain manipulations of the soft tissues of the body"(Beard and Wood 1964, 1). In his book, *The Art of Massage*, John Harvey Kellogg, MD, of the Battle Creek Sanitarium, describes massage as: "systematic rubbing and manipulation of the tissues of the body, (and) is probably one of the oldest of all means used for the relief of bodily infirmities" (Kellogg 1923). Kellogg goes on to say that the word "massage" is derived from the French, literally meaning kneading, as a baker kneads bread. It retains its French pronunciation, and is pronounced as though spelled *mas-sahzh*, and not as though spelled *massaj* or *massaje*, which is so frequently heard. *Masser* is a verb, and it has been used to mean the act of applying massage.

Possibly the best definition of massage therapy is the one developed in 2007 for a Policy of Therapeutic Massage published by Myklebust and Iler: "the systematic and scientifically based manipulation of the soft tissues of the body by a trained professional. It is organized intentional touch applied with sensitivity and compassion guided by a clearly formulated procedural plan" (2007, 3).

Common to many professions, the level of expertise of a practitioner develops over time and study. A reasonable analogy for professional competency is the necessary practice of completing annual taxes. Many people do their own bookwork, some try to get by with the help of a friend or family member who is good with figures, others employ an average bookkeeper, and then there are those who employ skilled, qualified, and experienced accounting professionals. Despite this wide variety of expertise and experience, the job gets done in some way or another. In addition, the job gets done in a less and less satisfying and effective way, as you move down the scale from the skilled practitioner to the handy person who gives it their best shot. Research has shown that massage can be beneficial at various levels of expertise, but, just with doing our taxes, the benefit varies in direct relationship to the practitioner's expertise, training, and experience (Porcino et al. 2013).

History and the Development of General Massage

Massage has persisted through human history. From cave paintings to formal art works and books, there is evidence of a fundamental appreciation that massage is beneficial to health, and also is an element of pleasure and even an expression of wealth. Massage for beauty and for anti-ageing was used by many ancient cultures such as the Egyptians, and it is still used by beauticians and barbers to apply oils and lotions to maintain a supple skin and

evoke relaxation (Paulson 2008). Massage has also played a significant role in the history of medicine, midwifery, nursing, and sporting activities. Among the Greeks and Romans, massage was used to relieve pain and encourage movement in bruised and injured joints and to hasten healing of injuries acquired in battle or by gladiators (Kamenetz 1985) (see Figure 4.1).

Massage as a healing art was developed and directly influenced in relation to interest in physical health. George H. Taylor's (1887) *New Movement Cure* was promoted and popularized as a treatment of disease. This interest in movement led to the development of gymnastics and manual manipulation of the body to stimulate the muscles. Doctors

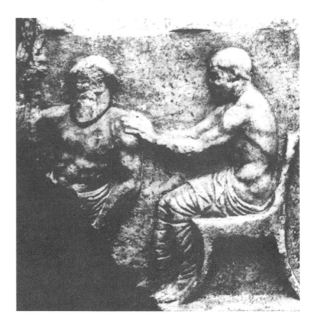

Figure 4.1
Gladiator massage.
Reprinted with permission of publisher. *The History of Massage* by Robert Noah Calvert published by Inner Traditions International and Bear & Company, ©2002. All rights reserved. http://www. Innertraditions.com

were divided in their application of these "physical treatments" for health and healing. Some relied solely on drug therapy, while others employed a prescription of more natural processes to promote health and healing. Consequently, a new interest developed in a process of hand movements used on the bare skin by a therapist. This eventually became known as *Swedish massage*.

The development of a set of organized soft tissue manipulations of massage was very important to contemporary massage, as it meant the system could be taught and studied as a stand-alone healing art. History, though blurred, seems to indicate this organization began with Professor Peter Ling (1776–1837) in Sweden with his system of "medical gymnastics" which demonstrated nineteen separate techniques. This laid the groundwork for the development of the four well-known categories of Swedish massage by the Dutch practitioner Johan George Mezger (1838–1909) (Kamenetz 1985). He used French terms *effleurage*, *petrissage, frictions*, and *tapotement*. In 1886, Mezger was probably the first to write a doctoral dissertation using those terms in relation to the treatment of injury and related pain, which was entitled "The treatment of foot sprain by friction" (Kamenetz 1985; Calvert 2002).

Early research into massage treatment was often written up as case studies citing symptoms of the presenting patient, the diagnosis, the treatment applied, and the results. The first clinical experiments were published in the *Archives of Medicine Journal* in 1880 by Drs. Jacobi and White. Dr. Kellogg also conducted experiments which he wrote in his 1895 book, *The Art of Massage*. Dr. William Murrell, in an article in the *British Medical Journal*, wrote about research conducted by Von Mosengeil and Zabludowsky (Murrell 1886a). These studies found massage most useful for chronic muscle pain conditions, joint pain, constipation, and ill health due to "obstinate" disease. "Swedish Massage" was used in these experiments. They ascribe the success of their treatments to the

strict adherence to the systematic process and the definite order of treatment: begin and end with *effleurage*, the palm of the hand, and sometimes the knuckles with a centripetal force, followed by *petrissage* as a more complex kneading movement, *friction* performed by the tips of the fingers, in conjunction with *effleurage* in treatment of the joints (Murrell 1886b).

> **Sidebar 4.1 Defining Massage**
> The National Institutes of Health's National Center for Complementary and Integrative Health's definition: Massage therapy encompasses many different techniques. In general, therapists press, rub, and otherwise manipulate the muscles and other soft tissues of the body. They most often use their hands and fingers, but may use their forearms, elbows, or feet (https://nccih.nih.gov/health/massage accessed July 2, 2015). Nahin et al. provide this definition in their National Health Statistics Reports (July 30, 2009): Massage—Therapy involving the manipulation of muscle and connective tissue to enhance function of those tissues and promote relaxation and well-being (http://www.cdc.gov/nchs/data/nhsr/nhsr018.pdf; accessed July 2, 2015, p. 13).

By the early twentieth century, massage was taught to nurses. The Society of Trained Masseurs started in England in 1894 and later became The Chartered Society of Massage and Gymnastics with 5,000 members. In the USA, Nurse Mary McMillan wrote *Massage and Therapeutic Exercise* (1925) as a teaching tool for practitioners in hospitals, the military, and private practice (Calvert 2002). Anatomy and physiology were taught along with the massage techniques. In 1943, the Chartered Society of Physiotherapists was formed to reflect the development of other techniques used in hospital care. Consequently, massage education shifted from the medical community into private schooling, where Swedish massage was retained as an important treatment approach.

Massage therapy today is a health care and wellness profession (Dryden and Moyer 2012). The practice of massage has a patient-centered focus, intended to support therapeutic goals. The major characteristics of contemporary massage therapy are based on touch and movement (Tappan and Benjamin 1998); massage therapists gather information to assess and judge the state of physiological and pathological conditions and parameters. This is called "palpation" (Chaitow 1997). Viola Frymann (1963, 1) wrote: "The first step in the process of palpation is detection, the second step is amplification, and the third step must therefore be interpretation. The interpretation of the observations made by palpation is the key which makes the study of the structure and function of tissues meaningful."

The basis of therapy is the application of massage techniques with intent and utilization (Baskwill 2011). Utilization is the selection of techniques in response to the therapeutic needs of the patient and the practitioner's intent to create beneficial change (Porcino et al. 2013). Though some massage can sometimes involve the learning of "recipes," or manualized protocols, by which to treat patients, massage *therapy* must include clinical reasoning skills (LeMoon 2008), and a patient-centered approach to individualizing care. This means that the massage therapist adapts to the environments, scenarios, and presentations of the patient (Andrade and Clifford 2001).

The individual utilization and variability of different massage treatments was recently

---

Sidebar 4.2 Patient Interviews

Authors in this book were given patient interview questionnaires and asked to distribute them among patients/clients in their practices. The results are interspersed throughout the chapters.

When asked, "Have your condition or symptoms or ability to function changed since receiving care?", a 54-year-old woman living with chronic pain for 20 years, replied: "I have never felt the same level of pain as I did before treatment, so I feel more in control of it. It's also reassuring that a massage therapist can locate areas of pain and work on making them better, whereas, for instance, a GP might not appreciate the level of pain or understand where it's coming from (i.e. it's all in your head!)."

When asked, "What information helped you decide to go to complementary treatment sessions or classes?", she replied:

"I had already tried most conventional treatments and some other complementary ones. As I was working through a list of things to try, it was pure luck that I found the treatment that helped long-term. The practitioners are highly skilled and professional and treat their clients with respect."

Sidebar 4.3 Research

Majchrzychi and colleagues (2014) investigated the effects of **deep tissue massage (DTM)** combined with non-steroidal anti-inflammatory drugs (NSAIDs) in the treatment of low back pain. The intervention included DTM alone, and DTM with NSAIDs: both groups had significant decreases in pain, suggesting that the most effective intervention tactic is DTM. The study authors went further to clearly define DTM as: "a form of massage used with 'the understanding of the layers of the body and the ability to work with tissues in layers to relax, extend, and unlock the persisting, incorrect tensions, in the most effective and energy-efficient manner'. Therapists working with this type of massage aim to change the soft tissues structure … The knowledge of anatomy of locomotor systems and the understanding of layer structure of tissues including fascia and muscles are needed. The therapist affects the tissues gradually until they respond with relaxation … The therapist affects the muscle belly as well as the tendon-to-bone attachment, trying to soften the tendon and to influence receptors of muscle extension (Golgi organs of tendons)" (Majchrzychi, Kocur, and Kotwicki 2014, 5).

researched by Porcino et al. (2011), investigating 791 Canadian practitioners. The research revealed that therapists used a combined-methods design which was influenced by the training they received, the number of techniques they were trained in, expertise, and the practice descriptors. Porcino and colleagues conclude that: "Practitioners individualize each patient's treatment through a highly adaptive process. Therefore, treatment provision is likely unique to each practitioner" (2011, p. 1).

Theoretical Approaches to Pain Management

In recent years, there have been developments in our understanding of the complexity of chronic pain. The standard medical treatment of chronic pain, however, is still hampered by inadequate personalization and by pharmacological side effects. Massage researchers propose that the total experience of a massage can have a complex physiological, mechanical, and psychological effect (Moyer, Rounds, and Hannum 2004; Field, Diego and Hernandez-Reif 2007). Although no single theory explains the complex response that is subjectively reported with massage therapy, mechanisms that have been suggested to facilitate, or are proposed to promote, the effects of massage on the experience of pain include the following items.

Touch

Massage is a direct contact with the skin. The skin is the largest organ of the body and has been shown to have an active interface with the endocrine, immune, and central nervous systems (Brazzini et al. 2003). Touch in humans has been shown to increase social bonds, decrease stress, and increase cooperative behaviors and relaxation (Uvnäs-Moberg 1997; Uvnäs-Moberg, Arn, and Magnusson 2005; Morhenn, Beavin, and Zak 2011; Rapaport, Schettler, and Bresee 2012). The relaxation brings about positive hormonal changes in cortisol levels, reducing inflammatory processes, increasing oxytocin, and calming the mental state, which can all have a positive impact on pain and the individual perception or expression of pain (Esch, Frichione, and Stefan 2003). MRI scans during a single session Swedish massage show an up-regulation in activity in areas of the brain that are specifically related to pain relief: the subgenual anterior cingulate cortex and the retrosplenal posterior cingulate cortex (Sliz et al. 2012). These areas are the targets for treating persistent chronic pain using deep brain stimulation (Kringelbach et al. 2007). This is a correlation that requires further research, but indicates that touch has more than just peripheral effects on tissue.

Improved Sleep Cycle

Massage therapy is often sought as a treatment for pain and sleep difficulties. Getting the right amount of sleep reduces pain perception and contributes to an individual's health and capacity to be positive in their approach to life (Sunshine et al. 1996). Insufficient sleep can lead to a lowering of mental and physical capacity or focus, which impacts the capacity of coping and resilience, and a reduced capacity to recover from sickness and stressful situations, which promotes inflammatory process and pain sensitivity (Richards, Gibson, and Overton-McCoy 2000).

Social Rejection and Pain

Eisenberger et al. (2006) showed that the **neural correlates** for pain and social rejection are expressed in the same brain region in the **anterior cingulate cortex (ACC)**. Massage therapy might often be doing more than just providing localized soft tissue relief and may also be satisfying social and mental health benefits while managing pain symptoms. It might be that the interpersonal patient–practitioner rapport that is achieved during massage therapy reduces activity in the ACC, creating a residual decrease in the experience of pain, although this hypothesis is yet to be tested.

Sidebar 4.4 Practitioner Interviews
When asked how massage therapy benefited their patients, replies included:

- "assists in treatment of physiological problems associated with the somatization of emotions"

- "very positive pain relief in a very whole body approach"

- "Our clients feel stronger, more confident in their physical movement and mental approach and aware of how it benefits their overall health and pain condition. They move from a patient identity to taking charge of their own health care."

Sidebar 4.5 Research
Barnes and colleagues (2008) reported from the National Health Interview Survey (NHIS) that pain in the form of back, neck and joint pain were the top three reasons Americans used complementary and integrative therapies in both 2002 and 2007. Meditation (9.4%), massage (8.3%), and yoga (6.1%) were among the most common in 2007. In 2012, the updated HNIS data, massage was used by 15.4 million (6.9%) Americans, stating promising evidence exists for massage for back pain, and improved quality of life for people experiencing depression, HIV/AIDS, and cancer (Clarke et al. 2015). The review also indicated massage therapy was found to be safe with very few adverse side effects. Adverse side effects were rare when massage was performed by qualified therapists and performed within the guidelines of the therapy (Ernst 2003; Ezzo 2007; Posadzki and Ernst 2013). The AAMT review recommends that care needs to be taken when considering site, intensity, and depth of massage with clients on anti-coagulation therapy, and with patients with prosthetic devices and cardiac defibrillators. Reviews of massage and mechanical neck disorders found side effects rare (Ezzo et al. 2007); however, case studies indicate care should be taken with neurovascular structures and vertebral artery compromise (Grant 2003). Cancer patients safely incorporate massage into their care and have shown positive benefits to quality of life (Corbin 2005). Minimizing of side effects and errors in treatment requires thoughtful and knowledgeable attendance to methods of practice.

Scope of Evidence for Effectiveness of Massage Therapy

In recent times, there has been an upsurge of interest and research into massage therapy. Certainly, there has been increased pressure for evidence-based treatments in the health industry and for healthcare insurance reimbursement. There has also been a galvanizing of practitioners into associations that seek to professionalize their profession. Massage therapy has been shown to be one of the most popular forms of complementary and alternative therapies (Xue et al. 2007) with beneficial physiological effects (Moyer et al. 2004). Studies show that massage improves symptoms of pain, anxiety, sleep difficulties, and depression, and improves quality of life (Wilkie et al. 2000; Cassileth and Vickers 2004; Wilkinson et al. 2007; Kutner et al. 2008). Adams, Lui, and McLaughlin (2009) report that massage therapy is commonly chosen by people in later life for chronic pain and stress reduction. In the recent review of some 740 studies and reviews of the effectiveness of massage therapy sponsored by the Australian Association of Massage Therapy (Ng 2011), moderate to strong evidence was found to support massage therapy for nausea and vomiting, anxiety, stress, chronic disease management, delayed onset muscle soreness, and pulmonary function.

Massage Therapy for Patients with Cancer-related Pain

Cancer is rapidly increasing throughout the world (WHO 2010). There are many newly diagnosed cancer cases, but there are also long-term active treatment cases and cancer survivors (WHO 2010). It is estimated that 25% of newly diagnosed and 75% of advance-stage cancer cases experience pain as their most debilitating symptom (American Pain Society 2008). Cancer pain is a complex, subjective, and medically challenging symptom that may be due to the cancer itself or to side effects of treatment regimens such as chemotherapy, radiation therapy, or surgery that can last for months or even years (Bajwa and Warfield 2007). Cancer pain is also considered one of the major causes of cancer-related fatigue (CRF), an ongoing distressing symptom experienced by most cancer patients after treatment (Berger et al. 2010).

Massage is a popular therapy that has been studied as a treatment to assist in the control of cancer-related symptoms. Yates et al. (2005), in their study into the prevalence of complementary and alternative medicine, found that massage was used by 75% of US cancer patients. Most of these patients specifically used massage for pain management. Other studies have shown that massage is also used to improve the quality of sleep and reduce anxiety

Sidebar 4.6 Research
In a 2011 evaluation of multiple studies, including international populations, 1,558 palliative cancer care patients were examined for pain, depression, and anxiety, prior to and post massage. Falkensteiner et al. (2011) found that massage therapy was useful in decreasing cancer-related pain with effects lasting up to 18 hours after the massage session. This synthesis found that depressive mood states were positively affected and anxiety was decreased. Of note, the context effects and the provider–patient relationship were found to be valuable contributors to decreases in perceived pain, anxiety levels, and depressive symptoms. In the United States, the National Cancer Institute stated that massage therapy is a safe and effective integrative approach to managing cancer pain and improving mood states on their About Cancer webpage http://www.cancer.gov/about-cancer/treatment/side-effects/pain/pain-pdq#-section/_240 (accessed September 9, 2015).

and distress. CRF is considered by many oncology specialists to be a result of increased inflammatory responses. Massage can improve immune function and reduce inflammatory processes (Field 2006). As an additional benefit, many cancer patients and survivors are benefitting from an array of pharmacological interventions that may continue for years. Massage is able to offer beneficial effects without increasing the patient's burden of pharmacological treatment (Corbin 2005).-

Methodology
Massage, in all its different forms and styles, practiced in different nations, and in the context of different cultures, is unified by an overarching goal and intention to create beneficial changes that help the body to achieve better health and well-being (Sherman et al. 2006). Generally, the basic philosophy of massage is predicated on:

- Wholism is the belief that all parts of the body work together to allow the body to work as a whole, and within the "whole" everything is connected and related.

- Muscles function by shortening and therefore a muscle that is in spasm will be unable to contract any further.

- Soft tissues of the body respond to a massage therapist's functional instrument of touch.

Gertude Beard (1887–1971), one of the most respected massage educators, explained that the "instrument of touch" is manipulated by the therapist through various "qualities of touch" that include direction, speed, rhythm, drag, frequency, duration, and depth of pressure. This is how a therapist achieves different goals and treats different people. The National Center for Complementary and Integrative Health (NCCIH), the United States Federal Government's lead agency for scientific research on complementary and alternative medicine (CAM), acknowledges the complexity of the industry and recognizes over eighty different massage techniques. The important point, however, is to note that it is not the plentitude of techniques, but the manner in which they are utilized to create the greatest treatment benefit. The three-leveled classification system developed by Sherman et al. (2006) is useful in clarifying some of the terminology used to describe treatments that are identified and practiced by massage therapists. Sherman and colleagues' classifications are: principal goals of treatment, styles, and techniques (see Figure 4.2) (2006, 3).

Four Principal Goals of Massage Treatments and their Common Styles and Techniques

These may be summarized as follow:

1. Massage for relaxation and promotion of wellness, designed to move fluids and promote circulation.
   a. Western massage therapists generally understand the style of Swedish massage as the basic relaxation massage that employs five basic techniques: effleurage (gliding strokes), petrissage (kneading and lifting), friction, vibration and percussion. There are other examples such as sports massage and spa massage.

2. Clinical or remedial massage used to address: chronic pain; muscular spasms or damage; **fascia**, lymph, circulation or nervous system care.
   a. Common techniques of clinical massage are **myofascial** trigger point therapy, **myofascial release**, neuromuscular therapy and structural integration. These therapies commonly use techniques of skin rolling, direct pressure, cross-fiber friction and manual stretching.

3. Movement re-education massage designed to increase awareness to improve posture and body movement.

   a. Generally used to improve quality and range of joint movement and to induce a sense of freedom and lightness of body. Styles many include proprioceptive neuromuscular facilitation, strain and counterstrain and muscle energy techniques. The techniques may include table work in which the therapists encourages, resists or assists movement.

4. Energy work (this may include mind/body therapies and/or subtle energy techniques) which are designed to encourage the flow of energy through "blockages."
   a. Styles include reiki, polarity and therapeutic touch from Western cultures and **acupressure**, Amma, Shaitsu and Tuina from Eastern cultures. These therapies use techniques involving an awareness of energy directions, smoothing, holding, rocking and traction.

Even though the classification creates a clear division of goals, styles, and techniques, in practice the goal of treatment may be achieved by utilizing a number of different styles and techniques as determined by the therapist in response to the client's needs. Porcino et al. (2013) explored practitioners' practice of styles and techniques of massage and found every treatment is individualized and evolving. Basic training of massage therapy typically includes a sample of styles. This basic training is expanded in ongoing continuing education training and in response to practitioner experience. Practitioners believe their underlying intent, experience, and knowledge guides the individualized treatment, based on the goal of treatment.

Massage, once historically taught through experience and apprenticeship, is now formally taught and government regulated or licensed. Education standards required from AMT are:

• knowledge of anatomy, physiology and biomechanics

Principal goals of treatment	Relaxation massage	Clinical massage	Movement re-education	Energy work
Intention	Relax muscles, move body fluids, promote wellness	Accomplish specific goals such as releasing muscle spasms	Induce sense of freedom, ease and lightness in body	Hypothesized to free energy blockages
Commonly used styles (examples*)	Swedish massage Spa massage Sports massage	Myofascial trigger point therapy Myofascial release Strain counterstrain	Proprioceptive neuromuscular facilitation Strain counterstrain Trager	Acupressure Reiki Polarity Therapeutic touch Tuina
Commonly used techniques (examples**)	Gliding Kneading Friction Holding Percussion Vibration	Direct pressure Skin rolling Resistive stretching Stretching – manual Cross-fiber friction	Contract–relax Passive stretching Resistive stretching Rocking	Direction of energy Smoothing Direct pressure Holding Rocking Traction

*While some styles of massage are commonly used in addressing one of the four principal treatment goals, some may be used to address several distinct treatment goals.
** By varying the intent (or purpose) of a technique, many of them can be used in massages with different principal treatment goals.

Figure 4.2
Proposed taxonomy of massage practice.
(Sherman 2006)

- well-developed assessment, observational, and palpation skills

- basic understanding of pathology and underlying dysfunction for contraindications and clinical reasoning

- expertise in a range of manual techniques and approaches

- an understanding of normal function in relation to soft tissues of the body and the ability to recognize dysfunction.

AMT, 2012

In the management of chronic pain, the massage therapist should be highly adept at examination, palpation, and assessment of the musculoskeletal system, and fully aware that this is only one aspect of the whole body. Co-morbidities, their connection and relationship are important in the focus of treatment in people with chronic pain.

Sidebar 4.7 Patient Interviews
When asked, "What have you learned about this treatment approach or self-care that you would like healthcare providers to know about?", a 54-year-old woman living with chronic pain for 20 years replied: "Massage therapy has been the one thing which has really worked for me, but I had to try a lot of other things before I discovered it. It has no adverse side effects! I didn't realize, before trying it, that the practitioners were so highly trained and knowledgeable. Had I known that, I may have tried it sooner."

Massage therapists usually try to provide a private, safe, comfortable, calm, soothing environment for both the client and themselves (Smith, Sullivan, and Baxter 2011). Massage therapists can, however, work in a variety of settings, including their own clinical space, business offices, hospitals, nursing homes, studios, sport and fitness facilities, and integrated healthcare settings. Some also travel to patients' homes or workplaces (Clay and Pounds, 2003).

Development of a Treatment Plan

As a general approach to the treatment of chronic pain, I follow this procedure:

- Assess the need for treatment; identify and measure the client's impairment.

- Educate the client regarding the massage process, behavioral and/or environmental risk factors of chronic pain disease. This may include identifying and explaining the possibility of referral to other healthcare practitioners.

- Assist the client to attain the clinical and individual goals in their pain experience and in their lifestyle.

- Give them support techniques to prevent recurrence and/or further damage.

While assessing the patient, I find that a template for a treatment plan begins to emerge in my mind. This will develop into a clear treatment plan. Although it is good to have a clear treatment plan, it is also important to be flexible and responsive to the client. I will not only utilize my knowledge and experience base, but I also think about possible referrals if I feel that the client will be better served elsewhere or with a team approach. Other therapists might follow different protocols, but all therapists are looking to find the best skill combination for the needs of the client.

Aspects of the Process of Clinical Care

The *first phase* is an evaluation phase, or client consultation, that includes an interview, physical assessment (range of movement, passive, and active movement), and the development of a treatment plan (see Figure 4.3) The treatment plan of care is

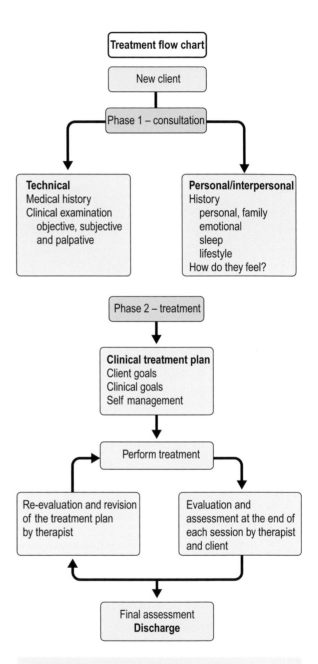

Figure 4.3
Basic flow chart of clinical care.

developed between the client and the therapist. The focus of the plan includes informed consent for treatment including: length of treatment, goals of treatment and treatment outcomes, frequency of treatment needed to reach the goals, location of therapeutic massages sessions, what area will be massaged, what techniques might be used initially, and what lifestyle changes will be suggested to support treatment (Andrade and Clifford, 2001).

The *second phase* is the massage treatment, which is guided by information from the first phase of assessment, plus sensitive palpation (Chaitow 1997) and "tissue dialogue" (Clay and Pounds 2003). "Tissue dialogue" is where the therapist gauges the response of the soft tissue and adjusts the pressure and utilization of techniques to achieve the desired tissue response.

Following these two phases of treatment, I usually provide the client with a self-management program that they perform at home. This program can vary greatly between clients and is specifically created in relation to the entire experience during therapy. This includes information from the initial assessment as well as information gathered during therapy. Lifestyle risk factors are considered, including diet, exercise patterns, ergonomic environment, and especially sleep patterns.

The length of treatment for massage is usually based on a sixty-minute session. I often find, however, that it is beneficial for chronic pain clients, at least on the first treatment, to increase this period to ninety minutes. This is in line with the natural ultradian cycle of 90–120 minutes as described by Nathaniel Kleitman (1982) as the *Basic Rest and Activity Cycle*, and by others (Rossi 2002). The longer time frame seems to help in the effectiveness of the treatment (Sherman et al. 2014).

Application of the massage treatment
Positioning and care
In the general application of massage therapy, it is usual for the client to undress and to be positioned prone or supine on a massage table covered with a

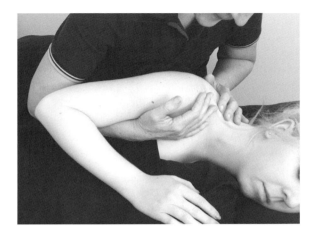

Figure 4.4
Massage positioning.

towel or sheet. The position of the client is guided by the aims of the treatment, information and preferences from the client, and areas to be accessed. I employ the use of pillows or bolsters to support the correct and comfortable positioning of the client (see Figure 4.4). An added benefit of bolstering is that it is possible to minimize pain and discomfort from over-extension or strain to damaged joint or muscular areas and assists the utilization of techniques during the massage. I have also found that the choice of position of the client on the massage table may be influenced by the capabilities of the client. For example, an older person with breathing difficulties may not be able to lie on the stomach, or a person with Parkinson's disease may be unable to turn easily. In these cases I would position them on their back and sides.

The client is always draped for warmth, modesty, safety, and comfort. Only the part being treated is undraped, and treatment, movement, and assessment can also take place through the sheet while draped.

Massage interventions and practice
In the therapeutic massage encounter, soft tissue layers are treated to achieve specific outcomes of

remediation of the impairment, reduce pain, and reduce functional restrictions. There are also many benefits that come from a positive interpersonal engagement. Evidence for this comes from a number of disciplines. Uvnäs-Moberg (1997) shows that there in an increase in oxytocin which acts in the brain to promote serotonin, which is known to calm mood and help create trust. The client–therapist relationship is complicated by both the needs and vulnerability of the client and the client's degree of dependence on the therapist. During my massage treatments, I also find it helpful to be mindful, constantly evaluating and reflecting on the person's soft tissue response at the time. I utilize my experience from palpation knowledge with previous tissue, my knowledge of the different techniques and their specific outcomes, and the interpersonal reaction and state of the client. Assessment and re-assessment is an ongoing process.

Evaluation of Treatment

Evaluation and recording of the massage treatment are usually completed straight after the treatment and before ongoing treatments. The evaluation might include:

- The therapist's evaluation: recording the therapy strategies, re-testing of objective range of motion (ROM) and re-evaluating subjective scores from the client with VAS scales (pain, sleep practices, and mood).

- The client's evaluation, usually reported before each treatment, which includes:

  - Information about the specific pain: How often are they now feeling the pain? How intense is it? How long are the breaks when there is no pain? If there is a relapse, how quickly are they able to get the pain under control again?

  - Information about their social experience. Some examples from my practice are: How well did they walk to the shops? Were they

able to sit longer at their bridge game or at a dinner outing? Did they play their sport of choice (tennis, golf or bowling)?

- Personal aspects of their lives: How are they sleeping? How grumpy were they with their partner or family since last visit? Were they able to enjoy a family outing?

These factors are all important for the re-assessment and evaluation which directs changes in the specific treatment process and self-management program.

Self-management Program

This may include:

- Breathing and relaxation exercises to assist in reducing pain (Phillips 2007).

- Sleep hygiene plan: an effective client program developed to assist longer and better sleep hours (Egger, Binns, and Rosser 2008).

- Pain diary: a record of pain score, anxiety score and activity during the day. This pattern of acknowledging and focusing on their body's sensations helps them to identify what seems to increase pain and what relieves, reduces, or affects the pain (Phillips 2007). This helps them to focus on the pain differently and they start looking at the activities that reduce pain. This takes about a month of monitoring.

- Exercise program, which might be organized by a rehabilitation or exercise physiologist.

Sidebar 4.8 Patient Interviews
When asked, "Do you do any regular self-care to relieve or prevent ongoing pain?", a 66-year-old registered nurse living with chronic pain for 20 years replied: "Complementary care has provided me with a range of options to manage pain other than resorting to medication … regular massage, practice Alexander Technique, yoga."

Case Study

Jane is a 56-year-old retired nurse, who presented for massage treatment in early 2013. Jane reported concerns about upper thoracic, right shoulder, and right arm pain.

History: Jane experienced multiple recent abdominal surgeries for diverticulitis — a condition in which small, bulging pouches (diverticula) in the digestive tract become inflamed or infected. During her hospital stay she experienced complications that resulted in painful infections, multiple surgical interventions, and daily intensely painful procedures. Jane also spent many weeks in the intensive care unit (ICU) as a result of the complications, which disrupted her sleep cycle. During her time in ICU, intravenous (IV) fluids were administered through a central IV catheter, positioned on the right side of her chest. Jane was positioned by the nurses in an attempt to reduce her pain: supine, the head of the bed elevated and her knees elevated. Jane reported she was unable to straighten out her body for many weeks, a result of her abdominal surgeries (wound and scar issues), the intense abdominal pain, and the nursing position. Though she had not experienced any additional injury, she reported intense pain across her shoulders and neck since recovering from the surgery (6 months). She reported pain that radiated down her right arm into her middle fingers as eight-out-of-ten on the pain scale. Her sleep scale was also eight-out-of-ten, which is considered a good result, but she also reported that her sleep was often disturbed. Jane described previous physiotherapy and a complex exercise program which she completed post surgery. She felt her pain had become progressively worse over the past 6 months. Jane was teary as she described her experiences in hospital and at home.

Client expectations and goals: Jane had chosen massage therapy because she wanted a treatment for her pain, but she "didn't want any more medical-based" procedures that "would cause more pain." She said she wanted something that was "relaxing" and not invasive. She had enough of being "poked, pushed and told to work harder." Jane was exhausted from struggling with the pain condition. She was worried that it would never go away and she would never be able to enjoy her life again. Jane was able to choose massage herself and this was important for her.

Observation and physical assessment: Jane presented with rounded or drooping shoulders and fatigued posture. She reported that her right arm felt heavy and it appeared slightly swollen. There was no discoloration in the skin. Being mindful of Jane's sensitivity to both touch and movement, her active range of motion (ROM) was tested carefully. Cervical movement tests revealed no restriction, though there were areas in the lower cervical spine that appeared to have lost their lordotic curve possibly due to muscle spasm restrictions. Passive ROM and strength tests did not reveal any numbness, tingling, burning. Jane's symptoms were consistent with thoracic outlet syndrome involving anterior or middle scalenes and insertion of the pectoralis muscle at the coracoid process. There was restriction in the ROM of her arm, which was consistent with teres major and infraspinatus muscle tightness. She demonstrated upper chest breathing, which was probably due to abdominal weakness and abdominal surgery.

Pressure considerations:

- Jane was very sensitive and fatigued; therefore, continual assessment and communication were made with client.

- Edema was noted in the upper arm, so gentle pressure was used.

- Though a light massage was used, where possible I increased the pressure to encourage movement, initially utilizing vibration and effleurage.

Positioning restrictions:

- Jane only wanted the areas of her pain massaged (upper body).

- She was unable to lie on her stomach for any length of time.
- When she laid on her back, she needed to have her knees bent and supported with a bolster.

Treatments: Initial treatments were focused on arms, upper thoracic, and neck. Jane was massaged supine to lateral or side-lying right and left. The massage revealed tightness, spasm, and restriction in the pectoral muscles, scalenus, coracobrachialis, infraspinatus, teres, middle trapezius, and sub-clavius muscles. Treatment focused on the upper body and with each consecutive massage I was able to apply more pressure and increase the variety of techniques used (skin rolling, kneading, compression). Jane was encouraged to commence breathing exercises and complete a pain diary, and she was shown how to do skin brushing to stimulate normal skin processes and improve lymphatic drainage.

Progress was made quickly with the increase of trust in the massage, and in circulation in the soft tissue which resulted in reduction in pain periods. Jane was given a dog by the family and she started to walk every day. By 2 months into her therapy, Jane was able to lie on her stomach and I was allowed to start giving her a full body massages. From the pain diary, Jane found that her pain was worse in the afternoon and when she was not busy. It also has indicated that, though she still has pain periods, they are less frequent, and she recovers from them more quickly. The diary has also helped her manage her day better. The breathing exercises helped Jane breathe with her abdominal muscles and this has improved her posture. She has also considerably reduced her pain medication.

Conclusion

Jane's experience with massage is representative of the many clients I have treated during my years of practice. Massage is a useful tool that integrates well with other treatments and consistently results in positive outcomes for clients. There is much we know, but also much we need to know. We cannot, however, halt or pause the utilization of therapies that can assist those who suffer while we wait for definitive research to prove effectiveness. Massage therapy creates beneficial change for many and it does so with very few side effects. If that is the nature of a broadly usable therapy across a population, then it seems wise to use massage therapy to relieve, manage, and sometimes even eradicate pain. What is equally important is that massage is practiced well to maintain effectiveness, and experienced often to reduce the impact of chronic pain in the population.

References

AMT (2012). Association of Massage Therapists Ltd, *Massage Therapy Code of Practice*, http://www.amt.org.au/downloads/practice-resources/AMT-code-of-practice-final.pdf (p.12). (accessed: January, 2015).

Adams, J., C.-W. Lui, and D. McLaughlin. 2009. The use of complementary and alternative medicine in later life. *Reviews in Clinical Gerontology* 19(4):227–36.

American Pain Society. 2008. *Principles of analgesic use in the treatment of acute pain and cancer pain*, 6th ed. Glenview.IL: APS.

Andrade, C.-K., and P. Clifford. 2001. *Outcome-based massage*. Philadelphia, PA: Lippincott, Williams & Wilkins.

Armstrong, A. R., S. P. Thiebaut, and L. J. Brown. 2011. Australian adults use complementary and alternative medicine in the treatment of chronic illness: a national study. *Australian and New Zealand Journal of Public Health* 35(4):384–90.

Bajwa, H. Z., and C. A. Warfield. 2007. *Overview of cancer pain* (online). Published online: 2007 (cited 2008 May). http://www.uptodateonline.com/online/content/topic.do?topicKey=gen_onc/12792&selectedTitle=1-150&source=search_result.

Barnes, P., E. Powell-Griner, K. McFann, and R. Nahin. 2004. Complementary and Alternative Medicine Use Among Adults: United States, 2002. *CDC Advance Data Report* #343, 1–19.

Barnes, P. M., B. Bloom, and R. L. Nahin. 2008. Complementary and alternative medicine use among adults and children: United States, 2007. *National Health Statistics Reports*; no 12. Hyattsville, MD: National Center for Health Statistics.

Baskwill, A. 2011. Changing the culture of clinical education in massage therapy. *International journal of therapeutic massage & bodywork* 4(4):33.

Beard, G., and E. C. Wood. 1964. *Massage: principles and techniques*. Philadelphia: Saunders.

Berger, A. M., A. P. Abernethy, A. Atkinson, A. M. Barsevick, W. S. Breitbart, D. Cella, B. Cimprich, C. Cleeland, M. A. Eisenberger, C. P. Escalante, et al. 2010. Cancer-related Fatigue: clinical practice guidelines in oncology. *Journal of the National Comprehensive Cancer Network* 8(8):904–931.

Brazzini, B., I. Ghersetich, J. Hercogova, and T. Lotti. 2003. The neuro–immuno–cutaneous–endocrine network: relationship between mind and skin. *Dermatologic Therapy* 16(2):123–31.

Calvert, R. N. 2002. *The history of massage : an illustrated survey from around the world*. Rochester, VT: Healing Arts Press.

Cassileth, B. R., and A. J. Vickers. 2004. Massage therapy for symptom control: outcome study at a major cancer center. *J Pain Symptom Manage*, vol. 28, no. 3, pp. 244–9.

Chaitow, L. 1997. *Palpation skills: Assessment and diagnosis through touch*. New York: Churchill Livingstone.

Cherkin, D. C., K. J. Sherman, J. Kahn, R. Wellman, A. J. Cook, E. Johnson, J. Erro, K. Delaney, and R. A. Deyo. 2011. A comparison of the effects of 2 types of massage and usual care on chronic low back pain: a randomized, controlled trial. *Ann Intern Med.* 155(1):1–9.

Clarke, T. C., L. I. Black, B. J. Stussman, P. M. Barnes, and R. L. Nahin. 2015. Trends in the use of complementary health approaches among adults: United States, 2002–2012. *National Health Statistics Reports;* no 79. Hyattsville, MD: National Center for Health Statistics. 2015.

Clay, J. H., and D. M. Pounds. 2003. *Basic clinical massage therapy: integrating anatomy and treatment*. Philadelphia, PA: Lippincott, Williams & Wilkins.

Corbin, L. 2005. Safety and efficacy of massage therapy for patients with cancer. *Cancer Control.* 12(3):158–64.

Dryden, T., and C. A. Moyer. 2012. *Massage therapy: integrating research and practice*. Champaign, IL: Human Kinetics.

Egger, G., A. Binns, and S. Rosser. 2008. *Lifestyle Medicine*. Australia: McGraw-Hill.

Eisenbeger, N. I., J. M. Jarcho, M. D. Lieberman, and B. D. Naliboff. 2006. An experimental study of shared sensitivity to physical pain and social rejection. *Pain* 126(1–3):132–8.

Ernst, E. 2003. The safety of massage therapy. *Rheumatology* 42(9):1101–6.

Esch, T., C. L. Frichione, and G. B. Stefan. 2003. The therapeutic use of the relaxation response in stress-related diseases. *Medical Science Monitor* 9(2):23–34.

Ezzo, J. 2007. What can be learned from Cochrane systematic reviews of massage that can guide future research? *J Altern Complement Med* 13(2):291–5.

Ezzo, J., B. G. Haraldsson, A. R. Gross, C. D. Myers, A. Morien, C. H. Goldsmith, G. Bronfort, and P. M. Peloso. 2007. Massage for mechanical neck disorders: a systematic review. *Spine* 32(3):353.

Falkensteiner, M., F. Mantovan, I. Müller, and C. Them. 2011. The use of massage therapy for reducing pain, anxiety, and depression in oncological palliative care patients: a narrative review of the literature. *ISRN Nursing,* 929868. doi:10.5402/2011/929868.

Field, T. 2006. *Massage therapy research*, 1st edn. Edinburgh, New York: Elsevier Churchill Livingstone.

Field, T., M. Diego, and M. Hernandez-Reif. 2007. Massage therapy research. *Developmental Review* 27(1):75–89.

French, H. P., A. Brennan, B. White, and Y. Cusack T. 2010. Manual therapy for osteoarthritis of the hip or knee – a systematic review. *Manual Therapy* 16(2):109–17. doi:10.1016/j.math.2010.10.011. PMID 21146444.

Frymann, V. 1963. Palpation: Its study in the wordkshop: parts I–IV, pp 16–31. Yearbook of selected osteopathic papers *Academy of Applied Osteopathy.*

Grant, K. E. 2003. Massage safety: injuries reported in Medline relating to the practice of therapeutic massage—1965–2003. *Journal of Bodywork and Movement Therapies* 7(4):207–12.

Kamenetz, H. L. 1985. History of Massage. In *Manipulation, Traction and Massage*, ed. John V. Basmajian. Baltimore, MD: William and Wilkins.

Kellogg, J. H. 1923. *The art of massage: a practical manual for the nurse, the student and the practitioner*, rev. edn. Battle Creek, Mich: Modern Medicine Publishing.

Kleitman, N. 1982. Basic rest–activity cycle – 22 years later. *Journal of Sleep Research and Sleep Medicine* 5(4):311–17.

Krieger, D. 1979. *The therapeutic touch: How to use your hands to help or heal*. Englewood Cliffs, NJ: Prentice Hall, Inc.

Kringelbach, M. L., N. Jenkinson, A. L. Green, S. L. F. Owen, P. C. Hansen, and P. L. Cornelissen, et al. 2007. Deep brain stimulation for chronic pain investigated with Magnetoencephalography. *NeuroReport* 18(3):223–7.

Kutner, J. S., M. C. Smith, L. Corbin, L. Hemphill, K. Benton, B. K. Mellis, B. Beaty, S. Felton, T. E. Yamashita, L. L. Bryant, and D. L. Fairclough, D. 2008. Massage therapy versus simple touch to improve pain and mood in patients with advanced cancer: a randomized trial. *Ann Intern Med* 149(6):369–79.

LeMoon, K. 2008. Clinical reasoning in massage therapy. *International Journal of Therapeutic Massage and Bodywork* 1(1):12–18.

McMillan, M. 1925. *Massage and Therapeutic Exercise*. Philadelphia and London: Saunders.

Majchrzycki, M., P. Kocur, and T. Kotwicki. 2014. Deep tissue massage and nonsteroidal anti-inflammatory drugs for low back pain: a prospective randomized trial. *The Scientific World Journal* 287597. doi:10.1155/2014/287597.

Morhenn, V., L. E. Beavin, and P. J. Zak. 2011. Massage increases oxytocin and reduces adrenocorticotropin hormone in humans. *Alternative therapies in health and medicine* 18(6):11–18.

Moyer, C. A., J. Rounds, and J. W. Hannum. 2004. A meta-analysis of massage therapy research. *Psychol Bull* 130(1):3–18.

Murrell, W. 1886a. Massage as a therapeutic agent. *The British Medical Journal* May 15:9267.

Murrell, W. 1886b. *Massotherapeutics or massage as a mode of treatment,* [1st] edn. London: Lewis.

Myklebust, M., and J. Iler. 2007. Policy for therapeutic massage in an academic health center: a model for standard policy development. *Journal of Alternative and Complementary Medicine* 13(4):471–5.

Nahin, R. L., P. M. Barnes, B. J. Strussman, and B. Bloom. 2009. Costs of complementary and alternative medicine (CAM) and frequency of visits of CAM practitioners, United States, 2007. *National Health Statistics Reports;* no 18. Hyattsville, MD: National Center for Health Statisitcs.

National Institute of Health National Cancer Institute About Cancer. http://www.cancer.gov/about-cancer/treatment/side-effects/pain/pain-pdq#link/stoc_h2_4 (accessed July 6, 2015).

National Institute of Health National Center for Complementary and Integrative Health. https://nccih.nih.gov/health/massage (accessed July 2, 2015).

Ng, K. C. W. 2011. The effectiveness of massage therapy: a summary of evidence-based research. *AAMT and RMIT, Melbourne, Australia.* http://aamt.com.au/wp-content/uploads/2011/11/AAMT-Research-Report-10-Oct-11.pdf (accessed March, 2012).

Paulson, S. 2008. "Beauty is more than skin deep." An ethnographic study of beauty therapists and older women. *Journal of Aging Studies* 22(13):256–65.

Phillips, M. 2007. *Reversing chronic pain: a 10-point all-natural plan for lasting relief.* Berkeley, California: North Atlantic Books.

Porcino, A. J., H. S. Boon, S. A. Page, and M. J. Verhoef. 2011. Meaning and challenges in the practice of multiple therapeutic massage modalities: a combined methods study. BMC *Complement Altern Med* 11:75.

Porcino, A. J., H. S. Boon, S. A. Page, and M. J. Verhoef. 2013. Exploring the nature of therapeutic massage bodywork practice, [electronic version]. *International Journal of Therapeutic Massage and Bodywork* 6(1):15–24.

Posadzki, P., and E. Ernst. 2013. The safety of massage therapy: an update of a systematic review. *Focus on Alternative and Complementary Therapies* 18(1):27–32.

Rapaport, M. H., P. Schettler, and C. Bresee. 2012. A preliminary study of the effects of repeated massage on hypothalamic–pituitary–adrenal and immune function in healthy individuals: a study of mechanisms of action and dosage. *The Journal of Alternative and Complementary Medicine* 18(8):789–97.

Rich, G. J. 2010. Massage therapy: Significance and relevance to professional practice. *Professional Psychology: Research and Practice* 41(4):325.

Richards, K. C., R. Gibson, and A. L. Overton-McCoy. 2000. Effects of massage in acute and critical care. *AACN Clin Issues* 11(1):77–96.

Rossi, E. L. 2002. *The Psychobiology of Gene Expression.* New York, NY: W. W. Norton.

Sherman, K. J., M. W. Dixon, D. Thompson, and D. C. Cherkin. 2006. Development of a taxonomy to describe massage treatment for musculoskeletal pain. *BMC Complementary and Alternative Medicine* 6(2):4. http://www.biomedcentral.com/1472-6882/6/24.

Sherman, K. J., A. J. Cook, R. D. Wellman, R. J. Hawkes, J. R. Kahn, R. A. Deyo, and D. C. Cherkin. 2014. Five-week outcomes from a dosing trial of therapeutic massage for chronic neck pain. *Annals of Family Medicine* 12(2):112–20.

Sliz, D., A. Smith, C. Wiebking, G. Northoff, and S. Hayley. 2012. Neural correlates of a single session massage treatment. *Brain Imaging and Behavior* 6:77–87.

Smith, J. M., S. J. Sullivan, and G. D. Baxter. 2011. A descriptive study of the practice patterns of Massage New Zealand massage therapists. *Int J Ther Massage Bodywork* 4(1):18–27.

Sunshine, W., T. M. Field, O. Quintino, K. Fierro, C. Kuhn, I. Burman, and S. Schanberg. 1996. Fibromyalgia benefits from massage therapy and transcutaneous electrical stimulation. *JCR: Journal of Clinical Rheumatology* 2(1):18–22.

Tappan, F. M., and P. J. Benjamin. 1998. *Tappan's handbook of healing massage techniques: classic, holistic, and emerging methods,* 3rd edn. Stamford, CT: Appleton & Lange.

Taylor, G. H. 1887. *Massage: principles and practice of remedial treatment by imparted motion: mechanical processes.* New York, NY: J. B. Alden.

Uvnäs-Moberg, K. 1997. Physiological and endocrine effects of social contact. *Annals of the New York Academy of Sciences* 807(1):146–63.

Uvnäs-Moberg, K., I. Arn, and D. Magnusson. 2005. The psychobiology of emotion: The role of the oxytocinergic system. *International Journal of Behavioral Medicine* 12(2):59–65.

Wilkie, D. J., J. Kampbell, S. Cutshall, H. Halabisky, H. Harmon, L. P. Johnson, L. Weinacht, and M. Rake-Marona. 2000. Effects of massage on pain intensity, analgesics and quality of life in patients with cancer pain: a pilot study of a randomized clinical trial conducted within hospice care delivery. *Hosp J* 15(3):31–53.

Wilkinson, S. M., S. B. Love, A. M. Westcombe, M. A. Gambles, C. C. Burgess, A. Cargill, T. Young, E. J. Maher, and A. J. Ramirez. 2007. Effectiveness of aromatherapy massage in the management of anxiety and depression in patients with cancer: a multicenter randomized controlled trial. *Journal of Clinical Oncology* 25(5):532–9.

World Health Organization. 2010. Cancer Fact sheet No 297. (online) Published online 2010. (cited 2010 October). http://www.who.int/mediacentre/factsheets/fs297/en/.

Xue, C. C. L., A. L. Zhang, V. Lin, C. Da Costa, and D. F. Story. 2007. Complementary and alternative medicine use in Australia: a national population-based survey. *Journal of Alternative and Complementary Medicine (New York, N.Y.)* 13(6):643–50.

Yates, J. S., K. M. Mustian, G. R. Morrow, L. J. Gillies, D. Padmanaban, J. N. Atkins, B. Issell, J. J. Kirshner, and L. K. Colman. 2005. Prevalence of complementary and alternative medicine use in cancer patients. *Support Care Cancer* 13:806–11.

Introduction

Anyone who has suffered a sprained ankle knows the pain and swelling associated with this injury. Pain can be attributed to the actual injury— whether sprained ligaments, strained tendons, or muscle tissue—or to the side effects of swelling. Within a short period of time after an injury, an accumulation of interstitial and lymph fluid, or edema, sets in. This abnormal fluid-filled enlargement of an injured area provides a casting effect. The forced immobilization protects the injured area but can also result in additional pain to the surrounding tissues and structures. Swelling as the result of an acute inflammatory response to a specific injury is something most people are familiar with, and the cause and effect of the condition can be easily identified. There are other kinds of edema—specifically lymphedema—where the cause may be more difficult to determine.

It is necessary to categorize the type of edema in order to identify the proper course of action. In most cases, edema is due to a condition related to a functional issue, such as a cardiovascular dysfunction where a weakened heart may not be able to supply enough blood to the kidneys, which then begin to lose their ability to excrete salt and water, causing the body to retain more fluid. Fluid also may accumulate in the extremities, resulting in edema (swelling) of the ankles and feet. A mechanical issue can be another reason for a back-up of fluid in the body, such as damage or obstruction (e.g. scar tissue) to the lymph nodes or vessels (Werner 2014).

Lymphedema is a different animal entirely. Edema is an accumulation of interstitial fluid, and lymphedema is an accumulation of protein-rich fluid. Lymphedema may be caused by a genetic condition, an injury or medical treatment that damages the lymph capillaries, an injury to or removal of lymph nodes, or a parasitic infection.

Surgical removal of even one lymph node can leave a client at risk for lymphedema. In my practice, I have seen this disruption to the lymphatic flow create mild lymphedema in the associated limb where the lymph node was removed. During an acute inflammatory episode, it is important to know if a client is at risk for lymphedema. Post injury, the acute edema should resolve itself, but lymphedema will not, and the client and the therapist will need to manage the chronic condition.

In the case of a sprained ankle, removing the excess fluid can relieve some of the pain and dysfunction. However, when complications arise, swelling persists and, in these situations, the use of **lymphatic techniques** can assist in resolving the dysfunction. These techniques involve gentle compression strokes, slight stretching of the skin, and manual stimulation of the lymph node clusters to help decrease fluid accumulation, increase lymphatic flow, and improve immune response (Stubblefield and Keole 2014).

In addition to its primary role in the immune system, the lymphatic system is the body's dynamic fluid regulator and its functions directly relate to the intricate workings of the cardiovascular system. A good working heart and valves help distribute blood, plasma, and water through the arterial network, and cellular debris is washed away and cleansed via lymphatic capillaries to and through the lymph nodes. In addition, wastes from other bodily functions are dumped into the lymphatic system and excreted through sweat, urination, and bowel movements. Lipids are also managed and distributed through the lymphatic system.

But what happens when the system has a problem? The lymphatic system is possibly the least understood of all the body's systems, and the history of how we came to understand it can be attributed to early scientists and their quest to understand the human body, initially through dissection of animals, then cadavers. We do not "see" lymph capillaries or lymphatic activity in the same way as we see veins or other cardiovascular flow. For this reason, it took time to identify the lymphatic system, and we are still trying to determine the capacity of its function.

History

Hippocrates (460–470 BCE) was the first person recorded to use the word "chyle" and list the "lymphatic temperament" as part of the four temperaments of blood, phlegm (including lymph/chyle), yellow bile, and black bile. Herophilus (4th–3rd century BCE) discovered the "milky veins" and mesenteric lymph nodes, and Gasparo Aselli (1581–1626) discovered the lymphatic system while dissecting a dog, where he noticed the white fluid within the lymphatic vessels (Chikly 2004, 6). He later confirmed the same observation in cats, sheep, calves, cows, horses, and goats but not in humans. However, 12 years after Aselli's discovery, Pierre Gassendi uncovered "white veins" in the mesentery of a dissected prisoner. In addition, John Pecquet (1622–1674) described the "receptaculumchile" (cysternachyle) in a dog and illustrated the thoracic duct and proliferation of lymph circulation under the left subclavian vein. He also recognized the lymphatic link to the large mesenteric nodes and made the connection between respiration and the circulation of chyle, as well as describing the presence of valves within the lymphatics. Later, Olof Rudbeck (1630–1708) clarified the lymphatic network throughout the body and its connection with the lymph glands.

Techniques specifically oriented to moving lymph fluid can be attributed to Per Henrik Ling (1776–1839), who created "Swedish massage," and Andrew Taylor Still (1828–1917), who noticed that body fluids and the lymphatic system in particular are a crucial part of an osteopathic treatment. In addition, Frederic P. Millard (1878–1951) put together specific work on the lymphatic vessels and nodes, and used the term "lymphatic drainage" for his manual technique. Further, Emil Vodder (1896–1986) founded **Manual Lymph Drainage (MLD)** which was originally used specifically for lymph work in relation to cosmetology, but was then tested clinically and established the medical effects, indications, and contraindications. Also, Vodder and his wife, Dr. Estrid Vodder, pioneered the medical specialty called "lymphology" (Chikly 2004, 13). More recently, Bruno Chikly developed **Lymph Drainage Therapy (LDT),** which improved some of the existing techniques via "mapping" of the superficial and deep lymphatic pathways, enabling assessment of the specific directions of lymph flow and areas of congestion and fibrosis (Chikly 2004, 13–15).

Lymphatic techniques to reduce pain and swelling include:

- decongestive techniques (light skin massage and gentle stretching of the skin)

- compression therapies and bandaging

- home care: gentle exercises, self-drainage, and dry brushing.

Decongestive techniques are used to ease areas of edematous congestion. There is an active (pressure phase) and a passive (relaxation phase) stage to each lymphatic stroke. During the active phase, the skin is stretched in the direction of lymphatic flow, which opens the gates of the lymphatic capillaries to allow lymph fluid to go through. The passive phase is the complete release of pressure on the stretched skin that allows the gateways to close. In addition, using very light pressure prevents further burden on an injured area and allows for the excess fluid to be drained out, which in turn results in an improved range of motion.

Compression therapies include garments and pneumatic compression devices to provide resistance to swelling and improve the function of drainage caused by muscular contraction. Compression therapy and lymphatic bandaging combined with the application of lymphatic techniques and gentle exercises (Stubblefield and Keole, 2014, 7–8) are the recommended treatments for lymphedema of the limbs. Compression garments are tube-like flexible fabrics that are tighter at the bottom than the top, which creates a pressure gradient that keeps lymph moving out of the affected area.

Sidebar 5.1 Research

In a Cochrane review (2015) summarizing six trials, Ezzo and colleagues sought to understand the efficacy and safety of manual lymphatic drainage (MLD) for breast cancer-related lymphedema (BCRL). The authors found that MLD, combined with intensive compressive bandaging, significantly decreased swelling compared to bandaging alone. These effects were most significant for women with mild to moderate lymphedema, compared to those with moderate to severe lymphedema. The reviewers also found that MLD was a safe intervention for BCRL (Ezzo et al. 2015).

Home care may consist of stretching and other light exercises, water therapy, dry brushing, and self-massage strokes to improve lymphatic flow. These are generally done daily as part of maintenance care.

Due to advancements in research, our understanding of the relationship between fascia and the lymphatic system has improved. It has therefore become more common to combine myofascial and lymphatic techniques to facilitate lymphatic flow.

Theoretical Approaches to Pain Management

Lymphatic fluid is made up of excess from the blood capillaries, with a high fat and protein content, white blood cells, toxins, bacteria, and extracellular debris (Chikly 2004). If the lymph drainage is inadequate, fluid accumulates in the interstitial compartments, and the resultant edema damages lymphatic capillaries, causing fluid back-up and further damage to the surrounding tissues. This slows the healing process due to the build-up of bacteria, which leaves the person prone to infections. A heaviness of the limbs can also cause the surrounding muscles to spasm and feel painful. As this casting of the area continues over time, postural and functional issues affect the person's general mobility and performance of activities of daily living. In addition, pain due to lack of movement may cause a more prolonged casting effect of the area, which can inhibit the normal contract/relax cycle of regular muscular activity (Zimmerman and Lerner 2014). The constant muscle tension results in a deficient blood supply to the affected area and an increased production and concentration of pain-producing substances such as histamine, prostaglandin E, and other metabolites (Zimmerman and Lerner 2014), which produce even more pain and discomfort. In turn, this can perpetuate the pain–spasm–pain cycle and a lack of movement due to edema in the area.

Edema vs. Lymphedema

Edema can be defined as excessive accumulation of extracellular or intracellular tissue fluid in the body. Pitting edema is when a finger impression remains on the skin after it has been pressed (Chikly 2004, 166).

Signs of edema are:

- a full or heavy feeling in an arm or leg
- the arm or leg starts to look swollen
- a tight or warm feeling in the skin
- less movement or flexibility in the affected joints
- tautness of the skin of the affected area
- pain in the affected area and/or joints
- discoloration of the surface area, e.g. redness or bruising if the swelling is related to an injury.

Lymphedema is different from edema in that it is an abnormal accumulation of protein-rich lymph in the extracellular fluid, resulting from damage to the lymphatic system. The protein-rich environment causes fluid retention in the soft tissue of the affected area and stimulates proliferation of fibroblasts and swelling of that quadrant of the body's extremity.

Some of the signs of lymphedema are:

- chronic swelling of an extremity (arm, hand, and fingers; or leg, foot, and toes) that lasts for 3 months or more
- chronic swelling of the face, genitalia, or torso
- fevers, chills, and generalized weakness due to the lack of drainage of bacteria, and other extracellular debris
- physical fatigue from the size and weight of the extremity
- severe impairment of daily activities
- recurring bacterial or fungal infections
- recurring episodes of cellulitis, lymphangitis, fissuring (the skin splits and lymph leaks out), ulcerations, and/or verrucous (wart-like) changes to the surface of the skin.

Lymphedema is a diagnosis of exclusion to rule out congestive heart failure, superior vena cava syndrome, or myxedema (Stubblefield and Keole 2014). It is a chronic condition, and most treatment is to assist the client with management. Lymphedema is categorized into stages:

- Stage 0–1 refers to mild lymphedema that can be reversed with timely treatment.
- Stage 2 is irreversible, as the lymphedema has been present for some time and fibrosity of the tissues is present. The skin will not move very much during treatment and skin fissuring as well as wart-like tissue may develop.
- Stage 3 is irreversible and the skin is very hard, with significant fibrosis. Also present is joint immobility and functional loss of the limb.

In the early stages of lymphedema, the tissues swell with protein-rich lymph that cannot drain properly. If this condition is not treated at this stage, the stagnant lymph becomes fibrotic (hardened) within the affected tissues as the disease progresses. As fibrosis develops, normal tissues are replaced by scar-like structures that create obstructions and severely compromise the ability of the lymphatic system to drain.

There are three types of genetic primary lymphedema:

- Milroy's syndrome, where the lymphedema is present at birth and generally seen bilaterally in the legs, but can also be seen in the face or abdomen.
- Meige's syndrome or praecox is seen at the onset of puberty and usually affects either one or both legs.
- Lymphedema tardum can appear after the age of 35 and, again, mostly in either one or both legs (Wheeler et al. 1981).

The type of primary lymphedema does not change the treatment protocol but provides information on the length of time the client has had the condition, development level, and any possible fibrosity of the area.

Areas of lymphatic fluid stagnation may be rife with bacteria, excess protein, lipids, and other extracellular debris. If left untreated, the fluid will leave the person at high risk of infection. By moving the fluid through the system, the lymphatic capillaries can reroute themselves around barriers (such as scar tissue) to intact lymph node areas. With continued sessions and self-care, these alternative pathways can assist in draining where the compromised lymph node or capillary areas cannot.

If the person is suffering from infection, lymphatic work is contraindicated and can be dangerous. If the skin is emanating heat, and there is redness around the swollen area, there could be an infection that would contraindicate any lymphatic or massage work until checked by the client's physician. Redness associated with swelling and pain to the touch can be a sign of cellulitis (a microbial infection of the tissue just underneath the surface of the skin).

Pain is not usually directly caused by lymphedema, but lymphedema can predispose the client to painful joint conditions such as adhesive capsulitis. In the case of genetic lymphedema, pain is related to the chronic swelling of the legs (or affected area). For breast cancer survivors, pain can be associated with lymphedema, as it affects the musculoskeletal area as well as the neurological system (i.e. neuropathies in the extremities caused by side effects from chemotherapy or radiation). A treatment plan consisting of lymphatic techniques, compression garments, and specific exercises can help manage the pain and discomfort of the condition.

> ### Sidebar 5.2 Patient Interviews
> In response to the question "What information do you wish your primary healthcare provider had given you to help make a better-informed decision to go to these treatment sessions or classes?" a 61-year-old woman post-double mastectomy replied: "[I would like to have known] that there are people out there doing specific lymph-targeted therapy that could make a world of difference in quality of life! While supportive of any alternative that helps, their only suggestion of PT fell way short of many ideas."

Methodology

Lymphatic techniques can be effective in most areas where there is congestion—such as nasal congestion due to allergies, post-event sports massage, or an overuse injury such as tendonitis—as long as infection is not present. For congested facial and nasal sinus areas, lymphatic techniques can clear the mucus membranes. In sports massage, lymphatic work can help with post-event healing of sore muscles by increasing the circulatory and lymphatic flow, and clearing any fluid retention. Lymphatic work is also used as an adjunct therapy post surgery to help bring down the swelling from surgical tissue trauma. Hospitals sometimes prescribe a lymphatic drainage machine rather than hiring a lymph drainage practitioner. These

machines can be effective in draining edema; however, they cannot determine whether the pathways are actually draining, nor can they regulate pressure and switch areas if the system is compromised and the drainage is not effective.

Lymphatic techniques aim to reduce excess fluid accumulation by stimulating the formation of physiological lymphatic shunts, alternative pathways, and/or lymph drainage. Typically, massaging the lymph nodes starting with the more superior part of the body (clavicular, then axillary, and then abdominal) encourages the flow of fluid through the lymph nodes and lymphatic capillaries, thereby, cleansing and detoxifying as the fluid flows through each lymph node area.

Combining lymphatic techniques with compression therapy can help lessen the volume of fluid for the client suffering from lymphedema. When clients have mild lymphedema (stage 0 or stage 1), a compression sleeve or garment may be the initial treatment. For stages 2 and 3 lymphedema, lymphatic techniques can bring down swelling (or "decongest" the limb) and a client will be advised to wear a compression sleeve or garment to maintain those results. Different garments may be needed for different activities (e.g. a firmer compression may be required for air travel or wearing at night).

Lymphatic bandaging is the art of creating compression for a lymphedematous limb or area by applying short-stretch bandages in overlapping layers, with a pressure gradient to assist the damaged lymphatic system decongest the area of excess fluid. In addition, exercises can be prescribed by a physical therapist for the client to do while wearing the bandages, which can help with the lymphatic flow and tone of the muscles.

Treating someone with chronic lymphedema requires proper training. A practitioner trained in lymphatic techniques can properly assess the area, ask very condition-specific questions, and apply sound judgments on treatment protocols. With this knowledge, the trained therapist can effectively decongest an edematous limb, without causing harm to the already compromised underlying tissues, and direct the fluid along the rerouted pathways. In some instances, the therapist may encourage the fluid to create these pathways with gentle movements in the direction of unaffected lymph node clusters. Some general, very light pressure massage in the direction that the lymph flows can have some pain-relieving effects for the lymphedema sufferer.

Treatment Planning

Treatment of acute injury-related edema requires more sessions that are scheduled close together to keep the swelling from recurring. These sessions should be short (e.g. 20–30 minutes of localized work) with the intention of clearing the excess fluid around an injured area. I check how the bruises are healing based on color: if they are very blue-purple, the sessions will be shorter to give the tissue time to heal properly. When the tissues turn a more yellowish color, I can work a little longer and start to include some range-of-motion movements into the session. This combination of movement and lymphatic technique allows more drainage by stimulating the "gates" of the lymphatic capillaries to move the fluid through the system. I also show the client how to do some basic drainage themselves, to keep the fluid from accumulating around the injury. As the injury heals, I add some light- to medium-pressure massage along with lymphatic techniques to assist the muscles in recovery. Then, depending on the health of the client and their ability to let the area rest and heal properly, there should be significantly less pain by 6–8 weeks and the client should be able to return to normal activity.

A client with lymphedema has a very different kind of intake and treatment protocol. Most clients find their way to me knowing they already have lymphedema, or that they are at risk. Other clients may be cancer survivors or are recovering from other types of surgery and have developed chronic swelling. The intake questions I ask help me determine the likelihood of lymphedema and center around how long the client has had the swelling,

> **Sidebar 5.3 Research**
> Butterfield and colleagues (2008) demonstrated the therapeutically beneficial effects of massage on the inflammatory response. These authors found decreases in inflammation and edema and increased function after massage. Building on this earlier work, Waters-Banker and colleagues examined the effects that massage therapy has on the inflammatory process and pain associated with acute injuries. The authors explain in detail the physiologic changes that **macrophages** undergo. Responding to environmental demands, macrophages can transition phenotypes, from an M_1 to an M_2 macrophage. For an acute injury, "promoting an anti-inflammatory condition with a higher concentration of M_2 macrophages versus aproinflammatory M_1-macrophage-dominated environment may be desirable" (Waters-Banker et al. 2014, 268). These authors found that the timing of and amount of pressure applied during massage were predictive factors in effectively treating the acute injury. They recommend that massage be applied early in the acute phase of inflammation. As part of their summary for the **immunomodulatory effects** of massage, these authors conclude: "[a]ttenuating the inflammatory and subsequent nervous response may allow clinicians to treat, manage, and prevent acute and chronic pain syndromes, as well as inflammatory-related diseases, with massage and without pharmaceutical intervention" (Waters-Banker, 2014, 271).

where it is located, and if there is lymph node or lymphatic system disruption (due to surgery or scar tissue, which can potentially cause blockage of the lymphatic capillaries). Palpating the area and measuring the limb circumference will provide information on where the fluid is accumulating or "pooling." Asking if this was the first time they have noticed the swelling, how long the swelling seems to last, and whether it ever lessens, gives me information to determine if the lymphedema might be reversible.

Treatment for the client with lymphedema involves a long-term regimen and dedicated self-care maintenance. Lymphatic techniques act as the lymphatic system should, by physically moving the excess fluid out of an area. Once the fluid has been evacuated, the client can do some gentle range-of-motion exercises to help reduce the pain from muscles and joint areas that have been unable to move due to the swelling. Wearing compression garments after a treatment session can also assist in keeping extra fluid from accumulating and allows the person to move more comfortably and with less pain.

Sidebar 5.4 Patient Interviews
When asked, "Have your condition or symptoms or ability to function changed since receiving care?", two massage therapy patients replied:

- "I have less lymphedema and pain and more energy."

- "The pain was making me feel depressed due to my inability to enjoy the physical activities important to me and that has been relieved by this treatment."

Interviews and Assessments

When clients come to my office for treatment for swelling, I begin by asking questions that will help me assess the underlying cause:

- Question: When was the onset of the swelling? For example, did the client have an accident, an injury or a skin issue, such as sunburn or a bug bite.

  - Reasoning: If the onset is due to an injury, the swelling is more temporary. If the area is swollen post injury, and the person is at risk for lymphedema, the treatment plan will be different. For example, the treatment for an injury could include ice or heat application, rest, and perhaps anti-inflammatory medications. However, for lymphedema none of these interventions would reduce the swelling.

- Question: Has the client ever had swelling in the same area in the past? (This could also be related to a genetic cause.)

  - Reasoning: If the swelling "comes and goes," this could be an indication of lymphedema.

- Question: Has the client had any surgery (recent or otherwise)?

  - Reasoning: Occasionally clients forget health issues that have happened in the past, or they may be under the impression that some health information is irrelevant to a massage session. Also, by identifying where a person has a scar or scar tissue can help the therapist determine what the treatment protocol should be and if lymphatic techniques are indicated.

- Question: Has the person ever had a lymph node removed? (Not everyone knows this post surgery.) Occasionally I ask for surgical notes to determine whether lymph nodes have been removed and, if so, how many.

  - Reasoning: Even having one lymph node removed can be the cause of episodic swelling in the area, as this procedure leaves scar tissue that can disrupt lymphatic flow. If all lymph nodes have been removed in the area, the risk for lymphedema, infection, and possibly loss of sensation in the associated quadrant of the body, including the limb, increases.

- Question: Does the client know of any relatives who have/had a lymphatic issue?

  - Reasoning: This will help determine if the lymphedema has genetic roots.

For the client who started life with an intact lymphatic system, but now has secondary lymphedema based on either damage to their lymphatic system from injury or surgery, or has had lymph node(s) removed or damaged due to surgery (most often from early-stage cancer treatment), the interview questions assist me in determining possible reroutes of the lymphatic fluid, areas to focus lymphatic techniques on, and the stage of their lymphedema. Some early-stage lymphedemas can be reversed through concentrated scheduling of sessions, compression garments, and vigilant homecare by the client. For stage 2–3 lymphedema, my work focuses on managing the client's condition and checking the quality of their skin—its movement, pliability, and casting effect on the joint area or muscles in the area of the lymphedema.

For a client with primary lymphedema, who generally knows their condition very well, has a homecare protocol that they follow, and is perhaps seeking help in maintaining chronic lymphedema, questions would include:

- How is your swelling today? In addition, I would measure the affected limbs or area.

- What kind of homecare are they doing for their lymphedema?

  - Reasoning: They may already be doing lymphatic techniques, dry brushing, or using a lymphatic drainage machine at home.

- When was the last time you had your compression garments checked/measured/replaced? With wear and laundering, the elasticity of the garment loosens, and the ability to compress is reduced. Ideally, garments should be replaced every 6 months to 3 years.

In addition to questions regarding swelling, I ask about pain and/or discomfort, and how the client rates their level of pain. A palpation assessment of the area will also help me determine the quality of the edema. For example, with a sprained ankle where the swelling is caused by an acute injury, I would be assessing where on the ankle the swelling is, what the quality of the skin feels like—is it moveable; does the swelling have a "watery" feel? If I do a slight stretch of the skin does it move and can I detect some movement of the fluid and underlying structures? In moving an affected joint area,

I am also feeling for where the pain begins and how close to or far away from the end range of the joint's movement does the client start feeling the pain.

I also need to determine whether there are any conditions where lymphatic techniques are contraindicated.

Contraindications for lymphatic work

Some considerations are:

- infection: lymphatic work may spread the infection

- open skin or wounds (if infected; local contraindication if no infection is present)

- renal failure (kidney disease, etc.)

- lymphedema caused by cardiovascular issues: lymphatic work could be dangerous to an already over-taxed cardiovascular system by overloading the heart with the excess fluid.

Treatment for the Client with Edema

For a client with an intact lymphatic system, I treat an acute injury by directing techniques along the typical lymphatic patterns of drainage. All lymphatic techniques begin by working the lymph cluster areas, starting with the clavicular nodes in area A of Figure 5.1, and then moving to the axillary nodes in area B. In the example of the sprained ankle, the lymphatic technique involves light pulsing moves starting in area A, and moving to area B in the direction of the lymph nodes that are responsible for clearing the proximal and distal areas. This should assist the flow of fluid, and a typical sequence would be:

1. Stimulating the lymph node clusters in the "big four": clavicular, axilla, supra-(abdominal) and infra-(legs) inguinal areas (A–D in Figure 5.1).

2. Effleurage in the direction of lymph flow (see directional arrows in Figures 5.1 and 5.2).

3. Specific techniques near the area of injury, treating proximal to distal, to open the pathway, then distal to proximal to flush the fluid.

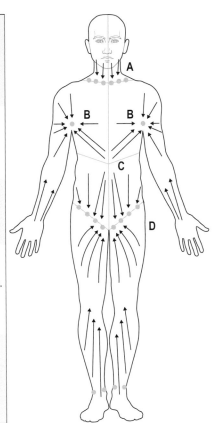

The body is divided into quadrants (A, B, C, D) and the arrows point toward the watershed areas, or lymph node clusters, indicating the direction of flow.

A The neck and head drain to the clavicular area (nodes and ducts).

B Most of the upper trunk and the arms drain to the axillary nodes.

C Part of the upper trunk and the entire lower torso drain to the inguinal nodes.

D The legs drain to the inguinal nodes.

Figure 5.1
Lymph drainage pathways of the anterior body.

Lymph vessels throughout the body open into larger ducts, e.g. the thoracic duct (which runs alongside the aorta) opens out into the neck veins that drain the right and left sides of the body (see Figure 5.3). After passing through lymph nodes and then larger collecting lymphatic ducts, lymph fluid is finally propelled to the thoracic duct that empties into the left subclavian vein (Scallan, Huxley, and Korthuis, 2010). Lymphatic techniques assist in this transport, and help the fluid reroute from the injured area and through the proper channels of lymphatic drainage.

For an acute injury, I would not spend a long time on the preliminary steps but would focus immediately proximal to the injury, and then move distally from the injury towards the original lymph node cluster areas, focusing on the nodes that are responsible for draining the injured part of the body. Once I have completed the techniques for that session, I set a plan for further sessions. I assess range of motion, amount of swelling, and progress of healing prior to and after each session.

Treatment for the Client with Lymphedema
After gathering background information, additional assessment is necessary. I assess the quality of the skin, and palpate to test the "texture" and density of the edema. I check to see if there are any fissures in the edematous area, or if there are any wart-like skin tags developing due to the stage of lymphedema. In physically palpating the density, I can test to see if the skin is moveable, and how advanced the fibrosity may be.

The body is divided into quadrants (A, B, C, D) and the arrows point toward the watershed areas, or lymph node clusters, indicating the direction of flow.

A The posterior neck (just above the superior trapezius) drains anteriorly to the clavicular area.

B The upper trunk and arms drain to the axillary nodes.

C Inferior to the watershed at the rib cage, and above the watershed of the inguinal line, the lymph drains anteriorly to the inguinal nodes.

D At the rectal area of the intergluteal fissure the lymph drains medially to the inguinal nodes.

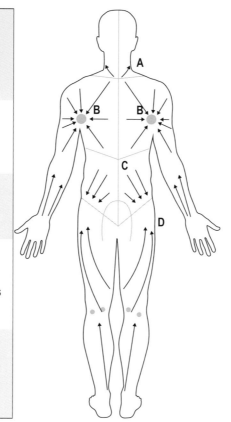

Figure 5.2
Lymph drainage pathways of the posterior body.

I take the client through range-of-motion exercises for the affected and non-affected areas in order to make comparisons and note the end ranges of movement. During movement, I check on their pain level to ensure comfort. I also take measurements of both limbs, noting the location of the highest level of lymphedema based on circumference and then repeat the measurements post session to ensure I am effectively moving the fluid. In my experience, drainage routes are rarely consistent with the known patterns of lymph flow, due to anatomical anomalies or damage to the lymphatic system. The dynamic lymphatic system runs along the path of least resistance, e.g. like a rock in the path of a stream where the stream finds a way around the rock. My goal is to help the system find an alternate pathway and support fluid flow.

Once the client is on the examination table, I begin by stimulating lymph nodes in "the big four" areas (see Figure 5.1), as with the client with edema, starting at the clavicular nodes (see Figure 5.2). By stimulating these areas first, I am clearing the path for the stagnant fluid to be able to find its way through the system. At the same time, I am attempting to determine if the flow is moving equally on the left and right sides of the body. With an edematous arm, when I move to the axillary area, I might feel stagnation or a "thickness" in the lymph node cluster area, and from there I palpate to see if I can determine which way the lymph *can* flow, if there might be some drainage going on in an alternative pathway, and if I can shunt some of the fluid towards an alternative route. After progressing through the four cluster areas, I then move to working in the area

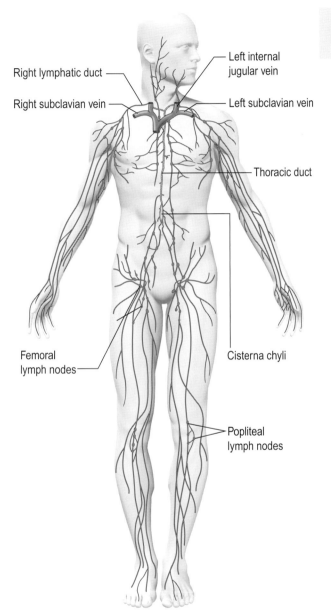

Right lymphatic duct

Right subclavian vein

Femoral
lymph nodes

Left internal
jugular vein

Left subclavian vein

Thoracic duct

Cisterna chyli

Popliteal
lymph nodes

Figure 5.3
Anatomy of the lymph system.

where there is lymphedema. In addition, I frequently check with the client to assess their comfort level, any pain associated with the fluid movement, and if they can feel where the lymph might be flowing. Lymphatic work begins proximal to the nodes, then distally to the affected areas, then back proximally towards the nodes again.

Post application of lymphatic techniques, I reassess to determine the effectiveness of treatment. Careful note taking is essential, particularly when working with healthcare teams, to document the effects of lymphatic work. Moisturizing the skin post lymphatic techniques promotes a healthy skin condition by preventing cracks or dry areas

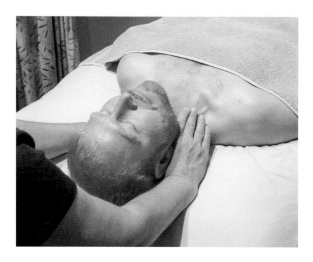

Figure 5.4
The gentlest pressure is used to stimulate lymph node cluster areas. The clavicular nodes drain the entire upper body and head, and stimulate better lymphatic flow for the whole body.

that can be an entry point for bacteria and increase the risk of infection. I also check range of motion and note any improvements after the session.

Self-care Techniques

At the conclusion of the hands-on session, the client is encouraged to put their compression bandages or compression garments on. In addition, there are some self-care techniques that I find extremely beneficial for clients when practiced on a regular basis:

- Dry brushing.

- Stretching and other light movements, as water exercise is quite beneficial due to the bonus of hydrostatic pressure to the entire body while submerged.

- Self-manual techniques focused on the main lymph node cluster areas, and light massage strokes that will encourage better lymphatic flow.

Dry brushing is an easy way for clients to help control mild versions of edema and lymphedema. This is generally done daily, and can be very helpful in stimulating lymph flow throughout the body. Dry brushing in the rerouted direction is encouraged and I recommend avoiding sensitive and broken skin areas, e.g. skin rashes (including those related to poison oak/ivy), wounds, cuts, and infections.

Case Study

Donna is a 56-year-old healthy female who works as an administrative assistant at a local hospital and was diagnosed with lung cancer in July 2008. Having never been a smoker, she noticed that she had a persistent cough, back pain, and could not sleep on her right side. She had an accident, in which she fell on her right arm and was sent for an X-ray; it was during this diagnostic test that the tumor was discovered.

She had fifteen axillary and right torso lymph nodes surgically removed. The right upper lobe of her lung was removed, and the tumor itself was determined to be too close to the larynx for it to be removed laparoscopically. Donna did not have chemotherapy or radiation, nor did she receive any physical therapy to deal with the aftermath of such a large scar on her upper back. Instead, she was prescribed pain medication, which she took as needed.

Donna noticed over the following years that her range of motion was diminishing, and that there was swelling in her underarm area beside her right breast, as well as her upper arm area. In the 4–5 years post surgery, she experienced severe pain in her right shoulder and upper back area and, although she had regular check-ups related to recovery from the removal of the cancerous tumor in her lung, she received no additional therapy for her pain or the possible lymphedema. When she did seek physical therapy, the therapist did not address any issues beyond improving the range of motion for her frozen shoulder.

Over the next year, Donna embarked on a weight-loss program and, after losing 20 pounds, she noticed that the area on her right side was still "puffy," and that her shoulder still had some range-of-motion issues. It was at this time that Donna sought my care to help treat her swelling and function.

Donna's goals were to make her arm look more "normal", ease her shoulder and upper back pain, and experience more comfort riding her bike. My goals were to find the most efficient way for her system to take care of the excess fluid, thereby lessening the amount of swelling in her arm, increasing her range of motion, and decreasing her shoulder and back pain.

Donna's treatment plan included five sessions in a short period of time, three times during the first week, and twice during the second week. Her treatment consisted of lymphatic techniques and massage to help relieve her pain and decrease the excessive fluid accumulation (edema) in her affected right arm. I measured the circumference of her arm and hand, and noted areas where the measurements for her right arm were markedly different from her left, with most of the fluid pooling towards the distal end of her forearm and wrist.

After stimulating the lymph node cluster areas, I focused on clearing the extra fluid in the right arm by stimulating the axillary nodes on the *opposite* side of the affected limb, and encouraging lymphatic flow proximal to these nodes and then distally towards the torso. In moving the fluid and clearing the opposing side first, this theoretically gave the excess fluid from the affected side a place to flow towards. Subsequently, I progressed through the first session, noting that her pain reduced from 8 to 6 as I did decongestive therapy on her affected right side. I then did some myofascial scar release work, testing her range of motion and lymphatic flow (using lymphatic mapping techniques) as I improved the pliability of

areas adjacent to the scar and then directly on the scar itself. This first session was short, as I wanted a sure diagnosis before proceeding further with lymphatic protocols.

Before going further down the path towards the full lymphedema treatment protocol, I asked that she consult her primary care physician to confirm my thoughts on the development of lymphedema in order to: (a) have the diagnosis in her medical record (which would then justify the course of lymphatic treatment) and (b) set her up for any further medical intervention that might be required due to the development of lymphedema. Donna's primary care physician corroborated my findings, diagnosed her with lymphedema, and prescribed compression garments.

Starting with the third session, I taught Donna some self-massage and lymphatic techniques. By the fourth session, Donna's lymphedema had improved enough that her measurements for the right arm were much closer to that of her left, unaffected arm. In addition, she noticed an improvement in how the sleeves of her clothing fitted, and felt more at ease in her swimming technique. As treatment progressed, I noticed that the lymphatic system seemed to respond more quickly to the rerouting.

Over the next 2 months and five additional treatments, Donna's pain in her right shoulder lessened from an 8 to a 5 out of 10. In addition, she uses regular movement (water aerobics and light weight-lifting) to maintain the swelling at a stage 0 level, massages to manage the pain and discomfort, and lymphatic sessions to manage the "puffiness" and fluid accumulation under her arm. Donna went on to report that the combination of lymphatic techniques, self-massage, regular dry brushing, exercise, and wearing her arm sleeve has significantly improved the swelling in her arm. Subsequently, she has also regained enough range of motion to regularly ride a bike.

Chikly, B. 2004. *Silent waves: Theory and practice of lymph drainage therapy: An osteopathic lymphatic technique*, 2nd edn. Scottsdale: I.H.H.

Ezzo, J., E. Manheimer, M. L. McNeely, D. M. Howell, R. Weiss, K. I. Johansson, T. Bao, L. Bily, C. M. Tuppo, A. F. Williams, and D. Karadibak. 2015. *Manual lymphatic drainage for lymphedema following breast cancer treatment*. Editorial Group: Cochrane Breast Cancer Group. Published Online: May 21, 2015. Assessed as up-to-date: May 24, 2013. DOI: 10.1002/14651858.CD003475. pub2.20 http://onlinelibrary.wiley.com/doi/10.1002/14651858. CD003475.pub2/ (accessed July 7, 15).

Lange, U., P. Oelzner, and C. Uhlemann. 2008. Dercum's disease (lipomatosis dolorosa): successful therapy with pregabalin and manual lymphatic drainage and a current overview. *Rheumatol Int* 29:17–22. doi 10.1007/s00296-008-0635-3.

Scallan, J., V. Huxley, and R. Korthuis. 2010. *Capillary fluid exchange regulation, functions, and pathology*. University of Missouri-Columbia, San Rafael, CA: Morgan & Claypool Life Sciences.

Stubblefield, M., and N. Keole. 2014. Upper body pain and functional disorders in patients with breast cancer. *The American Academy of Physical Medicine and Rehabilitation* 6:170–83.

Waters-Banker, C., E. E. Dupont-Versteegden, P. H. Kitzman, and T. A. Butterfield. 2014. Investigating the mechanisms of massage efficacy: the role of mechanical immunomodulation. *Journal of Athletic Training* 49(2):266–273. doi: 10.4085/1062-6050-49.2.25.

Werner, R. 2014. *A massage therapist's guide to pathology,* 5th edn. New York: Lippincott Williams & Wilkins.

Wheeler, E. S., V. Chan, R. Wassman, D. O. Rimoin, and A. Lesavoy. 1981. Familial lymphedema praecox: Meige's disease. *Plastic and Reconstructive Surgery* 67:362–4.

Zimmerman, S. I., and F. Lerner. 2014. Biofeedback and electromedicine: reduce the cycle of pain–spasm–pain in low-back patients. *American Journal of Electromedicine* June: 108–20.

Sidebar 5.5 Research

Lange and colleagues published a case study of a 58-year-old woman with Dercum's disease, or lipomatosis dolorosa, a rare and painful condition in which "the upper arms, elbows, stomach wall, buttocks, thighs and knees are predominantly affected showing painful subcutaneous adipose tissue deposits" (2008, 17). They reported that her "physical discomfort included intensive pain upon pressure on the adipose tissue and nodules, morning stiffness and paresthesia of the legs, a reduction of motion and function of the joints of the extremities, signs of depression, general weakness, allodynia, pain-induced mission of sexual life and finally social deprivation" (2008, 17). "Under periodical whole body manual lymphatic drainage two times a week for 60 min, a remarkable reduction of the diameter of the extremities could be achieved: upper legs 6 cm, lower legs 3 cm, upper arms 3 cm and forearms 2 cm" (2008, 19). These authors further reported a significant reduction of pain as reported on the Visual Analogue Scale from a 98 to a 4 (Lange, Oelzner, and Uhlemann 2008).

Conclusion

Lymphatic work is a very effective adjunct to physical therapy, general massage techniques, and other complementary practices, given its gentle application, thorough review of health conditions prior to application, and extraordinary benefit to those suffering from post-surgical or injury-related swelling. With proper assessment and adherence to lymphatic directional flow, a manual therapist can assist in decreasing the pain and dysfunction of an area by reducing the retention of extracellular fluid that can cause discomfort.

References

Butterfield, T. A., Y. Zhao, S. Agarwal, F. Haq, and T. M. Best. 2008. Cyclic compressive loading facilitates recovery after eccentric exercise. *Med Sci Sports Exerc* 40(7):1289–96.

Additional Resources

KLOSE Training (www.klosetraining.com).

Lymphatic Drainage Technique: LDT Training: Chikly Institute (www.chiklyinstitute.org).

Lymphology Association of North America: LANA (https://www. clt-lana.org).

Manual Lymph Drainage: MLD Dr. Vodder School (www. vodderschool.com).

National Lymphedema Network (www.lymphnet.org).

Introduction

Developments in medical technology have led to advancements in surgical techniques and emergency care (Blakeney 2002). Patients are now surviving injuries that would have been fatal 20 or 30 years ago, and many of these survivors are doing so with abundant scar tissue. Some 80–100 million people around the world possibly have scar tissue due to necessary or elective surgery or trauma (Gauglitz et al. 2011; American Association for the Surgery of Trauma 2014).

Scar tissue forms when our original tissue is damaged (e.g. from medical treatments, such as radiation and surgery, or from traumas, such as repetitive motion and burns) and is an attempt to maintain tissue integrity. The process of scar tissue formation follows a precise sequence of wound healing (inflammation, proliferation, and maturation/remodeling), and repair. When the wound repair process is complete, the new connective tissue is more fibrous than the original tissue. This scar tissue has a limited blood and oxygen supply, which results in changes in the pigmentation and density of the tissue. When the healing process is successful, the wound closes and the tissue is stable and blends cosmetically with the surrounding tissue in an attempt to restore the area to pre-injury function (Schleip et al. 2013). When the healing is less than ideal, the result is often complicated by pain and loss of function.

Mature scars resulting from trauma pose many problems: the scar may restrict joint movement or cause a feeling of drag or lack of mobility in one or more planes of movement. With edema modeling, there may be a feeling of decreased sensation in the area of the edema (Fitch 2014). After an injury, such as a hamstring or rotator cuff tear, scar tissue develops in the muscle as it heals, compromising the tissue—potentially making it more prone to re-injury. In the case of a fracture, bony scar tissue or callus will form on the bone, also contributing to the possibility of pain and decreased function.

Postoperative adhesion formation is the most common complication from surgery. Postoperative scars may cause discomfort or pain around the surgical incision due to edema modeling, nerve regeneration, or the formation of fibrotic "tentacles" under the surface of the skin. Four studies that followed patients who expressed postoperative pain after surgery found that 57% identified adhesions as the most likely cause of the pain. If fascia, muscles, and tendons are cut or repaired during surgery, scar tissue will develop, making movement more challenging, and some level of pain is present whenever movement is challenging (Broek et al. 2013).

Scars, adhesions, and fibrosis can lead to reduced function, integrity, independence, and structural uniformity in the surrounding tissue. Scar massage is useful in helping remodel scar tissue and reduce the resulting symptoms. Therapeutic massage is currently included as part of the care management of scars in integrative and conventional settings and has been shown to provide therapeutic benefits in pain management and scar healing (Kania 2012). In addition, with the current emphasis on healthcare treatments being cost-effective and outcome-focused, therapeutic massage for scar treatment is a natural addition to the recovery process (Kania 2012).

However, the protocols and patient-specific treatments vary with each individual, e.g. modalities used for dense burn scars may be too aggressive for less dense abdominal scars. A **degloving injury** (where the skin has been completely torn off the underlying tissue and there is a requirement for repairing with skin grafts or flaps) may take many more treatment sessions to sustain scar release than would be the case for a C-section scar. In addition,

Chapter 6

pain tolerance must also be considered when developing and administering scar massage protocols.

Pain is not just physically challenging but can be pyschologically damaging as well, and scars can therefore represent specific emotions. For example, pride may be associated with a scar gained as the result of a winning goal or may represent a loss of health or fear of death (Fitch 2014). Pain is a somatic and psychic experience and may be more intense when experienced in tandem with other symptoms or feelings, such as fatigue, anxiety, depression, isolation, fear, anger, and uncertainty. All of these will compound pain and must be addressed as part of a comprehensive approach to pain management (Fourie 2004).

We need only look as far as returning soldiers to understand how important scar work can be. Soldiers who experience disability and disfigurement often must reinvent themselves; they typically must find a new way of moving their bodies to complete tasks that once were accomplished with ease and without thought. This means they must find a new identity for their evolving body image, which can be a complex and difficult process (Blakeney 2002).

Therapeutic massage does not just treat the scar; it treats the person who has the scar. Massage therapists take into account the range of symptoms from pain and scarring, including a loss of function or shift in identity, and work together with the patient to encourage healing from the various sources of trauma (Fitch 2014).

Using therapeutic massage during any stage of recovery for scar patients will not only facilitate release of fascial restrictions and fibrotic tissue, but it will most likely also have a positive influence on pain and mood. For example, a study in 2005 revealed that cortisol decreases and serotonin and dopamine increase following massage therapy (Field et al. 2005).

Additional studies illustrate that therapeutic massage helps reduce depression, fatigue, and trait anxiety (Kennedy 2011). Improvements in pruritus (itching) and skin status (pliability and circulation) have also been demonstrated (Gürol, Polat, and Nuran Akçay 2010). These findings are powerful endorsements for including a skilled massage therapist in the healthcare team treating patients with scar tissue. The addition of massage therapy offers a safe approach to reducing the pain experienced by scar tissue patients (Gürol et al. 2010).

History of Scar Massage

In the fourth century BC, Hippocrates wrote that the "physician must be acquainted with many things and assuredly with rubbing" (Harper 2001–2015). The word "scar" was first mentioned in English in the fourteenth century and is derived from the French *escharre*, and Latin *eschara*, which is the latinization of the Greek *eskhara*. When used in medicine, it means "scab, eschar on a wound caused by burning or otherwise" (Harper 2001–2015). Excessive or traumatic scarring was first described in the Smith papyrus (approximately 1700 BC).

Based on the mechanistic effects of scar massage (Bond 2011) and current evidence gained from work with athletes, we can hypothesize that scar massage—mainly friction techniques—were likely used in the Olympic Games in 776 BC to clear somatic dysfunction for athletes prior to their events. Friction massage, although used for centuries, was not professionalized until 1903 when Edgar Cyriax, a physiotherapist, published *The Elements of Kellgren's Manual Treatment* (Cyriax 1903; Pettman 2007).

Massage continues to assist top athletes in recovering from overuse trauma and injuries, enabling them to compete at the highest levels. The 1984 Olympics in Los Angeles was the first time that massage therapy was televised during athlete treatments. Massage therapy was finally a sanctioned medical service and offered at the 1996 Atlanta Olympics, to the US Olympic team (Hussain 2011).

Scar massage has evolved over the last several decades with new research on the epidemiology, histology, and causation of excessive scar tissue formation. And research continues to shed light on the physiological mechanisms that support the many therapeutic effects (Goats 1994). Friction is identified as the standard and is widely used to assist in the release of scar tissue. More recently, and in my personal experience, **lymphatic facilitation** and myofascial release techniques are critical additions to scar massage.

Theoretical Approaches to Pain Management
Types of Scar
There are several types of scar tissue, based on various healing environments, and each has its own characteristics and complications. Mancini (in 1962) and Peacock (in 1970) differentiated excessive scarring into hypertrophic and **keloid scar** formation (Gauglitz et al. 2011).

Hypertrophic scarring (HTS) is raised above the skin level and remains within the confines of the original lesion (Hassan et al. 2014) (see Figure 6.1). This type of scar forms due to the overproduction of

Sidebar 6.2 Research
This research study included 146 participants; 76 were allocated to the usual care plus rehabilitative massage therapy group. The massage intervention, for hypertrophic scarring after burns, described in this study was a 30-minute session that included Swedish massage strokes such as effleurage, petrissage, and friction techniques. The researchers reported on pain, pruritus, and scar characteristics prior to and post intervention. The rehabilitative massage group had significant therapeutic benefits from the intervention, specifically the scar thickness, melanin, erythema, transepidermal water loss (TEWL), and elasticity of the scar improved when compared with standard scar therapy alone. Statistically significant decreases in scar pain and pruritus were also reported (Cho et al. 2014).

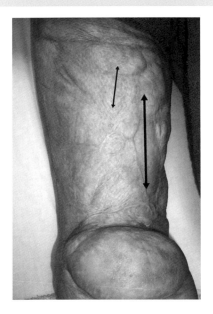

Figure 6.1
Hypertrophic and keloid scarring: left hamstring 4th-degree burn with skin grafts. THIN arrows line indicates hypertrophic scar. THICK arrow indicates keloid scarring along joined graft lines.

immature collagen in the last two stages of wound healing (Gauglitz et al. 2011). The collagen deposition and altered fibroblast activity result in repaired but not regenerated tissue that leads to formation of scar tissue. Complicating factors such as wound size and depth, method of injury, and tension on the wound contribute to the development of HTS (Hassan et al. 2014).

HTS generally forms in areas of high tension, such as the shoulder, ankle, neck, and presternal region, and may lead to reduced mobility and range of motion (ROM). The loss of function and the lack of pliability and moisture (also indicative of HTS) all contribute to the pain. Pruritus, or itching, is also a symptom of HTS and, when severe, has been associated with anxiety, sleep disturbance, and disruption in daily activities. However, recent studies have shown that therapeutic massage provided by trained professionals is more effective for reducing the effects of HTS than other methods, such as **acupuncture** and cold exposure (hydrotherapy) (Gürol et al. 2010).

Keloid scars are hypertrophic fibroproliferative scars that spread beyond the original boundary of the wound. Apart from this primary difference, keloid scars share several features with hypertrophic scars including increased and abnormal collagen deposition. Both hypertrophic and keloid scars cause significant quality-of-life issues because of decreased range of motion, pruritus, and pain. Keloid scars are more prevalent in populations with darker skin tones for reasons that remain unclear and suggest a hereditary component, which is supported by the observation that keloid predisposition can run in families (Hahn, McFarland, and Glaser 2014).

Pain from keloid scars is similar to the experience of pain with HTS. However, keloid scars are generally considered more disfiguring and take up to 1 year after injury to develop. They also may have more pruritus and pain associated with them due to abnormalities in the small nerve fiber

function, which suggest a small nerve fiber neuropathy (Lee et al. 2004).

A *contracture* is the pathological shortening of scar tissue that can lead to severe functional impairment during and after recovery and result in deformity. Unopposed scar contraction during healing can occur rapidly, leading to a loss of soft tissue extensibility and length, resulting in decreased joint motion and consequent disability (Godleski et al. 2013).

A *cicatricial* scar is one with considerable contraction. Scar contracture after an injury can lead to severe functional impairment during recovery and beyond, if not addressed. It may be necessary to divide the scar and graft on new skin, often the procedure for burns, if the scar massage is ineffective or not applied soon enough.

Pain from **cicatricial scars** is often complicated by habitual movement patterns developed to compensate for loss of function in the affected areas. The tissue, joints, and muscles are less pliable, and new movement patterns must be developed to achieve the same functional goals.

Adhesions/fixations are related to the scarring process and develop secondary to the normal healing process. They refer to the system of adhering or uniting two surfaces or parts, especially the union of the opposing surfaces of a wound (Merriam-Webster 2014).

Unlike scarring, adhesions are characterized by binding tissues that normally glide or move in relation to each other, and, once matured, may even be stronger than the tissue to which they adhere. Sometimes, scar tissue creates tentacles of adhesions that bind onto surfaces of muscles, joints, and organs (Schleip 2013). Adhesions can restrict tissue glide, resulting in dysfunctional movement and limited flexibility, and cause weakness, contributing to the experience of pain (Schleip 2013). They can also result in impaired muscle, joint, and connective tissue integrity. On organs, adhesions can inhibit or restrict their intended functions (Rodriguez 2013; Dalton 2014). The impact of the adhesion on normally sliding surfaces, and on normal organ or musculoskeletal function, ranges from negligible to debilitating.

Sidebar 6.3 Patient Interviews

When asked, "Have your condition or symptoms or ability to function changed since receiving care?", patient replies included:

- "[Massage] helped [me] feel better, feel less pain, especially work on scar tissue and adhesions."

- "[I] have better range of motion and less pain and helped with nerve pain in my foot all from burns."

- "I have noticed greater range of motion in my right ankle, which had been impaired by very thick scar tissue. I also have less swelling in that ankle, which I think is in part due to the lymphatic element of the massages."

Postoperative adhesion formation is the most common complication of abdominal or pelvic surgery, which is frequently performed by general, vascular, gynecological, and urological surgeons. Unlike other postoperative complications, such as wound infection or anastomotic leakage, the consequence of adhesion formation may comprise lifelong risks. The four most important complications of postoperative adhesion formation include: small bowel obstruction, difficulties at repeated abdominal surgery, female infertility, and chronic pain (Broek et al. 2013). This topic will be covered in more detail later in this chapter.

Sources of Pain

In general, scar tissue is weaker, less elastic, and more rigid than the tissue it replaced, creating a noticeable lack of movement compared to the original healthy tissue. Scar tissue does not facilitate

movements as the original healthy tissue did. This is where the pain process can begin. The pain can be transient or long lasting and include phantom sensations, sensory loss or changes (Junga 2003).

The pain associated with scars, regardless of type, manifests in a similar way. Pruritus, lack of pliability and mobility, the disruption of nerve, lymph, and blood pathways, and the adhering of unrelated tissues can create a host of painful complications (Chesire 2014). The intensity of the pain, while subjective, depends on a number of factors, such as the severity of the injury, location of the scar, and presence of disease or infection.

Complications of scar pain

Neuropathic pain results from a primary lesion or dysfunction in the nervous system, and scar tissue formation is a trauma recognized by the nervous system (Barral 1999). When scar tissue and/or adhesions compress a nerve ending, this can result in neuronal dysfunction, which can last indefinitely and is common with nerve damage after breast surgery (Schleip et al. 2013).

The resulting chronic pain can be constant if there is no release of the scar tissue that surrounds the nerve. For example, when the patient performs any activity that causes the tissues surrounding the nerve to tighten, (e.g. even sitting or walking), pain can be triggered (Buzzle 2014). Patients with scar tissue pain typically complain of neuropathic pain or neuralgia, during which continuous pain is present, alternating with spontaneous attacks of stabbing pain in the scarred area. This pain can sometimes occur after a complaint-free period lasting some months postoperatively (Maastricht 2011).

Neuromas can form whenever peripheral nerves are severed or injured. Macroneuromas consist of a palpable mass of tangled axons unable to regenerate to their target, whereas microneuromas contain small numbers of axons and may not be palpable. Clinical experience and animal models indicate that the formation of a neuroma in scar tissue can cause chronic neuropathic pain, and axons entrapped within these scars can cause spontaneous pain and severe mechanosensitivity (Junga 2003).

Visceral lesions or adhesions also complicate the pain associated with scarring. Fascia and ligaments that are attached to the viscera contain sensitive proprioceptors, which provide local and central sensory information by communicating with mechanoreceptors, volume receptors, and pressure receptors. These receptors can be under- or overstimulated by stretching during trauma. The overstretching begins the proprioceptive deprogramming, which disrupts the normal function of the organ. Consequentially, the organs, blood, and lymphatic flow become impaired, with resulting congestion, and the organ loses some of its function and vitality. Adhesions or lesions can then form, further complicating the original trauma (Barral 1999). Many cases of abdominal surgery have reportedly been associated with subsequent low back pain, myofascial pain syndrome, and compromised vascular anatomy of the abdominal wall (Schleip et al. 2013).

Psychosocial trauma and pain

I define excessive scarring brought about by a traumatic event as traumatic scars: a pathophysiological scar further compounded by traumatic emotional sequelae and other co-morbidities. Trauma is derived from the Greek word *traumat*, meaning wounding or piercing. Traumatic scars can occur as the result of accidents, acts of violence, and other catastrophic events (e.g. disease, burns, and surgery), but they can also be the result of medical treatment. Although cancer-related surgery (e.g. mastectomy) is a "planned" trauma, the accompanying emotional distress and body image-related issues place this type of wound within the description of traumatic scarring.

A traumatic event is any event that renders the patient helpless and causes a psychological and physical wound. Some of the characteristics of a traumatic event are (Colorado 2012):

- loss of control
- intense fear or horror
- helplessness
- the realization that one is about to die.

When excessive or traumatic scar tissue occurs, it is not only the soft tissue the therapist deals with, but also the effects from the trauma on the somatic system. Compassion is vital in scar management treatment. Recovery from such an injury is very likely associated with a good deal of pain along with many emotional and physical challenges (Badger 2013). Traumatic scar patients may incur life-changing events such as altered physical appearance, amputations, compromised functional abilities, changes in daily activities, and the need for increased social support. Larger scars can also result in psychological distress, particularly when there is an appearance alteration (Fauerbach 2007). "Survivors of physically disfiguring injuries require physical, psychological, social and occupational assistance to successfully rejoin society" (Blakeney 2002).

Depression can be a primary consideration when treating clients with traumatic scar tissue. Research has shown that a chronic inflammatory response

> **Sidebar 6.4 Research**
> In this small study from Korea, eighteen burn survivors received rehabilitative scar massage for hypertrophic scars over the course of 3 months. The pre-test, post-test design measured pruritus, subjective and objective scar assessments (Vancouver Scar Scale (VSS)), and depression. The findings included decreased depression and pruritus, and improvements in subjective and objective scar status (Roh 2007 Abstract (English), accessed July 14, 2015).

decreases serotonin levels (Kidd and Urban 2012; Kumar 2012). Most of the approximately 40 million brain cells are influenced either directly or indirectly by serotonin. This includes brain cells related to mood, sexual desire and function, appetite, sleep, memory and learning, temperature regulation, and some social behaviors.

Approximately 1 hour post injury, edema sets in. The vascular walls become more permeable and increased pressure within the vessels forces a plasma exudate into the interstitial tissues. This can last for a few minutes in cases of mild trauma, with a return to normal permeability in 20–30 minutes. More severe trauma can result in a prolonged state of increased permeability, or a delayed onset of increased permeability, with swelling not apparent until some time after the original injury. This possibility of a decrease in serotonin levels increases our need to recognize symptoms of depression and approach the patient with compassion and understanding.

Multiple studies have shown that therapeutic massage helps with depression, fatigue, and reduction of trait anxiety (Kennedy 2011). Additional studies have demonstrated reduced pruritus, improved tissue pliability, and a positive effect on mood after massage therapy (Gürol et al. 2010). In my own clinical experience with a wide variety of patients and scars, I have found that therapeutic massage during any stage of recovery will not only facilitate release of fascial restrictions and fibrotic tissue, but will have a positive effect on pain and mood.

Postoperative Scarring and Pain: Cancer

Postoperative pain, phantom sensations, and sensory loss or changes can be temporary or ongoing. Chronic pain following surgical procedures for breast cancer was once thought to be rare; however, recent studies suggest that it might actually occur in more than 50% of patients (Tasmuth 1995). In addition, adhesions, tissue fibrosis, and loss of tissue glide have been identified as sources of pain

and functional restrictions in up to 72% of patients after breast cancer surgery (Schleip et al. 2013).

Chemotherapy and radiotherapy (radiation therapy) can be additional sources of pain (Schleip et al. 2013). As more patients are surviving breast cancer due to advances in detection, diagnosis, and treatment, the population at risk for chronic pain and other late complications is expected to increase over the coming years (Junga 2003).

Chronic pain that is a direct result of breast cancer surgery can be either nociceptive (resulting from injury to ligament or muscle) or neuropathic in origin. Nociceptive pain usually resolves as damaged tissues heal, whereas pain from neuronal dysfunction can be unresolved or chronic. Neuropathic pain is considerably more common and has therefore been more of a focus of medical attention and research efforts (Junga 2003). Other sources of neuropathic pain following breast cancer surgery include damage to the pectoral nerves and the long thoracic or thoracodorsal nerves, which may be injured by scarring or by traction during mastectomy (Junga 2003).

Further complications from breast cancer surgery occur when scarring inhibits lymphatic flow. Impeding scars and adhesions disrupt the network of lymph capillaries that lie just under the skin. This disruption hinders fluid drainage and makes the removal of fluid in the affected area more difficult (National Lymphatic Network 2014). This can result from surgical incisions, trauma, or radiation therapy. Repeated episodes of infection can also cause progressive closure of the lymphatic system due to scarring, thus worsening the condition (see Figure 6.2).

Mobility issues are also associated with mastectomy surgeries. Findings show upper extremity limitations due to breast cancer surgery can be present 7 years after surgery (McClintick 2013). Research and clinical observation have demonstrated an increase in upper body dysfunction, decreased range of motion in the

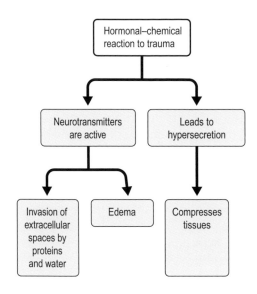

Figure 6.2
Trauma response.

shoulder girdle, and complaints of neck pain and headaches. These impairments may cause pain due to soft tissue fibrosis (scar tissue), deficits in muscle strength and pliability, neural hypersensitivity, and lymphatic insufficiency. Internal scar tissue and adhesions contribute to the chronic state of tissue hypertonicity, abnormal movement patterns, and pain (Fitch 2014).

Common among breast cancer survivors are: myofascial dysfunction, adhesive capsulitis, axillary web syndrome (AWS), post-mastectomy syndrome, brachial and cervical plexopathy, and neuropathy. Breast cancer surgery can also lead to scapula internal rotation due to pectoralis muscles shortening, elevating the risk of rotator cuff compression (McClintick 2013). These issues lead to a decreased function of the upper extremity that influences activities of daily living (ADLs) and lowers quality of life.

Dana Zakalik, MD, Director of the Cancer Genetics Program at Beaumont Hospital in Michigan, says of oncology massage: "Many patients can benefit

significantly from massage therapy, both for symptom management and improvement of well-being, which plays a critical role in the patient's recovery from cancer treatment" (Cancer Consultants 2014).

Pain and scar management techniques can assist in reducing pain and edema and improving lymph fluid drainage and scar tissue release (Bove and Chappelle 2012). The integration of scar management massage for pain treatments to standardized care might lead to greater pain management and might offer a safer approach for reducing pain and procedural anxiety (Gürol et al. 2010).

Scar Massage: Addressing the Pain
Take objective knowledge and make it human.

Ania Kania, BSc, RMT

Well-structured massage therapy sessions can assist in pain reduction, edema and lymph fluid drainage, and scar release (see Figure 6.3a,b). In rehabilitation centers specializing in scar management, therapeutic massage is used in 52% of the treatment protocols (Kania 2012).

One effective approach to minimize postoperative edema and pain is to provide manual lymphatic drainage in the early post-operative period (Wagh 2013). Manual therapy, including myofascial release and trigger point therapy, directly targets the scarred fascial layer and addresses the trigger points that may lie just under the surface of the scar (Jung, Smoot, and Prater 2012).

I find that manual lymph drainage (MLD) combined with myofascial release is the best modality to use when treating any type of scar tissue.

Note that before cancer research effectively demonstrated the positive effects of massage therapy, massage was thought to be a contraindication for cancer patients. Now more is known of the benefits of massage for these patients and there is an increase in the number of massage therapists trained in oncology massage. Current theories purport massage treatments will *not* create lymphedema

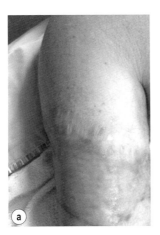

Figure 6.3 a
Keloid scar on 3rd-degree burn along deltoid/bicep junction on left arm, Spring 2014.

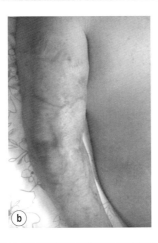

Figure 6.3 b
After bi-monthly treatments, Spring 2015.

individually based protocols that address all complications of cancer surgeries, including fascial restrictions, pain, LE, and scarring.

Methodology
Assessment and Interviews
My goal in working with scar tissue, be it physically limiting, emotionally traumatic, or relatively minor, is to reduce pain and restore proper function. I have a holistic approach to each client, and consider not just the fibrotic tissue itself, but the underlying structures, functional changes, and client's emotional and physical discomfort. I note postural changes if the patient is compensating to handle the scar restrictions. It is also important to check with the referring physician for psychological symptoms arising from the pain or the treatment of the scar (Kania 2012).

(LE), mobilize a deep vein thrombosis, compromise the patient's possible immunosuppressed state, or send chemotherapy through the body more quickly than intended (Cancer Consultants 2014). However, it is important to seek therapists with training in scar management, MLD, and oncology massage to ensure proper assessment and development of

Development of a treatment plan for a scar tissue client involves several important factors, and I evaluate and assess the following:

- Current scar condition: What is the age of the scar, is there any weeping, are bandages still involved?

- Inflammation: Edema or LE, is there a temperature, and what is the volume?

- Patient tolerance: Is there sensitivity to touch? Tracking the patient's pain is of extreme importance at this phase. On many occasions patients may think they need to "take it" when too much pressure is being applied. However, this is counterproductive due to the stress it puts on the tissue and nervous system, and the effects it has on the patient's attitude to treatment. Some discomfort and pain may be experienced during a session, but my clinical experience has shown that longer-lasting results and patient compliance with home care come with the "less is more" approach.

Additional questions and answers about the patient's scar experience also contribute to the development of the treatment plan. For example:

- How does it affect quality of life? ROM?

- What other treatments have they tried? Were those treatments successful? Why/Why not?

- Is it possible to get the surgical report or speak to their doctor?

- What medications, if any, are they currently taking? More specifically, are they on any pain medication and how frequently are they taking this?

- Identify the goals of the client.

I find obtaining a copy of the surgical report very helpful for understanding the possible scar formation, adhesion patterns, and subsequent pain derived from the surgery. The extent of tissue dissection and the fascia structures supporting the tissue during surgery can assist in designing a proper sequence of treatments and outcomes.

At the initial assessment, I take photographs to establish a baseline for the client's restrictions and compensation patterns. I then refer to these photographs to gain an idea of how the patient's body has incorporated the treatment, looking at tissue, ROM, and structural changes. Depending on the type of scar and the desired outcomes or goals for treatment, I take additional photographs pre- and post-treatment, at least every third session.

By measuring the length, width, and volume of the scar pre- and post-treatment, I have a base from which to show improvements. This assists in making proper protocol changes for the next session and helps in demonstrating progress to the client. I also repeat the intake questions each session to determine if the treatment plan is appropriate for the day. For example, a change in medication (i.e. dosage, new drug, elimination of medication, etc.) might affect the depth of pressure tolerated. Medications that a effect tissue response, vascularity, and pain provide information on how to proceed with pressure, depth of palpation, and any changes noted in the tissue response.

If the client is receiving additional physical or occupational therapy, I find that collaborating and coordinating treatment is beneficial. In addition, a minimum of 24–48 hours between sessions, including other manual therapy modalities, facilitates the best outcomes.

Treatment Planning

Healing rates vary depending on tissue type, severity of the injury, age of the scar, and individual health status. All surgeries carry a risk of dysfunctional scarring and adhesions resulting in restricted tissue glide, muscle weakness and imbalance, and loss of flexibility. In addition, disturbed patterns of adhesions may be evident centimeters from the initial scar (Schleip et al. 2013).

I consider tissue realignment, hydration, and mobility when attempting to restore function and diminish pain associated with scarring. Myofascial release used in conjunction with MLD is a key component of my scar massage protocols, with the intent to decrease congestion and initiate the release of the fascial restrictions. Upon decongesting the area, I typically notice a change in pallor and a reduction in pain due to the reaction of the mast cells entering the area.

Positive hydration to the scarred area by elimination of the congestion will make the tissue more pliable. In addition, clearing the inflammation from the distal area of the scar promotes a healing environment and assists in ongoing drainage during the session.

After the inflammation is cleared, other manual therapy techniques can be used directly on and around the scar, taking the pain tolerance of the patient into consideration. As discussed, depth of the scar may affect the pain tolerance experience of the patient. Therefore, constant evaluation of changes in tissue density, pallor, and response helps to minimize the patient's pain experience.

Adhesions, tissue fibrosis, and loss of tissue glide can be identified as the source of pain and movement restriction in scars (Fourie 2012). Some scars may entrap nerves, ligaments, or tendons and can cause pain to the client. Myofascial release, when applied slowly and distal to the scar line during initial treatment, helps to relieve scar adhesions that have formed on adjoining tissues or structures from the initial scar formation, making it easier to restore function. I also use effleurage and petrissage, stretching, and cranial sacral therapy when appropriate. Cross-friction can address adhesion release. While each requires an educated therapeutic approach, the intended outcome is to facilitate optimal healing and reduce risks to fragile tissues.

Treatment Outcomes

Treatment outcomes should be directed towards regaining some or all of normal pain-free movement to the scarred area. This can sometimes be a long

and arduous process for the client in pain. However, continued discussions on goals will focus the treatment goals around a patient-centered outcome.

I have found that incremental goals will help the client mentally and physically, and usually aid in compliance with home care.

A common goal of treatment is to reduce the appearance of the scar. Photographs are another valuable means to measure progress.

Patient Education and Self-care

Knowledge changes attitude. Attitude changes intent.

Anonymous

Medical advances mean more people are living after serious scar-producing injuries than in prior years (Church 2006; Stroke 2014). These accomplishments have created a paradigm shift from focusing on short-term mortality to long-term enhancement of quality of life for the scar client. While therapeutic massage is a benefit at any phase of the scar healing process, assisting patients with their home care protocol has become crucial for realizing successful outcomes.

Sidebar 6.6 Patient Interviews

When asked, "Do you do any regular self-care to relieve or prevent ongoing pain?", replies included:

- "I learned a way to stretch the scar tissue, massage helped immensely with healing and the pain in the skin healing."

- "I feel confident that I am doing all I need to do. My therapist Nancy Smith provides me with the info and the best possible care—for both the mastectomy scar and lymphatic drainage. I wear full-length compression stockings on my legs 23 hours/day. I also perform simple scar massage while I apply lotion to my legs twice/day. I also exercise almost daily: mostly running, walking, and biking, and I try to stretch my legs to maintain range of motion and prevent the skin and muscles from getting too tight or stiff."

The following are guiding principles that I use in home care for scar tissue clients with pain:

- Education: Muscle charts are great visuals to provide a deeper understanding of the mechanics of the trauma, the healing process, and how self-care can affect change.

- Hydration: Teach the patient to apply an oil-based or water-based lotion to keep the scar hydrated. Using a lotion with alcohol or peroxide may dry out the tissue.

- Progress: Go over the measurements and photographs to help maintain perspective. They may only see the scar is still there, or feel that the pain persists. Acknowledging progress may help them see the bigger picture.

- Journal: Ask the client to note changes in ability to perform daily activities, changes in pain levels, etc.

- Hydrotherapy: Pain relief between sessions might be possible using ice or heat. Simple safety guidelines are necessary and easy to provide.

- Discuss side effects: If a scar has released around muscle tissue or a structure, the client may feel soreness in an area that was previously numb. Help them understand that this is a positive reaction, that nerve flow, lymphatic fluid, and blood supply may be re-entering the area.

After the initial session and assessment, I communicate with the client and referring physician within 24 hours. I note changes in tissue, ROM, pain, and overall comfort, as this information will help to shape a proper protocol for the next session.

Case Study

No one ever turned me over.

Ann, a 62-year-old breast cancer survivor and scar tissue client.

Subjective

Ann is a 62-year-old female breast cancer survivor who was first evaluated at my clinic 4 years after her subsequent right latissimus flap breast reconstruction (which she received 6 years after her initial diagnosis).

A latissimus flap is a muscle-transfer reconstruction that consists of an oval flap of skin, fat, muscle, and blood vessels from the upper thoracic region. This flap is removed beneath the skin layers to the anterior chest wall to rebuild the breast. The artery and vein of the latissimus dorsi flap are left attached to their original blood supply in the back.

Ann had periodic MLD treatments from four separate therapists due to her travel schedule and reported that the LE was affecting her quality of life. She stated that her back on the surgery side "felt like there was a large bandage covering much of the area" with "pain in my back near the spine." Ann commented that her physician sent her for X-rays to determine the cause of the pain but these proved inconclusive, with no other explanation for the discomfort. In addition, her physician felt the scarring was unlikely to cause pain.

For Ann, the pain in her back was constant and she rated it at 5 out of 10 with a "full feeling" in the upper thoracic, right shoulder girdle, right arm, and phalanges. In addition, Ann had difficulty "twisting her trunk" and had developed headaches.

Objective Assessment

Ann presented with a rounded right shoulder held in a guarded position. Her right posterior and anterior deltoid, pectoralis minor and major, latissimus dorsi, serratus anterior and posterior, abdominal muscles, scalenes and sternocleidomastoid were all hypertoned. In addition, Ann stated that areas were tender to the touch.

The right upper extremity including phalanges showed LE modeling and slight independent movement on inhalation and exhalation. The trapezius and anterior scalene attachment on the right clavicle was thick and non-pliable, and her levator scapula presented hypertoned bi-laterally. Visual presentation of the right and left arms showed a larger volume of fluid on the right. On assessment, Ann's ROM, abduction, and lateral rotation of the right shoulder were limited. In addition, AWS was noted during testing.

Assessment of the scar on the posterior right upper extremity (RUE) determined that it was closed, non-pliable, dense, and magenta in pallor with puckering along the edges. The scar contracture showed no mobility along the distal and proximal ends. Pre-treatment measurements of the right arm fluid volume, scar length, and width were taken on the latissimus flap scar on the posterior thoracic area near Ann's spine:

- Pre-treatment measurements:
  right arm, volume of deltoid = 33.4 cm;
  scar length = 42 cm; scar width = 0 .9 cm.

Treatment
Ann received a 75-minute session during which MLD, myofascial release, and specific trigger point therapy were included in the protocol and the release of the scar was achieved.

Reassessment
At reassessment, Ann stated that the "bandage feeling" was gone and she rated her pain as 0 out of 10. Her post-treatment measurements indicated that the fluid volume had decreased by 1.6 cm, scar length had decreased by 5 cm, and scar width had increased by 0.3 cm.

Conclusion
In the developing world, approximately 100 million patients acquire scars each year as the result of 55 million elective operations and 25 million operations after trauma (Gauglitz et al. 2011). Excessive or traumatic scars form as a result of physiological irregularities with wound healing and may develop following any injury to the deep dermis, including burn injury, lacerations, abrasions, surgery,

piercings, and vaccinations. Traumatic or excessive scarring can cause pruritus, pain, and contractures that may dramatically affect a client's quality of life, both physically and psychologically.

Therapeutic massage is a benefit during any phase of the scar healing process. Through the therapeutic scar management provided by a well-trained body worker, it is possible to restore function and assist in normalizing cellular and organ metabolism. Integrating manual therapy, focused on scar management treatment, can play an essential role in an individual's pain management.

References

American Association for the Surgery of Trauma. 2014. *Trauma Facts.* http://www.aast.org/TraumaFacts.aspx.

Badger, K. 2013. Describing compassionate care: The burn. *Journal of Burn Care Res* 33(6):772–80.

Barral, Jean-Pierre A. C. 1999. A tissular approach to trauma. In *Trauma An Osteopathic Approach*, 105–6. Seattle: Eastland Press.

Blakeney, P. 2002. *Psychological and Physical Trauma: Treating the whole person.* http://www.jmu.edu/cisr/journal/6.3/focus/blakeneyCreson/blakeneyCreson.htm.

Bond, E. A. 2011. Wound contraction is attenuated by fasudil inhibition of Rho-associated kinase. *Plastic and Reconstructive Surgery* 128(5):438–50.

Bove, G. M., and S. L. Chapelle. 2012. Visceral mobilization can lyse and prevent peritoneal adhesions in a rat model. *J Bodywk Mov Ther* 16(1):76–82. doi: 10.1016/j.jbmt.2011.02.004. Epub 2011 Apr 9.

Broek, R, I. Yama, J. Evert, R. Kruitwagen, J. Jeekel, E. Bakkum, M. Rovers, H. van Goor, and N. Bouvy. 2013. Burden of adhesions in abdominal and pelvic surgery. *British Medical Journal* 3 October, pp. 1–15.

Buzzle, 2014. *Scar Tissue Pain.* http://www.buzzle.com/articles/scar-tissue-pain.html.

Cancer Consultants, 2014. *Massage Therapy and Cancer: Is Your Therapist Trained to Address Your Needs?.* http://news.cancerconnect.com/massage-therapy-and-cancer/.

Chaitow, L., T. W. Findley and R. Schleip. 2012. *Fascia research III: Basic science and implications for conventional and complementary health care.* Munich: Kiener.

Chesire, A., 2014. *Trauma Recovery Clinic-Pain Conditions.* http://www.traumarecoveryclinic.com/pain-conditions/scar-tissue-and-adhesions.

Cho, Y. S, J. H. Jeon, A. Hong, H. T. Yang, H. Yim, Y. S. Cho, D. H. Kim, J. Hur, J. H. Kim, W. Chun, B. C. Lee, and C. H. Seo. 2014. The effect of burn rehabilitation massage therapy on hypertrophic scar after burn: a randomized controlled trial. *Burns* 40(8):1513–20. doi: 10.1016/j.burns.02.005. Epub 2014 Mar 12.

Church, D. 2006. *Burn Wound Infections.* http://www.ncbi.nlm.nih.gov/pmc/articles/PMC1471990/.

Colorado, M. H. A. 2012. *Colorado Mental Health Advocates' Forum – Trauma.* http://www.colorado.gov/cs/Satellite?blobcol=urldata&blobheadername1=Content-Disposition&blobheadername2=Content-Type&blobheadervalue1=inline%3B+filename%3D%22Consensus+Statement+on+Trauma+Informed+Care.pdf%22&blobheadervalue2=application%2Fpdf&blobkey=id,

Cyriax, E. 1903. *The Elements of Kellgren's Manual Treatment.* New York: William Wood and Company.

Dalton, E. 2014. Scar remodeling adhesions and nerve pain. *Massage and Bodywork* January/February: 107–8.

Fauerbach, J. A. 2007. Psychological health and function after burn injury: setting research priorities. *Journal of Burn Care* 28(4):587–92.

Field, T., M. Hernandez-Reif, M. Diege, S. Schanberg, and C. Kuhn. 2005. Cortisal decreases and seratonin and dopamine increase following massage therapy. *International Journal of Neuroscience* 115(10):1397–413.

Fitch, P. 2014. Life Passages: Secrets, pain and mourning. In *Talking Body Listening Hands: A Guide to Professionalism, Communication and the Therapeutic Relationship* ed. J. Goucher, 199–201. Upper Saddle, New Jersey: Pearson.

Fourie, W. 2004. *Widening our treatment options: understanding the role of connective tissue in post mastectomy pain.* Manchester, England: The Chartered Society of Physiotherapists.

Fourie, W. 2012. Abstract, *Journal of Bodywork and Movement Therapies* 12:3.

Gauglitz, G. G., H. C. Korting, T. Pavici, T. Ruzicka, and M. G. Jeschke 2011. Hypertrophic scarring and keloids: pathomechanisms and current and emerging treatment strategies. *Molecular Medicine* 1:113–25. Available at http://www.ncbi.nlm.nih.gov/pubmed/20927486 (accessed November 2014).

Goats, G. C. 1994. Massage: the scientific basis of an ancient art: part 2 physiological and therapeutic effects. *British Journal of Sports Medicine* 3:153–6.

Godleski, M., A. Oeffling, A. K. Bruflat, E. Craig, D. Weitzenkamp, and G. Lindberg. 2013. Treating burn-associated joint contracture: results of an inpatient rehabilitation stretching protocol. *Journal of Burn Care and Research* 34(4):420–6.

Gürol, A. M., S. P. Polat, and M. M. Nuran Akçay. 2010. Itching, pain, and anxiety levels are reduced with massage therapy in burned adolescents. *Journal of Burn Care and Research* 31(3):429–32.

Hahn, J. M. B., K. L. M. McFarland, and K. B. Glaser. 2014. Inhibition of hyaluronan synthase 2 reduces the abnormal migration rate of keloid keratinocytes. *Journal of Burn Care And Research* 35(1):84–92.

Harper, D. 2001–2015. *Etymology Dictionary.* http://www.etymonline.com/index.php?term=scar (accessed November 2014).

Hassan, S. B., G. Reynolds, J. Clarkson, and P. F. P. Brooks. 2014. Challenging the dogma: relationship between time to healing and formation of hypertrophic scars after burn injuries. *Journal of Burn Care and Research* 35(2):118–24.

Hussain, T. 2011. Modern times. In *Sports Physiotherapy.* New Delhi: Pinnacle Technology.

Jung, M., A. Smoot, and H. Prater. 2012. *A case report of chest wall pain in the superficial fascial layer treated with ultrasound-guided injection and manual therapy.* Vancouver: Fascia Congress.

Junga, B. 2003. *Neuropathic pain following breast cancer surgery: proposed classification.* http://www.elsevier.com/locate/pain.

Kania, A. B. L. 2012. Scars. In *Massage Therapy: Integrating Research and Practice*, Chapter 15. Champlain, IL: Human Kinetics.

Kennedy, A. 2011. *Massage can reduce symptoms of depression.* http://www.amtamassage.org/approved_position_statements/Massage-Can-Reduce-Symptoms-of-Depression.html (accessed June 2014).

Kidd, B. L., and L. A. Urban. 2012. *Mechanisms of inflammatory pain.* http://bja.oxfordjournals.org/content/87/1/3.full (accessed June 2014).

Kumar, V. 2012. Inflammation and repair. In *Robbins Basic Pathology*, Chapter 2. Philadelphia: Elsevier.

Lee, S. S., G. Yosipovich, Y. H. Chan, and C. L. Goh. 2004. *Pruritus, pain, and small nerve fiber function in keloids: a controlled study.* http://www.ncbi.nlm.nih.gov/pubmed/15583600/ (accessed November 2014).

Maastricht, U. P. C. 2011. *Scar Tissue Pain.* http://www.pijn.com/en/patients/cause-of-pain/diagnoses-per-body-region/upper-back-chest/scar-tissue-pain? (accessed November 2014).

McClintick, K. 2013. *Critical Analysis of Occupational Therapy Practice.* http://spahp.creighton.edu/sites/spahp.creighton.edu/files/basic-page/file/McClintick_Critically_Appraised_Topic_December_2013.pdf (accessed June 2014).

Merriam-Webster Dictionary. 2014. *Merriam-Webster-adhesion.* http://www.merriam-webster.com/dictionary/adhesion (accessed November 2014).

National Lymphatic Network, 2014. *Scar Therapy and Lymphedema.* http://www.lymphnotes.com/article.php/id/31/ (accessed 14 November 2014).

Pettman, E. 2007. A history of manipulative therapy. *The Journal of Manual and Manipulative Therapy,* 165–74.

Rodriguez, G. d. R. 2013. Mechanistic basis of manual therapy in myofascial injuries. sonoelastographic evolution control. *Journal of Bodywork and Movement Therapies 17.* http://www.bodyworkmovementtherapies.com/article/S1360-8592(12)00188-X/fulltext (accessed November 2014).

Roh, Y.S., H. Cho, J.O. Oh and C.J. Yoon. 2007. Effects of skin rehabilitation on massage therapy on pruritis, skin status and depression in burn survivors. *Taehan Kanho Hakhoe Chi,* Mar; 37(2):221–6.

Schleip, R., T. W. Findley, L. Chaitow, and P. Huijing. 2013. *Fascia: the tensional network of the human body: the science and clinical applications in manual and movement therapy.* Philadelphia: Elsevier.

Stroke, Office of Communications and Public Liaison National Institute of Neurological Disorders and Stroke National Institutes of Health. Bethesda, MD 20892014. 2014. Spinal cord injury: hope through research. http://www.ninds.nih.gov/disorders/sci/detail_sci.htm

Tasmuth, T. 1995. *Oxford textbook of palliative medicine,* 837. New York: Oxford University Press.

Wagh, V. 2013. Unfavourable outcomes of liposuction and their management. *Indiana Journal of Plastic Surgery* 377–92.

Structural bodywork and fascial balancing

Introduction

Pain relief is a common reason that people seek our care. A clinical challenge we face daily is that pain mechanisms are not always clear, and diagnostic tools are often inconclusive. MRIs and X-rays do not always identify pain generators, just as blood screens reveal some types of inflammation (one source of significant pain) but not others. Given the physiological complexity of pain, we may not be able to identify the root cause, which can be:

- local tissue damage firing nociceptors

- reliable referral patterns via **myotomes**, **dermatomes**, or **viscerotomes**

- diffuse inflammation or mechanical pressure somewhere along the length of a nerve (nervi nervorum excitation or ectopic disruption)

- dysfunction in centralized pain modulation at spinal segments, brainstem, or higher centers (Butler and Moseley 2003).

All clinicians work with partial information and treat according to what is most likely. In complex cases (fibromyalgia or centralized pain dysfunction), clinicians may confirm a diagnosis only after seeing which treatments are effective.

Sidebar 7.1 Research
In a 2014 meta-analysis of nonpharmacological treatments for pain, massage showed a medium effect size for decreasing pain in fibromyalgia patients (Perrot and Russell 2014).

In our practice, we see that people with severe or chronic pain likely have more than one pain generator, but even that is unpredictable. Clients with similar screening results (imaging or diagnoses) can have extremely divergent experiences of pain or limitation. Because the experience of pain is subjective and varies dramatically from person to person, structural bodywork does not use pain, per se, as a primary guide to treatment. In our field, following pain is often referred to as "chasing the dragon." Pain, like other symptoms, is not a reliable locator of dysfunction. "Where you think it is, it ain't!" is an aphorism of Ida Rolf, originator of **Structural Integration** (T. W. Myers, August 12, 2003, personal communication).

Structural bodywork practitioners are mainly guided by alignment; to improve it, we free and balance soft tissue. With some clients, this approach may treat the root of their pain (thoracic outlet syndrome or false sciatica); with others, our treatment relieves symptoms of a condition that is concurrently being treated in other ways (muscle spasms associated with migraines or temporomandibular dysfunction). From this perspective, our work can be central, alternative, or complementary, depending on circumstances.

Structural bodywork, in its diverse forms, rests on the premise that better organization (whether we call it alignment, balance, or posture) leads to better function, increased well-being, and less pain. Within manual therapy, what is distinctive about structural bodywork is its focus on optimizing *fascial* mobility. Because fascia is everywhere in the body, our work can be directed to any layer, as needed—from superficial fascia to the deepest interfaces between bone and soft tissue.

In our opinion, the critical element in making fascially oriented bodywork clinically effective is refined assessment skills. Our version includes both overall evaluation of each client's alignment pattern and moment-to-moment palpatory re-evaluation as treatment unfolds. This immediate feedback allows the work to remain focused on what is happening in real time (rather than assuming that one person's low back pain will respond as the last person's did). Our goal is to evoke ongoing improvement in alignment, function, and the client's well-being, which includes pain relief as well as empowered self-care and body use.

Sidebar 7.2 Patient Interviews

When asked, "What information do you wish your primary healthcare provider (PCP) had given you to help make a better-informed decision to go to these treatment sessions or classes?", a 43-year-old female with neck, shoulder, and hip pain replied: "I wish they had encouraged me to do this 15–20 years ago! Also, if my PCP at the time had known the benefits of this work not only for structure and function of myofascial/structural conditions but benefits for overall health, emotional and mental well-being, I would have gone sooner."

History and Overview of Related Modalities

In many ways, contemporary methods of structural bodywork can be traced to Ida P. Rolf, PhD (1896–1979). Her work, which she called Structural Integration (SI; others dubbed it "Rolfing"), centered on two innovative ideas: that gravity is the organizing principle for our structure, and that fascia, as the "organ of support," is an appropriate primary target for manipulation (Rolf 1989). She was influenced by early osteopathic principles and yoga, as well as her personal experience with chronic back pain. Ahead of her time, Rolf emphasized treating the whole system, rather than localized injuries. She created a systematic ten-session treatment "series." This protocol for organized whole-body change is one of the hallmarks of her approach. Two other notable characteristics of SI are: an emphasis on educating the client about posture, and the client's active involvement during treatment, through active movement and repositioning. Although Rolf's work long ago acquired the reputation of being painful to receive, current teaching emphasizes versatility of touch, allowing practitioners to work within clients' pain tolerance.

Some who trained under Rolf went on to create their own SI schools in the USA and internationally; graduates of these schools are collectively known as Structural Integrators. Some of the better-known SI schools include the Rolf Institute for Structural Integration, the Guild for Structural Integration, Hellerwork, and Kinesis Myofascial Integration. These schools teach manual techniques and treatment strategies based on Rolf's work. In 2002, the International Association of Structural Integrators (IASI) was established, along with an independent certification exam. This community was pivotal in establishing the Fascial Research Congress, first gathered in 2007.

Sidebar 7.3 Research

In the Fascia Research III publication (Chaitow, Findley, and Schleip 2012), section 8 is dedicated to pain and innervation (2012). Tesarz and colleagues (Chaitow et al. 2012, 170–1) sum their discussion by stating: "Our study demonstrates that the rat thoracolumbar fascia (TFL) and the subcutaneous tissue (SCT) overlying the fascia are densely innervated tissues … and may play a role in lower back pain" (170). They conclude that the TFL contains a dense network of nociceptive fibers and, "Therefore, the TFL may well be an important source for low back pain" (171). In another abstract from the Fascia Research III publication, Blanquet and colleagues provide the results of their human study on ultrasound measurements of the TFL after a myofascial release intervention. These authors found that the myofascial release approach can change the TFL and surrounding tissues, as measured by ultrasound and this can explain the effectiveness of myofascial release for treating chronic low back pain (Chaitow et al. 2012, 181). Other important research on fascia includes promising results from sonographic features/distinctions of connective tissue in persons with and without lumbopelvic pain (Chaitow et al. 2012, 191), and core dysfunction (intrinsic and extrinsic myofascial systems) and the clinical significance (Chaitow et al. 2012, 184).

Judith Aston, who originally trained as a dancer, worked closely with Rolf to develop movement work to complement the SI series. Feeling that her insights into alignment, movement, and manipulation went beyond Rolf's paradigm, Aston moved away from the SI community and developed her own work, Aston-Patterning, starting in the late 1970s. Her approach is characterized by a focus on detailed and ongoing assessment and by a deeply integrated model of balance and movement. Because her work does not utilize a "series" format, it is not technically considered SI, but the goals of the two methods are very much in harmony.

Some Structural Integrators took what they learned from Rolf and began teaching elements of the work within the wider massage community. The teaching and writing of Carole Osborne, Art Riggs, and Erik Dalton, for example, have strongly contributed to what is known as Deep Tissue. Deep Tissue tends to be more muscle-specific, addressing fascia within individual bellies or muscle groups. This method tends not to address systemic patterns, focusing instead on local or regional restrictions that limit function. Like SI practitioners, Deep Tissue practitioners often use knuckles, forearms, and elbows to create slow, steady, and compressive contact. Many practitioners blend this style with Swedish massage to offer clients a treatment that is both freeing and relaxing.

Another major contributor to the field is John Barnes, PT, who developed Myofascial Release® (MFR). Barnes began his exploration in the 1960s and has since trained a large number of practitioners. MFR is characterized by gentle, broad, and sustained (90 seconds or more) contact. Barnes's work is often associated with emotional release, in which clients experience a discharge of physiological stress and emotional content accompanying fascial change. Often practiced by physical therapists, MFR has been integrated into mainstream clinical settings to a greater extent than other approaches.

The overall field of structural bodywork contains many subcategories—Structural Integration, Aston-Patterning, MFR, Deep Tissue, and more. Each has its own emphasis and style, and many practitioners are trained in more than one method. In this chapter, we offer a description of our particular style and expertise, as well as information common to the overall field.

Theoretical Approaches to Pain Management

The premise of structural bodywork is that improving alignment and soft-tissue mobility helps to improve balance and overall function, which may lead to pain relief. Other members of a client's care team may take a similar approach, such as:

- a physical therapist who focuses on balanced strength of muscles or joint range

- a chiropractor who emphasizes balanced alignment and mobility of spinal facets

- an athletic trainer who focuses on balanced, efficient movement patterns.

In this section, we look closely at some elements of our rationale:

- Posture is best understood as a dynamic pattern of neutral and non-neutral alignment of body segments. This fundamental pattern of organization, in turn, underlies and sometimes constrains our movement options.

- Posture is, and is meant to be, largely subconscious and automatic; nevertheless, restoring awareness of postural patterns is a valuable aspect of treatment.

- Fascia, in its various forms, plays a primary role in organizing tissue and movement; as such, fascia can maintain imbalances of alignment and shape, which play a role in pain generation. Increased mobility of fascial interfaces is a logical premise for the mechanism of our work.

Posture as Neutral and Non-neutral Alignment

It is easy to believe that "better" alignment is "better for us," but what defines "better?" One reasonable definition is that, in good alignment, any given weight-bearing segment of the body rests on top of the segment below so that their centers of gravity align. (We're thinking of simple weight-bearing activities here—standing, walking, and the upper body in sitting.) We refer to this kind of alignment as *poise* or *neutral*. When we start to think about neutral and non-neutral alignment, some interesting properties emerge.

A segment in neutral alignment is, in fact and feeling, *poised* in its highest position. Non-neutral alignment, conversely, is accompanied by a sense of *sinking* and *falling off* the supporting segments. Non-neutral alignment naturally forms a pattern of counterbalances; when one segment falls back, another must fall forward, and so on (see Figure 7.1). As segments drift further from neutral, the body begins to lose efficiency and to struggle in weight-bearing, sometimes to the point of pain.

This struggle represents both an imbalance of muscle tone and a strain on the connective tissue network. The three-dimensional distortion of the fascial web is, in our experience, more easily understood in terms of alignment patterns than individual muscles being short, long, loose, or tight (terms often used in general massage). Furthermore, our movement patterns are, by necessity, built on this foundational alignment pattern—neutral or not.

Posture and Awareness

Posture, like breathing, is a persistent body function that lives in both the voluntary and involuntary realms. Once we learn to stand as infants, we don't concentrate on *how* to stand (unless we are in unstable environments: "getting our sea legs" or recovering from a temporary loss of function). Our neuromotor system naturally learns new gestures and converts them into habits. The advantage of habit formation is that our waking awareness is freed to engage in other activities; the disadvantage is that not all habits are good ones.

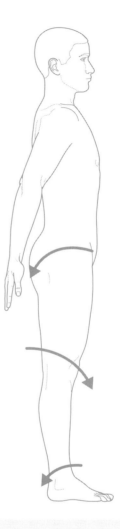

Figure 7.1
Body outline with arrows.

Less-than-optimal postural habits have both biomechanical roots (slouching in a chair, for example) and expressive ones (such as "depressed" or "aggressive" posture). The subconscious nature of postural and movement patterns means that our systems actively stabilize or habituate *any* pattern we create, whether they are optimal or suboptimal, even if they contribute to pain.

An additional component of our work involves encouraging clients to see their postural habits with

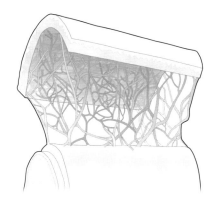

Figure 7.2
Fascial matrix.
(Adapted from Guimberteau videos, 2005, 2010.)

fresh eyes. Framing these habits in a nonjudgmental, descriptive way (e.g. "a pattern of compensatory relationships" vs. "slouching") is helpful. We find it especially useful when clients focus on simple, automatic relationships between alignment and stability; this increased awareness brings new opportunities to use postural strategies that are more efficient and less likely to cause pain or effort.

Fascial Interfaces

Appreciation of fascia as a unifying and coordinating tissue has grown since Rolf's time. Current best thinking about the mechanism of fascial bodywork is that tissue manipulation alters the fluid balance within fascial interfaces, allowing freer movement between structures. This idea draws, in part, on the work of Guimberteau, a French hand surgeon who conducted microvideographic *in vivo* studies (Guimberteau 2007) (see Figure 7.2). The camera shows a surprisingly dynamic matrix in which collagen fibers shift and glide independently. This *multi-microvacuolar collagenic absorbing system*, as Guimberteau terms it, is highly responsive to mechanical stressors, fractal in organization, and dependent on hydraulics to function well. Given that fascial interfaces occur throughout the body, current thinking assumes that dysfunction in this matrix generates restrictions in tissue mobility. Local tissue restriction decreases movement between structures, decreasing overall range, limiting coordination, and possibly participating in local inflammatory cycles.

Compensation, Force Transmission and Biotensegrity

Appreciating fascia as the primary tissue of global force transmission helps to explain coordination of movement (Huijing2007; Zorn et al. 2007). Notably, Thomas Myers's Anatomy Trains concept shows how myofascial chains can coordinate regional and systemic force transmission in predictable ways. Each myofascial meridian, as he calls them, includes many muscles and crosses multiple joints (Myers 2014) (see Figure 7.3). With these lines, we track relationships between local injuries and other areas of the body. A right ankle sprain, for example, can have

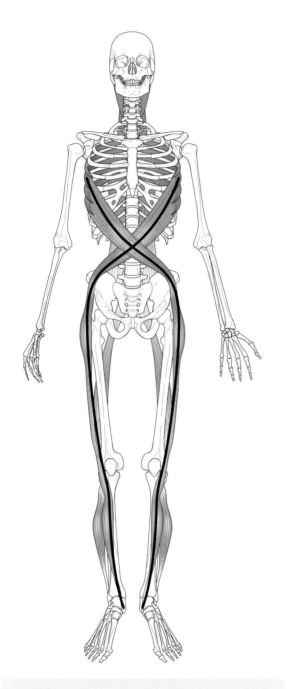

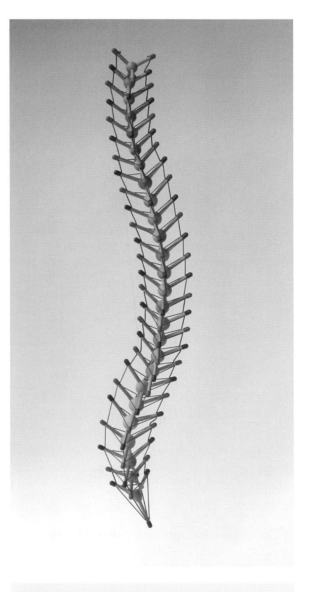

Figure 7.4
Tensegrity structure with definition.
(Copyright T. Flemons, 2006, www.intensiondesigns.com)

Figure 7.3
Spiral line.
(Used with permission Lotus Publishing.)

mechanical effects that ripple upward to the right ribcage or left shoulder, depending on each person's compensation strategy. Over time, distal effects can generate new, related areas of dysfunction or pain.

This matrix of fascial continuity is even more meaningful when we see the body as a **biotensegrity** structure (see Figure 7. 4). Many scientists have explored biotensegrity as an organizing principle, from the cellular level (Ingber and Chen 2007) to the gross functional level (Levin and Martin 2012). Biotensegrity enriches our understanding of balance in a number of ways. First, tensegrity structures lose volume in all dimensions under compression, and gain it in all dimensions when that compression is released. Thus, in practice, we see that people with poor alignment are not only "crooked," but also *shorter*, as multiple segments sink into compression. Likewise, as segments regain poise in treatment, clients get taller; the effect is so commonplace that we use it to assess client progress. Second, well-functioning biotensegrity displays evenness in fascial tension and a neutral shape. The presence or absence of these qualities is an immediate measure of alignment, and a primary guide in our treatment. As alignment neutralizes, pain and other symptoms often quickly improve, both at the site of an intervention and more globally.

In summary, less-than-ideal alignment patterns are driven by unconscious habits *and* held in soft tissue limitations. Does it make more sense to change the habit or the tissue? Divergent modalities, such as Rolfing (tissue mobilization) and Feldenkrais (movement education), each achieve success; so the answer is yes—current research points to a convergence of these treatment options. Fascia is now appreciated as a component of the neuromotor system (Schleip et al. 2012; van der Waal 2012) and free nerve endings found in fascial interfaces are understood to be *mechano* receptors (as well as **chemoreceptors**) contributing to pain generation (Schleip et al. 2012). Those of us who are tissue manipulators are primarily experts in *doing something* to the fascia, and our everyday clinical experience shows us that mobilizing tissue can change alignment, and eventually change habits—all of which likely improves symptoms, and most importantly in this context, pain.

Methodology
Introduction and Session Flow

In our practice, we see a wide range of problems, but most people have acute or chronic pain. Many clients have clear-cut orthopedic conditions such as frozen shoulder or hip arthritis; others have pain without an obvious mechanical source or clear onset. In practice, structural practitioners treat local problems while concurrently addressing non-neutral systemic patterns, all of which are particular to each client.

Here is a brief outline of how a client moves through our practice:

- *Intake:* At the first session, we interview clients to learn their history: injuries, diagnoses, previous treatments, symptoms and treatment goals. At subsequent visits, we check on how they have been doing since the previous session.

- *Assessment:* We assess the client's postural pattern in standing, and perform any relevant functional and orthopedic tests.

- *Treatment goals and strategy:* We use our findings to generate treatment goals and strategies for one or more sessions.

- *Client education:* If a client is new to this work, we explain our findings and treatment strategies to lay the foundation for client education.

- *Treatment methods:* At the table, we manipulate soft tissue, gently mobilize bones, and engage the client in exploration of those changes. Intermittently, we ask them to stand briefly so they can notice specific changes as they occur.

- *Client self-care:* Building on changes that occur during the session, we take clients through simple sensory awareness exercises that emphasize poise.

- *Monitoring client outcomes:* We constantly reassess alignment and tissue mobility while we work, honing treatment. Between sessions, we monitor overall progress through observable changes in alignment and function as well as the client's subjective reporting.

To understand the richness of structural bodywork and how it differs from other manual approaches, several aspects of clinical practice warrant a closer look.

Global and Local Assessment Methods

Clinicians who work with systemic alignment think globally: about the overall pattern of the body. Clinicians who treat pain investigate local imbalances: a compressed or misaligned joint, an irritable tendon, or muscle spasm. Both skills are critical, and we tend to move back and forth between examining global and local imbalances.

Weight-bearing palpation (WBP)

We evaluate and describe the postural pattern by quickly palpating the junctions between segments, noting the directional bias of each segment (see Figure 7.5). With WBP, our understanding of segmental relationships becomes more vivid than with static visual assessment: this assessment method allows us to immediately feel which segments are poised (neutral) and which are sinking.

In this process, postural patterns that relate to pain often become obvious. Those who suffer from low back pain, for example, often have lumbar spines that are quite compressed in standing. Commonly, we find these people sink into their heels, and the pelvis settles behind the femoral heads. In this "down" pattern, the lumbar spine is pulled down by its surrounding musculature. Decompressing this pattern—helping the lumbar spine regain poise—often relieves pain.

Visual assessment

A standard approach to assessing posture is to view a minimally dressed client from several angles. Some practitioners hang a grid on the wall behind

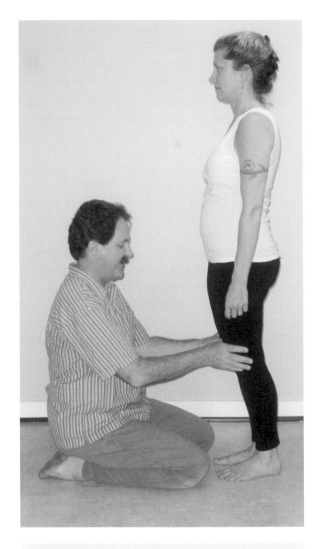

Figure 7.5
Palpation.

the client or a plumb line to establish a norm; others take photos before and after sessions to track alignment changes; and some use a mirror to show a client their observations.

Using bony landmarks, the practitioner deduces the spatial relationships between segments. For example, the sternal angle and pelvic landmarks illuminate the relative position of the ribcage, pelvis, and lumbar spine. Throughout his work, Myers promotes a consistent, simple language to describe bony position (Myers 2014). We describe these terms as follows:

- *Tilt* refers to displacement off vertical, where the top of a segment falls to one side.

- *Shift* refers to horizontal displacement, where the center of gravity no longer rests directly on the segment below.

- *Rotation* refers to displacement on a vertical axis, and simply means "turned to one side."

- *Bend* refers to a series of tilts, usually for side-bends in the spine.

These easily understood terms demystify our work and aid in client education. They also emphasize bony position rather than actions at the joint, which illuminates postural pattern rather than muscular length or strength.

Global functional assessment

Practitioners often ask the client to perform simple movements such as walking, bending forward to touch the ground, or rotating the trunk. We look for signs of asymmetrical range of motion, undue effort, or soft tissue restriction; the movements are not performed to evoke pain or assess local injury. For example, watching a client accomplish a forward bend reveals not only overall range, but also whether they emphasize flexion of the hips or of the spine (global strategy), and which spinal sections flex more and less evenly (local pattern). Initially, the client may or may not be aware of these limitations, but functional assessments can give clear evidence of progress.

Soft tissue assessment at the table

Under ideal circumstances, soft tissue should have well-balanced mobility and a pliable end-feel. ("End-feel" refers to the quality in tissue at its end of easy movement.) Our simple assessment method explores how tissues vary from this ideal. Sometimes,

restrictions at fascial interfaces closely correlate with anatomical structures: a single muscle, a septum between muscles, or a tendon. At other times, the restriction's shape is harder to identify, either because it is small enough to be within a single muscle, for example, or because it spans several muscles and/or joints. Our findings organize our treatment priorities: harder end-feels represent more robust restrictions.

Specialized orthopedic tests

One thing that separates a purely "structural" practice from a "clinical" one is the use of tests that identify particular pathologies, the so-called "special" orthopedic tests. For example, we evaluate capsular patterns of joint limitation (Cyriax and Cyriax 1996) to screen for arthritis, particularly in the hip, knee, and shoulder, and we use careful passive testing to screen for shoulder impingement (Lowe 2006) as distinct from biceps tendonitis or bursitis. Some, but not all, structural

---

Sidebar 7.5 Research

In a 2006 Archives of Internal Medicine trial of Swedish massage for osteoarthritis of the knee, Perlman et al. (2006) found statistically significant decreases in pain, stiffness, and physical limitations, and range of motion increases, when analyzing results reported on the Western Ontario and McMaster Universities Arthritis Index (WOMAC) and visual analogue scale (VAS). In the comments section, these researchers state: "The potential importance of massage as an adjunct to or even an alternative to pharmacotherapy is self-evident. Current pharmacological treatments for OA are associated with high rates of adverse effects, such as cardiovascular, gastrointestinal, renal, and hepatotic toxic effects. Many patients are already adding or trying massage as a therapy for OA" (Perlman et al. 2006, 2537). Although this study employed Swedish massage, the effects of both approaches can have common results and the assessment tools used are aligned well with structural bodywork and fascial balancing treatment goals and approaches.

practitioners use specialized tests; if a client has an orthopedic condition, inquiring about a practitioner's skill set is helpful. Each of these assessment methods gives immediate information that guides our treatment strategy as we work with individual clients.

Treatment Goals and Strategies

After completing the intake and initial assessments, we create an overall strategy for one or more sessions. These strategies are responsive and flexible, taking several factors into account:

- Clients' goals: Clients seek our treatment for various reasons: to relieve pain or recover from injury, to optimize the ability to perform particular activities, as a strategy for healthy aging, or to improve posture.

- Overall alignment pattern: Many clients present with pain associated with common alignment patterns (e.g. head-forward posture is part of particular back-and-forth systemic patterns associated with headache, neck, or shoulder pain). Others present unique structural challenges and complex symptomatology, such as a client with scoliosis who is navigating recovery from the asymmetrical challenge of knee surgery.

- Phase of healing: Our first session has different goals from our fifth or tenth. Initial sessions generally focus on freeing tissue and balancing a client's structure, while later sessions emphasize client education and self-care. Continual reassessment and monitoring outcomes informs the overall trajectory and focus of care.

- Client's age: Because their tissue and cognition are so malleable, children often require fewer sessions than adults. Our work is precise and gentle enough to use even with infants who have torticollis or club foot, for example.

- Our place in their overall care: Some people come intermittently as a complement to

physical therapy, chiropracty, or acupuncture. For others, we may be their primary or only treatment. This may stem from the client's beliefs about alternative or allopathic care, or from the nature of their concerns and limitations.

With the above considerations in mind, we use principles, rather than protocols, to guide our treatments. Practitioners utilize these principles one at a time or in combination, in one or more sessions. Here are some examples:

- Hardest end-feel: Upon palpation, the strongest fascial bias and hardest end-feel represent a simple way to prioritize our work. Once that restriction eases, there will be a next "most restricted" place to treat. We work through local, regional, and global patterns, assessing, treating, and reassessing. It is easy to assume that the earliest or most severe injuries govern the body's pattern; this is not always the case. Organizing treatment by end-feel is an effective strategy.

- From the ground up: Given the role of gravity in our approach, many practitioners work "from the ground up." If the body is busy balancing one segment on top of another, it makes sense to treat lower segments before attempting to balance upper ones. Taken to an extreme, every session would start with the feet and "build" upward—and, in fact, that is how many people assume that Rolf worked. Actually, SI session strategy is more complex: the "recipe" moves through a treatment sequence that addresses superficial compensations, then deeper "core" patterns, concluding with sessions that reintegrate and educate the client in their new, freely moving structure (Myers 2004). In our experience, most SI practitioners use the "recipe" more formally early in their practice and later transcend its specific protocol.

- Start one segment below: Taking gravity into account *locally* means "starting one segment below." To balance the shoulder girdle, we begin treatment on the upper rib cage; to balance the pelvis, we first address the femurs. Within the context of gravity, we appreciate that support is optimized when a segment is in neutral alignment on the segment below.

- Outside-in: Given multiple fascial layers, especially in the trunk, it is often useful to free outer layers before addressing deeper tissue. Rolf discriminated between "core" and "sleeve" components of a postural pattern. "Sleeve" refers to superficial myofascia, particularly the appendages, while "core" relates to the deepest layers of tissue, particularly in the trunk. Working in this way, we release restrictions in the legs and abdominal wall (sleeve) before addressing the deep paraspinals, quadratus lumborum, and psoas (core) in a client with chronic pain from scoliosis.

- Inside-out: Working "inside-out" addresses the bones themselves, freeing bones within the deepest soft tissue layer. Though not a common approach, this strategy is particularly useful in areas where reaching the deepest layer requires significant force or where more delicate structures (e.g. organs, nerves, glands) limit our access. For example, if a client has hip pain with a unilateral pelvic inflare, we gently engage the ilia; the bone begins to glide through surrounding tissue as tissue mobility eases in the adjacent iliacus and glutei. This method of tissue change is effective, quick, and more comfortable than many approaches.

Clients come with their goals (explicit) and current compensation strategy (usually unconscious). To assist them toward better function, we disturb their status quo, which must be done with consideration. We do not want to destabilize them so much that they cannot find new, improved balance. This range of treatment strategies allows practitioners to customize their treatment for each client, and accounts for the variety of approaches within structural bodywork.

Treatment Methods

Our interventions fundamentally have two components: tissue mobilization at interfaces of soft tissue, bones, and joints; and client education to optimize their posture and usage habits.

Tissue mobilization

In treatment, we directly balance soft tissue mobility, while at the same time keeping in mind overall segmental alignment. The mechanics of treatment (hand positions and degree of force applied) are similar to those of palpatory assessment. Because of this, the cycle of assessment–treatment–reassessment is quick and seamless. Ongoing re-evaluation ensures that the work is effective and efficient.

Our soft-tissue assessment leads to identifying relevant restrictions as determined by hard end-feel. Restrictions also have a *direction* in which the end-feel is found. In treatment, we either distract (move away from the restriction) or compress (move towards the restriction) to engage a barrier to motion. Specifically, tissue manipulation consists of smoothly gliding the tissue through that barrier, which generally takes a few seconds and decompresses tissue that has been held in a compressed and/or contracted condition.

The details of our work differ from the general field in several ways:

- Contact: Our work uses fairly gentle force (often, just a pound or two). The degree of pressure used is a significant variable in the field, with Deep Tissue and classic SI work being at the vigorous end.

- Lubrication: We usually do not use oils or creams, and so often work through clients' clothes. Most fascial release practitioners use lotion, waxes, or creams.

- Draping: Because we work through clothes, we use draping for warmth as needed. It is more conventional for the client to partially undress for visual assessment and direct tissue contact.

Tissue mobilization is our most concrete intervention and one that provides clients with immediate improvement. Whether or not those changes are lasting often depends on how the client uses their body in daily life.

Client education

To realize the full potential of structural bodywork, clients need to participate in changing their habits. Our work affords several avenues for client education:

- Awareness of restrictions: Clients may have this awareness, or we may point out limitations of which they were unaware. This process usually begins during our initial assessment.

- Changes during the session: When clients stand periodically during a session, changes in balance and movement (as well as improvement in symptoms) are often immediately obvious.

- Coaching and homework: We help clients with simple postural strategies that improve segmental support, to clarify awareness of alignment (how it *feels* to be more neutral), and to find appropriate degrees of control and surrender in body usage. This kind of homework emphasizes internal exploration, and can be combined with stretching or stabilization exercises.

- Empowerment during the healing process: For those with severe or chronic conditions, it is easy to become discouraged. We track client progress in concrete ways, reviewing changes in their symptoms, activities, and treatment. Sometimes, simply educating the client about weight-bearing dynamics and postural compensation allows them to change long-held self-judgment and see new options for improved posture. At other times, educating clients about pain as a complex phenomenon (with distal, ectopic, and centralized mediators) helps them reinterpret their symptoms (Butler and Moseley 2003).

Our goal is to balance the body objectively and to improve the client's subjective well-being in immediate ways that instill confidence in the healing process.

Client Self-care

Along with coaching clients to be more aware of their posture, we give specific home care to reinforce changes achieved during sessions. Self-care often includes postural strategies for accomplishing daily tasks, such as engaging the whole foot while standing, or perching on the edge of a chair to align the pelvis and spine.

We often give clients specific stretches to sustain fascial mobility or to assist in injury recovery,

---

Sidebar 7.6 Patient Interviews

When asked, "Do you feel different about yourself or your pain as a result of getting this care?", replies included:

- "I always feel there's hope of not being in pain and I know there's a way to both manage it and not have to live with it."

- "Since the treatments and exercises I am more in control of what I can do to help the healing process and the specific treatments have zeroed in on the biggest pain and muscle/bone challenges."

- "Lauren is very knowledgeable, and freely shares her insights. Knowing more puts me at ease."

for example, stretching the rotator cuff and triceps for shoulder impingement. These stretches may use props (balls, rollers, wedges) and can easily complement physical therapy, yoga classes, or self-directed exercise.

Becoming more aware of our body, its aches, pains, and holding patterns, can be challenging; for some clients, it evokes strong emotions. Their home care may include self-directed journaling or conversations with loved ones, or we may suggest more formal support through professional counseling. This is particularly true for those with debilitating persistent pain or survivors of significant physical or emotional trauma. We see our work as complementary to other healthcare practices and advocate for our clients to have a strong and varied healthcare team.

Monitoring Clinical Outcomes

We consistently monitor the immediate effects of our treatment through reassessment during the session. To track the client's overall progress, we use several indicators:

- Overall alignment pattern: Through charting and/or photographs, we track the client's overall alignment. It is common for patterns to improve significantly during a session and then re-establish somewhat between sessions (this speaks to the role of postural habit). With "two steps forward, one step back," the pattern gradually eases over time. In our experience, when a "critical mass" of change in tissue and habit has occurred, the client's system begins to stabilize their new postural pattern.

- Change in symptoms: The severity, frequency, duration and location of pain changes with treatment. Changes in the location of pain are often a result of muscles working in new ways to stabilize better alignment; these changes are generally diffuse and transient, resolving as the myofascia regains appropriate tone and stamina.

- Increase in activities: Often, increased function will occur prior to resolution of pain; people do as much as possible within their pain threshold. As people's tissue becomes freer, they are often able to accomplish tasks that were previously limited. "Now I can reach the cans on the upper shelf!" People resume ordinary tasks with more ease (laundry, housecleaning, getting in/out of cars), as well as hobbies and pleasurable activities (gardening, exercise, playing with children).

- Increased resilience: As people resume activities, we often see increased resilience as a measure of progress. They stand for longer periods without pain, they meet the challenge of moving house without a relapse, or they move through a stressful family situation without reverting to old postural habits rooted in emotional guarding.

As progress occurs, clients' goals may change. As one area of discomfort resolves, they may have new discomforts that become priorities (Butler and Moseley 2003). Often their goals shift from seeking pain relief from us as providers to optimizing their ability to take care of themselves through postural strategy, stretching, or exercise.

With significant progress, we taper our work, usually seeing clients for shorter sessions or at greater intervals. Some practitioners, particularly in SI, have a "closed" approach to treatment: they work within a set number of sessions and when that protocol ends, treatment concludes. Others work with an ongoing approach, allowing goals to shift organically without a set end to treatment. In our practices, we work both "open" and "closed" sequences, depending on the client's needs and circumstances. Our overall goal is to empower each client to self-manage via better postural habits, self-care routines and, hopefully, only minimal maintenance care.

Case Study

Erin, a 27-year-old barista, first came to me 4 years ago, after 3 months of shooting pain down her leg. She had a history of chronic low back pain, significant athletic activity, and a prior rotator cuff surgery. (The surgery was successful, though her work as a barista often aggravated this area and resulted in residual stiffness and modest pain in her left shoulder and forearm.) She was already receiving chiropractic care and physical therapy for her low back; chiropractic adjustments, or spinal manipulative therapy (SMT), alleviated the most severe symptoms and her physical therapy exercises supported her return to work. She hoped that adding a soft tissue approach would bring further improvements in daily function and pain relief. Erin came for weekly treatments as consistently as possible.

My initial assessment revealed a functional genu valgus; left hip and shoulder compression; lateral shifts between pelvis, rib cage, and shoulder girdle; a diminished thoracic curve; and significant neck strain.

Initial treatments focused on increasing mobility in the fascia of the affected leg; decompressing the hip, knee and subtalar joints; and increasing pliability in the dural membrane at the lumbar and cervical regions. Because Erin presented with acute neural symptoms (tingling and shooting pain down the length of her leg), our work together progressed gradually to avoid flaring her pain by keeping pressure within her comfort threshold and taking time to integrate changes.

Erin responded well to treatment: her alignment pattern improved at the lumbosacral joint, sacroiliac joints, and knees. She began to experience less pain in her hip and leg, and more ease in her low back and shoulders. She reported improved range of motion and better sleep after treatments. Her homecare included gentle stretching, selected exercises she learned in physical therapy, and taking over-the-counter (OTC) pain relievers as needed. As treatment progressed over 4 months, Erin no longer needed pain relievers (ice or OTC medication) and was able to return to her accustomed level of physical activity and range of tasks at work, which included bending, lifting, and carrying heavy loads. After this initial phase of treatment, she elected to come in on a monthly basis for general maintenance and well-being.

In the following 3 years, Erin has experienced modest recurrence of her symptoms, often after unusual or extreme activities: a long hike on a steep trail, twisting for prolonged periods while working under her car's engine, or days of inventory at work. Though her alignment pattern reverts toward earlier imbalances, her symptoms have not been as severe as the initial flare that prompted her to seek treatment. Working in conjunction with her chiropractor, we are able to restore Erin's alignment and decrease her symptoms with fewer and fewer sessions. Throughout working together, Erin impressed me with her tenacity, sense of humor and patience; her challenges, courage and eventual success have taught me much about healing.

Conclusion

A structural bodywork session, at its best, provides a "preview" of improved balance. By freeing soft tissue restrictions and providing the client with new awareness of alignment and postural mechanics, to set the stage for improved balance and well-being. The reality that the body is able to stabilize improved alignment is, for us, a profoundly optimistic idea: habits and prior injuries need not create persistent pain and limitation limitation.

References

Butler, D., and G. L. Moseley. 2003. *Explain pain*, 2nd edn. Adelaide: Noigroup Publications.

Chaitow, L., T. W. Findley, and R. Schleip. 2012. *Fascia research III. Basic science and implications for conventional and complementary health care.* Munich: Kiener.

Cyriax, J. H., and P. J. Cyriax. 1996. *Cyriax's Illustrated manual of orthopaedic medicine,* 3rd edn. Oxford, UK: Butterworth Heineman.

Guimberteau, J. C. 2005. *Strolling under the skin*. Vanves, France: Service du Film de Recherche Scientifique (SFRS).

Guimberteau, J. C. 2007. Human subcutaneous sliding system. In *Fascial research*, ed. T. Findley and R. Schleip. Munich: Elsevier.

Guimberteau, J. C. 2010. *Muscle attitudes*. Pessac, France: Endo Vivo Productions.

Huijing, P. 2007. Muscle as a collagen fiber reinforced composite: a review of force transmission in muscle and whole limb. In *Fascial research*, ed. T. Findley and R. Schleip. Munich: Elsevier.

Ingber, D., and C. S. Chen. 2007. Tensegrity and mechanoregulation: from skeleton to cytoskeleton. In *Fascial research,* ed. T. Findley and R. Schleip. Munich: Elsevier.

Levin, S., and D. C. Martin. 2012. Biotensegrity: The mechanics of fascia. In *Fascia: Tensional network of the human body*, ed. R. Schleip, R., Findley, L. Chaitow, and P. Huijing. Edinburgh: Elsevier.

Lowe, W. 2006. *Orthopedic assessment in massage*. Sisters: Daviau Scott Publishers.

Myers, T. 2004. Variation in Ida Rolf's "Recipe". *Journal of Bodywork and Movement Therapies* 8(2):131–42.

Myers, T. 2014. *Anatomy trains: Myofascial meridians*, 3rd edn. London: Churchill Livingstone Print and DVDs.

Perlman, A. I., A. Sabina, A. Williams, V. Njike, and D. L Katz. 2006. Massage therapy for osteoarthritis of the knee: a randomized controlled trial. *Arch Intern Med* 166(22):2533–8. doi:10.1001/archinte.166.22.2533.

Perrot, S., and I. L. Russell. 2014. More ubiquitous effects from non-pharmacologic than from pharmacologic treatments for fibromyalgia syndrome: A meta-analysis examining six core symptoms. *European Journal of Pain Special Issue: Fibromyalgia* 18(8):1067–80, September 2014. Article first published online: 19 Aug 2014 doi:10.1002/ejp.564.

Rolf, I. 1989. *Rolfing: Reestablishing the natural alignment and structural integration of the human body for vitality and well-being*. Rochester, VT: Healing Arts Press.

Schleip, R., T. Findley, L. Chaitow, and P. Huijing, eds. 2012. *Fascia: Tensional network of the human body*. Edinburgh: Churchill Livingstone.

Schleip, R., H. Jäger, and W. Klinger. 2012. Fascia is alive: How cells modulate the tonicity and architecture of fascial tissues. In *Fascia: Tensional network of the human body*, ed. R. Schleip, T. Findley, L. Chaitow, and P. Huijing. Edinburgh: Elsevier.

van der Waal, J. 2012. Proprioception. In *Fascia: Tensional network of the human body*, ed. R. Schleip, T. Findley, L. Chaitow, and P. Huijing. Edinburgh: Elsevier.

Zorn, A., F. J. Schmitt, K. Hodeck, R. Schleip, and W. Klinger. 2007. The spring-like function of the lumbar fascia in human walking. In *Fascial Research*, ed. T. Findley and R. Schleip. Munich: Elsevier.

Additional Resources

Books and DVDs

Chaitow, Leon, ed. *Journal of bodywork and movement therapies*. Oxford, UK: Elsevier.

Earls, J. and T. Myers. 2010. *Fascial release for structural balance*. Berkeley: North Atlantic Books.

Guimberteau, J. C. 2010. *Strolling under the skin* and *Muscle attitudes*. DVD.

Porter, K. 2013. *Natural posture for pain-free living*. Rochester, VT: Healing Arts Press.

Smith, J. 2005. *Structural bodywork*. London: Elsevier.

Websites (as of February, 2014): Find A Practitioner and Current Research

Anatomy Trains/KMI: anatomytrains.com

Aston Patterning: astonkinetics.com

Guild for Structural Integration: rolfguild.org

International Association of Structural Integrators: theiasi.net

Myofascial Release/Barnes: myofascialrelease.com

Research: fasciacongress.org

Research: somatics.de

Rolf Institute for Structural Integration: rolf.org

Introduction

Musculoskeletal conditions have the fourth greatest impact on the health of the world's population and are the second greatest cause of disability (Murray et al. 2013). The burden of musculoskeletal disease has increased by 45% over the past 20 years and will continue to do so. The prevalence of many musculoskeletal conditions increases markedly with age, and with lifestyle factors (Woolf and Pfleger 2003). Musculoskeletal conditions have diverse pathophysiology but are linked anatomically and by their association with pain and impaired physical function. More than ever, patients are searching for effective treatments for their musculoskeletal pain. For over 140 years, osteopathic practitioners have developed assessment, treatment, and pain management methods to address somatic pain and limitation of function of their patients. Osteopathic practitioners provide treatment for patients of all

---

Sidebar 8.1 Patient Interviews

In response to the question, "What have you learned about this treatment approach or self-care that you would like healthcare providers to know about?" a 71-year-old male with central cord syndrome replied: "My preference is for non-drug approaches to pain control. We have different types of nerves that send signals to our brain (temperature, pressure, stretch, sharp/smooth). Since I have spinal cord damage, those signals are weaker by the time they get to my brain, which causes some numbness in my arms and legs. The motor control nerve signals from my brain to my muscles are also weaker. I don't want to further block the nerve signals with pain medications.

"My muscles are subject to spasticity and cramping, so starting a massage with light pressure and gradually increasing to deep tissue massage works best. Stretching feels good, but sometimes causes spasms so has to be done very slowly."

---

ages for pain management and improvement in mobility, function, and quality of life.

This chapter provides a brief history of osteopathy, an explanation of osteopathic principles, the therapeutic models of health and treatment, and an overview of some commonly used osteopathic techniques employed by a variety of manual therapists to address patients' pain and disability.

History
Origins of Osteopathy

From the 1850s, Dr. Andrew Taylor Still MD started developing his philosophy and practice of what would become osteopathy, with significant development and refinement over the following decades. It was not until the 1880s that Still gave his style of practice a name (Fossum 2004, 2; Lewis 2012, 130). Although not thinking it a descriptive enough term (Lewis 2012, 130), Dr. Still named his new philosophy osteopathy using words from Greek; "*osteo*" from *os*, meaning bone and "*pathy*" from pathos, an incoming impression.

Still first articulated his osteopathic concept to improve the medical practices of his day (Still 1899). The style of medicine that Dr. Still learned was "heroic" medicine, known for its extensive use of bloodletting, emetics, purgatives, alcohol, mercury based compounds, and morphine (DiGiovanna 2005a, 6; Lewis 2012, 58). During the 1800s, medicine was undergoing a shift away from the Galenic basis of medicine (an "unnatural accumulation of humours") to one based on scientific method, new methods of investigation (compound microscope and staining techniques), a new theory of evolution, and a germ theory of disease. Dr. Still read the latest literature by Darwin, Virchow, Haeckel, Spencer, and Pasteur on evolutionary biology, medicine, and natural history (Lewis 2012, 66), combining the latest scientific information of the time with intensive anatomical study via dissection and study of the bony skeleton (Lewis 2012, 88).

Still developed a medical philosophy designed to facilitate natural healing processes of the body. With a thorough mental image of normal functioning anatomical structure, Still examined his patients for deviations from this ideal to locate areas of altered fluid circulation and tissue health. The techniques he developed were designed to correct altered mechanics to improve fluid circulation and tissue health. Still was reluctant to document his treatment methods, emphasizing that a full understanding of structure and function would guide the practitioner to develop the appropriate technique.

As news of Still's successes spread, he was encouraged to teach his new method and the first class of students commenced study at the American School of Osteopathy in Kirksville, Missouri, in 1892 (Peterson 2011, 26). From these early beginnings, osteopathy developed into two distinct professional streams and spread to 50 countries around the world (OIA 2013, 2).

Scope of Practice: Osteopathy Around the World

It is important to note that scope of practice and practice rights accorded osteopathic practitioners differ from country to country and even between jurisdictions within countries.

The evolution and development of osteopathic training and practice has been subject to the specific cultural, economic, and political factors of individual countries in which it was established, resulting in two distinct branches; full scope of medical practice osteopathic physicians, primarily in the United States; and non-physician manual medicine osteopaths primarily in British Commonwealth and European countries (OIA 2013, 2). For the purposes of this book, the term "osteopathic practitioner" encompasses all professional applications of osteopathic techniques.

In addition, some osteopathic techniques that form the basis for osteopathic manipulative treatment (OMT) have gained popularity in other manual therapy professions. For example, **muscle energy technique (MET), counter strain (CS)** and **functional technique (FT)** are used by chiropractors, massage therapists, physical therapists, athletic trainers, physiatrists, and sports medicine physicians in clinical practice.

Some osteopathic techniques have been adapted and transmitted in modified forms. As such, osteopathy has served as a deep font from which many therapies have developed, for example, Myofascial Release® craniosacral therapy, manual lymphatic drainage, **Ortho-Bionomy®, structural relief therapy, zero balancing®,** Rolfing® and others (Harris and McPartland 1996, 683; McPartland and Miller 1999, 594).

Sidebar 8.2 Research

In a 2012 systematic review of seven **craniosacral therapy (CST)** studies, three randomized controlled trials (RCTs) and four observational studies, all using trained craniosacral therapists, were summarized. The most common outcome measures were quality of life and pain. All three studies that measured pain reported significant decrease after the CST intervention, compared with control groups. Other findings included significant improvements in duration of sleep for people with fibromyalgia. The authors conclude that CST has clinical benefit for patients in pain and other important outcomes (Jäkel and Hauenschild 2012).

The emphasis of this book, however, is on techniques that may be safely performed by nonphysicians, and therefore this chapter will not address all osteopathic manipulative techniques. In some countries, the term manipulation has become synonymous with a specific kind of technique— high-velocity, low-amplitude (HVLA) thrust techniques—while in others, manipulation refers to all kinds of tissue manipulation techniques (Eck and Circolone 2000). In certain jurisdictions, the use of HVLA thrust techniques is restricted to particular professions. This chapter will use the term manipulation in the wider sense to describe any active or passive movement initiated or assisted by the practitioner.

Theoretical Approaches to Pain Management—Principles, Models, and Methods

There are four osteopathic principles incorporated into courses of osteopathic philosophy (ECOP 2011, 33).

- The human being is a dynamic unit of function.
- The body possesses self-regulatory mechanisms that are self-healing in nature.
- Structure and function are interrelated at all levels.
- Rational treatment is based on these principles.

Kuchera and Kuchera (1994, 4) further elaborate on these principles by stating **osteopathy** encompasses all recognized tools of diagnosis, including osteopathic palpatory and manipulative treatment methods. Embedded in osteopathic philosophy is the rationale for the incorporation of manual manipulation.

As a guiding principle on treatment, "Find it, fix it, and leave it alone, Nature will do the rest" is an oft-quoted Still aphorism (Lewis 2012, 164). This statement expresses osteopathy's two complementary principles: structure and function are interrelated, and nature's inexorable drive to express health. Osteopathy places the 75% of the human body that is the neuromusculoskeletal system—and its intimate relationship with the viscera—at the forefront of its "lens" of assessment and treatment. Osteopathic practitioners see this system as the "primary machinery of life" (Korr, in Seffinger et al. 2011, 15), the ultimate instrument for carrying out human behavior and action. Through this system we communicate, express emotion, move through the world, and interact with our environment.

Manipulation is a tool used by the osteopathic practitioner to influence the patient's body

function. Korr (1997, 12) has put forward four reasons that osteopathic practitioners direct their attention to the musculoskeletal system. First, the vertical human frame is highly vulnerable to gravitational, torsional, and shearing forces. Second, because of this vulnerability, the musculoskeletal system is a common source of impediments to the function of other systems by virtue of its rich two-way communication with these other organ systems. Third, these impediments exaggerate the physiological impact of other detrimental factors in the patient's life and via the convergence of the central nervous system to impact on specific organs and tissues. Fourth, these somatic dysfunctions are accessible to the hands of the osteopathic practitioner and responsive to manipulative treatment. Through the use of manual manipulative techniques, the osteopathic practitioner seeks to optimize body mechanics for the fullest expression of health in the patient (DiGiovanna 2005a, 3).

Osteopathy is not focused solely on musculoskeletal structural aberrations as the cause of pain and disease. Poor diet, alcohol intake, bereavement, loss of property or finances, and exposure to toxins, poisons, and microorganisms can all be stressors to the system. The importance and power of emotions, thoughts, and psychology were also factors considered in Still's system.

Over time, osteopathy has evolved to a system of manual medicine with a patient-centered biopsychosocial approach with an orientation toward health, rather than disease or dysfunction. Evidence-based practice and use of modern diagnostic imaging (MRI, US, CT, X-ray) have been incorporated into modern osteopathic practice.

Models of Health

Scientific validation for the use of manual manipulation approaches is limited. As a consequence, manual medicine practitioners must rely on theoretical and clinical models to justify the use of manual manipulation techniques in clinical practice (Tehan and Gibbons 2010). Based on the coordinated body functions required for human function and health, five models have been developed to give the osteopathic practitioner perspectives by which to view the patient and guide clinical reasoning and treatment (Seffinger et al. 2011):

- biomechanical

- respiratory-circulatory

- neurological model (including autonomic nervous system, pain, neuroendocrine)

- metabolic

- psychobehavioral.

Biomechanical model
The biomechanical model entails approaching the patient from a structural or biomechanical perspective via observation and assessment of muscles and joints of the trunk and extremities that are primarily involved in posture and motion. The model suggests that because of the interdependence and interaction of the musculoskeletal system with neurological, respiratory-circulatory, metabolic, and behavioral functions of the body, a structural problem can comprise vascular or neurological structures and affect metabolic processes or behavior (Seffinger et al. 2011). From observation and physical assessment of muscles and joints of the trunk and extremities, the somatic dysfunction can be identified. The goal of treatment is to optimize the patient's adaptive potential through restoration of structural integrity and function, restoring motion and function to joints, ligaments, muscles, and fascia.

Respiratory-circulatory model
"Approaching the patient from the perspective of the **respiratory-circulatory model** entails focusing on respiratory and circulatory components of the homeostatic response in pathophysiological processes" (Seffinger et al. 2011, 5). Consideration is given to central neural control of respiration and circulation, cerebrospinal fluid flow, cardiovascular function, arterial supply, and venous and lymphatic

fluid drainage in maintaining homeostasis. A. T. Still's aphorism "the rule of the artery is supreme" can be broadened to cover the various fluid transport systems of the body. As venous and arterial blood accounts for just 8% of total body fluid, the importance of acknowledging other fluid systems is vital (20% of total body fluid is extracellular fluid, 40% intracellular).

Research from Hodge and co-workers has investigated the commonly used group of osteopathic techniques called **lymphatic pump techniques (LPT)** thought to improve lymphatic fluid circulation and enhance immune system function. Hodge et al. (2010) identified the gastrointestinal lymphoid tissue (GALT) as a tissue that releases immune cells into lymphatic circulation during LPT and enhanced immune function in the treatment of pneumonia as a result of these techniques (Hodge 2012). A more recent study has shown a combination of antibiotics and LPT can reduce bacterial load in cases of acute pneumonia in a rat model (Hodge et al. 2015).

Neurological model
The neurological model views the patient through the "lens" of neurological function. Dysfunctions that cause or are caused by responses in the structural, respiratory-circulatory, metabolic process and behavior activities are investigated. Attention is paid in particular to the head, as the location of the special senses, brain, cranial and peripheral nerves to the head, neck and upper limbs; the spinal cord; and autonomic nervous system. The relationship between the visceral autonomic system and the somatic system is of particular importance. Treatment influences the sensory, motor, or autonomic systems or reflexes associated with them, in particular in the thoracic and upper lumbar spine, which contain the sympathetic chain ganglia.

Metabolic-energy model
A key homeostatic function of the body is the generation and maintenance of adequate energy demand and consumption. Efficient posture and

motion is key for energy conservation and efficient metabolic functions. The mass of the neuromusculoskeletal system comprises 75% of human body; therefore, improving the functioning of the largest system of the body aids total body energy economy.

Psychobehavioral model

Assessment of mental, emotional, psychosocial, socioeconomic, hereditary, and environmental factors is included in the psychobehavioral model of health. Emotions and stress manifest in the musculoskeletal system as heightened sympathetic arousal increasing muscular tension. In conjunction with their listening skills and compassion, the practitioner uses both manual treatment and education to help patients adapt, manage, or compensate for these biopsychosocial stressors.

Theoretical Approach to Pain

Osteopathic philosophy emphasizes a patient-centered approach to health. In practice, this mean evaluating not just the painful area but also "the whole person who is in pain." Osteopathic practitioners assess locally and globally, acknowledging the biomechanics of the musculoskeletal system, which can implicate tissues "distant" from the patient's reported location of pain as the cause of symptoms, as well as the importance of the patient's environment, general health, and family relationships. Dr. Still was quoted as saying, "To find health should be the object of the doctor. Anyone can find disease" (Still 1899, 28).

Pain is a powerful motivating symptom that influences patients' treatment-seeking behaviors (Bialosky, Bishop and Price 2009) and, as such, osteopathic practitioners gather pain history as part of the patient intake process. However, pain can be a "liar." This is not to diminish the pain experience of the patient but to highlight the fact that, because pain is a complex multifactorial experience with multiple mechanisms for nociception, pain referral, and radiation, using measures of pain may not always be a good indicator for the success of treatment (Comeaux 2009).

Pain can be both protective and maladaptive. Pain is an expected symptom of acute tissue damage and is expected to abate as tissue heals and returns to normal. However, tissue damage is not necessary for the experience of pain; the threat of potential tissue damage may trigger the experience of pain. There is a distinction here that nociception and pain are separate but related entities; people can feel pain without physical trauma and vice versa.

Osteopathy acknowledges that noxious peripheral stimuli can have a profound effect on the musculoskeletal, immune, and endocrine systems. The neurological system is both plastic in its response to these stimuli and can be damaged or become dysregulated and facilitated to become a source of nociception itself. Through manual manipulation, the osteopathic practitioner seeks to effect change in the tissues of the patient that might generate noxious stimuli. The tissue dimension of skin, muscle, fascia, ligaments, joint structures, and fluid systems are directly affected by the practitioner's hands, which can assist tissue repair, fluid flow, and tissue adaptation. More remote changes occur at the neurological level to the autonomic nervous system, pain reflexes, and the neuromuscular (motor) system.

The effects of touch and manual techniques on the mind and emotion offer some of the more potent but less understood effects in the psychological dimension. Via verbal and non-verbal communication, the osteopathic practitioner seeks to affect the behavioral and psychological dimensions of the patient's pain. Complex mind–body interactions may result in a wide array of psychological responses affecting every system of the body. These include changes in pain perception and neuroendocrine and autonomic responses.

In the cases of chronic pain, where actual tissue damage is absent or long since healed, the pain experience may be due to a variety of higher cortical functions.

In chronic pain cases, more time may be spent addressing the tissue adaptation process, together with an educational strategy addressing neuro-physiology and neurobiology of pain, which has been shown to have a positive effect on pain, dis-ability, and physical performance (Louw et al. 2011).

Some of the effects of massage and other bodywork systems have been thought to be due to a release of neuropeptides, in particular endor-phins (Pert, in McPartland et al. 2005). McPartland and co-workers investigated whether osteopathic manipulative treatment and other healing modal-ities associated with the endorphin system—such as acupuncture, chiropractic, massage, and meditation—might actually be mediated by the body's endocannabinoid system (McPartland 2008). The mean blood levels of one of the meas-ured endocannabinoids in participants in this dual-blind, randomized controlled trial assigned to the OMT treatment group (myofascial release, muscle energy, joint articulation, and high-velocity, low-amplitude thrust techniques) increased 168%. The authors suggested: "healing modalities popu-larly associated with changes in the endorphin sys-tem, such as OMT, may actually be mediated by the endocannabinoid system" (McPartland et al. 2005, 283). This study suggests that the mechanisms of pain are as yet poorly understood, yet skilful bod-ywork may yield powerful pain attenuating effects.

Methodology

The practice style of osteopathic practitioners is het-erogeneous according to practice environment, areas of interest, scopes of practice, treatment modalities employed, and the divergent practice styles of non-physician osteopaths and osteopathic physicians.

Many patients who present to osteopathic practi-tioners have little knowledge of what an osteopath does or what osteopathy is (Osteopathy Australia 2014, 3). The primary avenue by which patients learn of the benefits of osteopathic treatment is a word-of-mouth recommendation from friends or family (Peachey 2011). Occasionally their medical practi-tioner or family medicine doctor may refer them.

Osteopathic practitioners work with patients of all ages; one-quarter were 18 or younger, one-third between 31 and 50 years old. More than half of all patients were seeking help with either acute or chronic pain (Orrock 2009a). While some present due to a specific trauma or injury or orthopedic issue such as osteoarthritis of the hip or lumbosacral pain, others many have pain without an obvious mechani-cal source or clear onset. Typically, osteopathic prac-titioners will use a range of techniques with a single patient such as rhythmic techniques, joint position-ing techniques, soft tissue manipulation, stretching, and, in regions where scope allows, high-velocity and non-high-velocity thrusts (Johnson and Kurtz 2003; OIA 2012; Orrock 2009b), and may integrate other complementary therapies alongside the osteopathic techniques. In addition to manual treat-ment, exercise prescription, stress management, and dietary intervention may be included as part of patient management and education.

Sidebar 8.3 Patient Interviews

In response to the question, "Have your condition or symptoms or ability to function changed since getting care?" a 53-year-old woman with a trau-matic brain injury replied: "I believe a confluence of treatment has contributed to reducing my pain:

- Learning and applying meditation I learned in [a mindfulness] workshop.

- Commencing treatment with an osteopath and receiving periodic adjustments.

- Starting a new medication that treats nerve pain.

- Starting a new medication to help brain function.

- Having an ergonomic evaluation and implementing its suggestions.

- Realizing that I have to pace myself and proactively take care of myself."

The following is an outline osteopathic consultation and treatment session that I typically conduct as a nonphysician osteopath in clinical private practice.

- *Intake*: Patients complete an intake form, which, along with the medical history taken by the practitioner, records their medical details. I ask about the presenting problem and symptom chronology, aggravating and relieving factors, and any medications taken. Patients are encouraged to bring along any X-rays, scans, or test results that may relate to their presenting complaint.

- *Consult*: Duration of consultation varies in the profession from 10 minutes to 1 hour but is typically 25 to 40 minutes in my practice.

- *Assessment*: I conduct a physical examination that may include orthopedic or neurological testing and postural assessment or range of motion testing. Patient comfort and privacy during this assessment are important, so patients are encouraged to wear comfortable loose clothing. Depending on the area of the body requiring treatment, I may ask the patient to undress to underwear with a gown provided. The examination may include passive and active movements. Osteopathy takes a whole-body approach to treatment so I examine the area that is troubling the patient as well as other parts of the body. For example, if the patient presented with a sore knee, I also examine and assess the ankle, pelvis, and back for dysfunction that may contribute to the knee pain.

- *Treatment goals and strategy*: I consider the information from the patient's history and physical examination findings to determine if osteopathic treatment is appropriate or if they need to be referred to another practitioner, and discuss this with the patient. Successful treatment is based on an accurate assessment and diagnosis of the complaint. Determining if the complaint is within my scope of practice is vital.

- *Client education*: With the informed consent process and the dialogue during the physical examination between the patient and practitioner, there is opportunity to educate the patient about osteopathic treatment, management, and to discuss options available and any concerns they may have.

- *Treatment methods*: I often use a range of techniques with a single patient, so the treatment might include rhythmic techniques, joint positioning (e.g. **Strain-CounterStrain®** (**SCS**) techniques, soft-tissue manipulation, stretching, and muscle energy techniques. Technique selection is made according to patient preference, the target tissues, and the nature of the patient's complaint and general health, among other factors.

- *Patient self-care*: I may also provide advice to help manage the condition between treatments. This may include exercise prescription, ergonomic advice, and physical activity modification during the course of treatment.

Assessment
Osteopathic physical examination
There are several textbooks devoted to the many osteopathic physical examination assessment methods and treatment procedures. Readers interested in further information are directed to texts listed in the resources section at the end of this chapter (Chila 2011; Hartman 2001; DeStefano 2011).Here, we shall discuss a basic outline of the structural exam and treatment.

The structural examination may contain all or some of the following elements. It should be noted that osteopathic practitioners might use alternative assessment methods that are relevant to the technique approach of their choice.

Static postural examination
The patient is examined from three viewpoints in a standing position, assessing their posture from anterior, lateral, and posterior aspects. Relationships of the major body segments and bony landmarks are noted.

Regional range of motion testing

The aim of this component of the screening structural examination is to locate any region with decreased or increased ranges of motion (ROM) as well as assess asymmetry of paired movement of side bending and rotation. Both passive and active ROM testing is ideally performed in the neck, thorax, lumbar spine, pelvis, and hips to add further data to the clinical reasoning process.

Segmental motion testing

Segmental motion testing is the detailed motion testing of the vertebral segments of the spine. A vertebral unit is defined as two adjacent vertebrae with their associated disc, ligamentous, myofascial, and neural structures, and associated fluid networks (lymph, arterial, and venous supply).

Palpatory assessment

Palpation is fundamental to osteopathic structural and functional diagnosis. Traditionally, four components guided the location of dysfunction tissues in the palpatory assessment (Kuchera and Kuchera1994, 19). These are: Tissue texture changes, Asymmetry, Restriction of motion, and Tenderness (resulting in the acronym TART). Tehan and Gibbons (2010) argue that pain provocation and reproduction of the patient's familiar symptoms should also be incorporated into palpatory assessment ("S" for reproduction of symptoms, creating the acronym START) to locate somatic dysfunction. Chaitow (2012) reviewed recent studies investigating the accuracy or inaccuracy of the various components of the TART model. While some recent studies have cast doubt on the reliability of practitioners assessing tissue texture changes, restriction of motion, and tenderness, it was found that manual palpation could be made more reliable by the level of training and confidence of the practitioner.

Evidence of acute and chronic changes

Investigation of the skin might give important clues about the nutrition of local tissues and the influence of local and distance neural tissues during palpatory examination.

Fascial assessment

Fascial assessment can provide a wealth of information on the patient's fluid health, preference for motion, and tissue health (Findley and Shalwala 2013). In addition to assessment of the presence of the common compensatory pattern (CCP), assessment of terminal lymphatic drainage sites and the presence of excess lymph fluid at posterior axillary fold, supraclavicular, inguinal, popliteal, and Achilles tendon areas of the body indicates where fascial restriction is impeding fluid circulation (Kuchera 2005, 2011).

Other examinations

Orthopedic tests, blood pressure measurement, gait assessment, and physical examination of the cardiovascular, respiratory, neurological, and digestive systems may be conducted if indicated by the patient's signs, symptoms, or history.

Classification of Osteopathic Techniques

Osteopathic techniques can be classified as direct or indirect (Fossum 2004; DiGiovanna 2005b, 78; Modi and Shah 2006, 7). Direct techniques are methods that move the restricted joint or tissue against the restriction to motion. An indirect technique is one in which the restrictive barrier is disengaged and the dysfunctional joint or tissue is moved away from the restrictive barrier until the tissue tension is equal in one or all planes and directions (ECOP 2011, 30). Some techniques incorporate movements both away from and towards the restrictive barrier; these techniques are termed combined. Figure 8.1 illustrates this classification of techniques and assists the clinician in technique selection for appropriate treatment. The following section outlines three osteopathic techniques that are widely used by manual therapy professions: muscle energy technique (MET), Strain-CounterStrain® (SCS) and functional technique (FT).

Muscle Energy Technique (MET)

MET is a form of osteopathic manipulative treatment developed by Fred Mitchell Sr. DO, later refined and expanded by his son Fred Mitchell Jr.

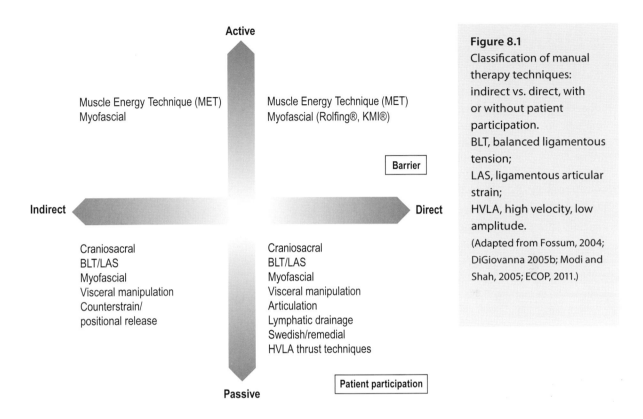

Active

Muscle Energy Technique (MET)
Myofascial

Muscle Energy Technique (MET)
Myofascial (Rolfing®, KMI®)

Barrier

Indirect   **Direct**

Craniosacral
BLT/LAS
Myofascial
Visceral manipulation
Counterstrain/
positional release

Craniosacral
BLT/LAS
Myofascial
Visceral manipulation
Articulation
Lymphatic drainage
Swedish/remedial
HVLA thrust techniques

Patient participation

Passive

Figure 8.1
Classification of manual therapy techniques: indirect vs. direct, with or without patient participation.
BLT, balanced ligamentous tension;
LAS, ligamentous articular strain;
HVLA, high velocity, low amplitude.
(Adapted from Fossum, 2004; DiGiovanna 2005b; Modi and Shah, 2005; ECOP, 2011.)

DO (Fryer 2011), used by osteopathic practitioners, massage therapists (Hamm 2006), physical therapists (Reddy and Metgud 2014), athletic trainers (Moore et al. 2011), chiropractors (Mehdikhani and Okhovatian 2012) and other manual medicine practitioners.

The approach relies on active patient effort, via muscular contraction, from a precisely controlled position, in a specific direction against a practitioner's firm resistance to effect changes in structural muscle balance (Chaitow and DeLany 2008, 218). This technique is "active," whereby the patient is making a contribution to the treatment and therefore MET requires clear communication between the practitioner and patient not only to perform the technique correctly but also to promote trust and cooperation.

There are four main variants of MET (isometric, isotonic, pulsed, and isolytic). The isometric version is most widely used and more extensively studied in research (Chaitow and Franke 2013, 40). In an isometric MET, the practitioner's counterforce matches that of the patient, and is repeated three to five times. Light contractions recruit postural (type I) muscle fibers, which are postulated to have caused a restrictive barrier to normal motion.

Chaitow and DeLany (2008) recommend different applications for acute and chronic conditions. In acute conditions, the treatment aim is to promote fluid drainage and hypoalgesia by repeated mid-range, isometric muscular contractions and placing the tissues in a position of ease to reduce the secretion of pro-inflammatory cytokines to minimize pain and inflammation (Fryer 2011). The characteristics of chronic tissue conditions necessitate a different approach. Thickened tissue that restricts range of motion with minimal localized pain and tenderness suggest that stretch and mobilization of tissue will be most appropriate.

Strain-CounterStrain® (SCS)

The origins of SCS are based in the observations of Lawrence H. Jones DO treating a patient with acute psoasitis. The patient saw a number of physicians, and Jones's own usual treatment methods had failed to relieve the pain and discomfort that prevented the young man from sleeping. Jones spent one office visit finding a comfortable pain-free sleeping position upon Jones's treatment table. He left the man propped up in that position, while he went to go to see another patient. He returned 20 minutes later and, to the surprise of them both, the patient was able to stand erect without pain (Jones 1995). Jones found the position of ease for the patient was an exaggeration of the position that the spasm was holding him (Chaitow and DeLany 2008, 198). Subsequently, Jones identified tender points that were related to particular strain patterns and that, with appropriate positioning, the tenderness of the tender point would reduce.

SCS is a positional release technique which is both indirect and passive but does require constant communication with the patient to monitor

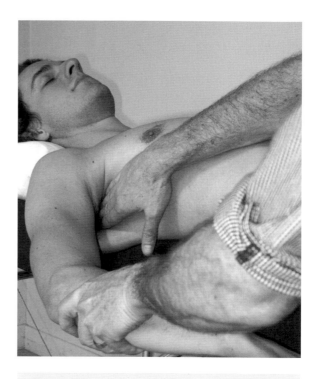

Figure 8.2
Patient positioning for strain-counterstrain of the subscapularis muscle, a common site of somatic dysfunction in computer workers. The forearm is medial rotated to initiate a position of ease and the tender point is monitored during the 90-second position of ease.

the tenderness of the associated tender point and maintain patient relaxation. Positional release techniques, despite the term "positional," actually take practitioners away from assessing and focusing on structure, and into the realm of function—how tissues feel, how they behave, and how they react to different stresses and loads (McPartland, 2002, 6).

The gentleness of SCS makes it a good choice for treating pain conditions in fragile, elderly, and pregnant patients. The technique is gentle on practitioner and patient alike, the patient being moved slowly in non-painful directions that are within their limited range of motion. SCS is also useful for reducing local pain as a sole treatment modality or in conjunction with other techniques, preparing tissues for other treatments if required.

Although several hypotheses have been proposed for the therapeutic mechanism of SCS, they remain largely theoretical (Wong 2012). Emerging clinical research suggests that SCS is effective in relieving pain and tenderness in various body regions (Meseguer et al. 2006; Wong 2012; Wong et al. 2014).

Functional technique

Functional technique refers to osteopathic manipulative procedures that apply palpatory information gained from tests for motor function (Johnson 2011) to resolve "dysfunctional function" (McPartland 2002). The approach was first described by osteopathic physicians Hoover (1958), and subsequently elaborated by Bowles, and Johnston (2011). The technique focuses on reducing palpated tone in stressed tissues as the body is being positioned in

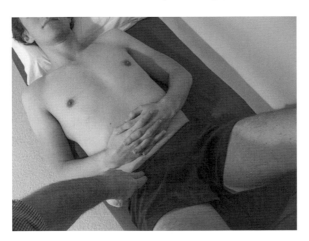

Figure 8.3
Patient positioning and location of the tender point for monitoring the iliacus muscle for strain-counterstrain treatment.

relation to all available directions of movement (Chaitow and DeLany 2008, 228). Like SCS, functional technique is an indirect technique, but differs from SCS by monitoring muscle motor tone rather than monitoring tender points. Functional technique treatment seeks a "dynamic neutral," a bilateral balance of tension while always moving, whereas with SCS the practitioner identifies a position of ease and remains in that position for 90 seconds. While the mechanisms for the therapeutic effect of functional technique have not been identified, these indirect techniques subtly allow the body to 'correct' and heal itself.

Treatment Goals and Strategies

There are two main therapeutic aims that osteopathic manual treatment can address (Lederman 2005): the repair process, and the adaptation process. The patient's complaint and history will indicate whether the treatment will be directed primarily at assisting the repair process or the adaptation process, or a combination, as the patient is treated over time or in more complex cases.

There are a finite number of ways to load tissue with therapeutic manual therapy. Tissues can be tensioned, compressed, sheared, bent, and torqued when twisted about its long axis (Wells 2011, 95). Some techniques may use a combination of these forces or attempt to reduce these forces, such as indirect techniques. A further two variables are the magnitude of the forces and the dose (duration of application). The combination of the method of the forces applied, the magnitude of the forces applied (technique), together with the dose (duration of the treatment session) and frequency of treatment, form the basis of treatment planning. In addition, the patient's age, acuteness or chronicity of the pain, general health, response to previous treatment, and time and financial resources will factor into the final form of the treatment and management plan.

A patient presenting with a swollen ankle after a fall a few days prior would be best treated with techniques that assist the tissue repair process. A patient who presents with a history of several months of hip stiffness is presenting with a dysfunctional adaptation process in the tissues so the aim of the therapeutic techniques would be to provide the appropriate stimulus to the tissues to encourage adaptation. However, there is more than the tissue domain to address, as suggested by the five models of health outlined previously.

Measurement Tools

For motor vehicle accident insurance claims, I typically use paper-based pain and function assessment tools such the Neck Disability Index (Feise and Menke 2001) and the Functional Rating Index (Vernon and Mior 1991) for documenting progress. With other patients, I will use visual or verbal analogue scales for pain, and monitor function with activities of daily living (ADLs) such as brushing hair, putting on a jacket or bending to put on shoes.

Case Study

Yolanda, a 52-year-old office worker, first presented with a history of chronic pain around the left lateral hip and posterior thigh at rest that increased with walking. She required assistance to the appointment due to limited mobility, stability, and pain in her left hip, thigh, and knee regions, and difficulty with forward bending and removing her shoes.

This first visit was 7 months after a series of falls and the sequelae of the injuries sustained during these incidents. After a second fall within days of her first, Yolanda was admitted to hospital for further investigations, as she had chest pain in addition to injuries to her left knee. These investigations cleared her of any cardiovascular pathology but MRI scans revealed a tear of a previous gastric band operation for weight management and a full-thickness tear of her left posterior cruciate ligament. An X-ray of her left knee showed no bone injury as a result of the fall. Yolanda sought my care on the recommendation of her co-worker.

Yolanda has a family history and diagnosis of Charcot-Marie-Tooth disease (CMT), which is the most commonly inherited musculoskeletal disorder (Pareyson and Marchesi 2009, 654) with prevalence of 1 in 2,500 (Martyn and Hughes 1997, 311). The hereditary, motor, and sensory neuropathy of CMT affects both motor and sensory nerves, typically resulting in weakness of the foot and lower leg muscles, which may contribute to frequent tripping or falls.

My initial assessment included a neurological, vascular, and musculoskeletal examination. Further passive range of motion and palpatory examination indicated the tissues causing her pain symptoms. Yolanda said that her pain was worsened when her "foot turned out"; once that happened, she also experienced some puffiness around her left ankle.

The goal of the treatment was to address her acute hip pain to allow Yolanda to return to her exercise program and maintain as much mobility and function as possible. My treatment was part of a multimodal, integrated approach to her health that included a tailored exercise program with a personal trainer to maintain strength and coordination, and reviews by her family doctor, endocrinologist, surgeons, and neurologist for medical management.

In the initial treatment, I focused on improving tissue health via identifying and treating impediment to lymphatic and venous drainage due to fascial or muscular restriction. During physical examination, I found restriction at the left thoracic outlet area, the lower thoracic spine including the lower four ribs bilaterally, and posteriolateral hip muscles. Having addressed the muscular hypertonicity in the lower leg with soft tissue manipulation and counterstrain on the deeper posterior compartment muscles, I worked through treating the thoracic and pelvic diaphragms with myofascial techniques. Yolanda's left lateral hip was very tender, so I decided to use muscle energy technique to address the tissue barrier and improve the pronounced external rotation of her left lower extremity that was evident as she lay in supine position on the table. I finished the treatment by encouraging lymphatic drainage with lymphatic pump techniques at thoracic outlet, lower six ribs, and pelvis. At the conclusion of the treatment, Yolanda was able to put on her shoes and walk to the reception area unassisted and reported less pain in her left thigh and hip and that her left foot was not feeling as swollen.

The first two sessions were directed at symptomatic treatment of Yolanda's painful and functionally overloaded left posterior leg, thigh, and hip muscles. At the start of these monthly sessions, I would question Yolanda about updates to her general health as her multiple health issues required ongoing review. Despite requiring thyroid surgery, which resulted in disruption to her exercise program, she has continued to improve with greater walking distance, duration, and continued weight loss. While ongoing monthly treatments to address the myofascial adaptations associated with her ruptured PCL and CMT, Yolanda has not regressed to the state of impaired mobility and hip and leg pain she experienced at her first visit and her mobility has improved such that she has resumed her passion for adventure travel.

Conclusion

For 140 years, osteopathy has offered a system of health care that emphasizes at its core the importance of the integrity of the patient's musculoskeletal system in total health. With the number of osteopathic practitioners growing in both professional streams of osteopathy, and new osteopathy schools opening worldwide, an increasing number of patients can experience for themselves this patient-centered, evidence-informed, treatment modality to manage pain, increase mobility, and improve quality of life.

References

Bialosky, J., M. Bishop, and D. Price. 2009. The mechanisms of manual therapy in the treatment of musculoskeletal pain: A comprehensive model. *Manual Therapy* [Electronic] 14(5): 531–8. doi: http://dx.doi.org/10.1016/j.math.2008.09.001.

Chaitow, L. 2012. The ARTT of palpation? *Journal of Bodywork and Movement Therapies* [Electronic] 16(2):129–31.10.1016/j.jbmt.2012.01.018, (accessed April 30, 2014).

Chaitow, L., and J. DeLany. 2008. *Clinical application of neuromuscular techniques: The upper body.* New York: Churchill Livingstone.

Chaitow, L., and H. Franke. 2013. *Muscle Energy Techniques.* New York: Churchill Livingstone.

Comeaux, Z. 2009. Second International Fascia Research Congress (Basic Science and Implications for Conventional and Complementary Healthcare), Clinical Demonstration Session, Disc 1, [DVD] USA: A/V Mix Studios, NYC.

DiGiovanna, E. L. 2005a. Introduction. In *An osteopathic approach to diagnosis and treatment*, ed. E. L. DiGiovanna, S. Schiowitz, and D. J. Dowling, 3rd edn. Philadelphia: Lippincott Williams & Wilkins.

DiGiovanna, E. L. 2005b. Goals, classifications, and models of osteopathic manipulation. In *An osteopathic approach to diagnosis and treatment*, ed. E. L. DiGiovanna, S. Schiowitz, and D. J. Dowling, 3rd edn. Philadelphia: Lippincott Williams & Wilkins.

Eck, J. C., and N. J. Circolone. 2000. The use of spinal manipulation in the treatment of low back pain: a review of goals, patient selection, techniques, and risks. *Journal of Orthopaedic Science* [Electronic] 5(4):411–17.

Educational Council on Osteopathic Principles (ECOP). 2011. *Glossary of terminology.* Chicago, IL: American Association of Colleges of Osteopathic Medicine (AACOM), [Electronic]. http://www.aacom.org/resources/bookstore/Documents/GOT2011ed.pdf (accessed Apr 15, 2014).

Feise, R. J., and J. M. Menke. 2001. Functional rating index: a new valid and reliable instrument to measure the magnitude of clinical change in spinal conditions. *Spine* 26:78–87.

Findley, T. W., and M. Shalwala. 2013. Fascia Research Congress evidence from the 100 year perspective of Andrew Taylor Still. *Journal of Bodywork and Movement Therapies* [Electronic]17(3):356–64.10.1016/j.jbmt.2013.05.015 (accessed September 3, 2013).

Fossum, C. 2004. *History and evolution of osteopathic techniques.* Maidstone, Kent: European School of Osteopathy.

Fryer, G. 2011. Muscle energy technique: An evidence-informed approach. *International Journal of Osteopathic Medicine* [Electronic] 14(1):3–9. http://www.sciencedirect.com/science/article/pii/S1746068910000301 (accessed December 12, 2014).

Hamm, M. 2006. Impact of massage therapy in the treatment of linked pathologies: Scoliosis, costovertebral dysfunction, and thoracic outlet syndrome. *Journal of Bodywork and Movement Therapies* [Electronic] 10:12–20.

Harris, J., and J. McPartland. 1996. Historical perspectives of manual medicine. *Physical Medicine and Rehabilitation Clinics of North America* 77:679–92.

Hodge, L. M. 2012. Osteopathic lymphatic pump techniques to enhance immunity and treat pneumonia. *International Journal of Osteopathic Medicine* [Electronic] 15(1):13–21.10.1016/j.ijosm.2011.11.004 (accessed April 16, 2012).

Hodge, L. M., M. K. Bearden, A. Schander, J. B. Huff, A. Williams, H. H. King, and H. F. Downey. 2010. Lymphatic pump treatment mobilizes leukocytes from the gut associated lymphoid tissue into lymph. *Lymphatic Research and Biology* [Electronic] 8(2):103–10. http://www.ncbi.nlm.nih.gov/pmc/articles/PMC2939849.

Hodge, L. M., C. Creasy, K. Carter, A. Orlowski, A. Schander, and H. H. King. 2015. Lymphatic pump treatment as an adjunct to antibiotics for pneumonia in a rat model. *The Journal of the American Osteopathic Association* [Electronic] 115(5):306–16. doi:10.7556/jaoa.2015.061.

Hoover, H. V. 1958. Functional technique. *Academy of Applied Osteopathy Yearbook* 1958:47–51.

Jäkel, A., and P. von Hauenschild. 2012. A systematic review to evaluate the clinical benefits of craniosacral therapy. *Complementary Therapies in Medicine* 20(6):456–65. doi: 10.1016/j.ctim.2012.07.009. Epub 2012 Aug 22.

Johnson, S., and M. Kurtz. 2003. Osteopathic manipulative treatment techniques preferred by contemporary osteopathic physicians. *Journal of the American Osteopathic Association* 103(5):219–24.

Johnson W. L. 2011. Functional Technique. In *Foundations of Osteopathic Medicine*, ed. A. G. Chila, 3rd edn. Philadelphia: Lippincott, Williams & Wilkins.

Jones, H. 1995. *Jones Strain-Counterstrain*. Boise, ID: Jones Strain-Counterstrain Inc.

Korr, I. M. 1997. An explication of osteopathic principles. In *Foundations of osteopathic medicine*, ed. R. C. Ward. Philadelphia: Lippincott, Williams & Wilkins.

Kuchera, M. L. 2005. Osteopathic manipulative medicine considerations in patients with chronic pain. *The Journal of the American Osteopathic Association* [Electronic] 105(9):29–36. http://www.ncbi.nlm.nih.gov/pubmed/16249364 (accessed August 7, 2011).

Kuchera, M. L. 2011. Lymphatics approach. In *Foundations of osteopathic medicine*, ed. A. G. Chila, 3rd edn. Philadelphia: Lippincott Williams & Wilkins.

Kuchera, W. A., and M. L. Kuchera. 1994. *Osteopathic principles in practice*, revised 2nd edn. Columbus, OH: Greyden Press.

Lederman, E. 2005. *The science and practice of manual therapy.* Edinburgh: Elsevier Churchill Livingstone.

Lewis, J. 2012. *A. T. Still: from the dry bone to the living man.* Gwynedd, Wales: Dry Bone Press.

Louw, A., I. Diener, D. S. Butler, and E. J. Puentedura. 2011. The effect of neuroscience education on pain, disability, anxiety, and stress in chronic musculoskeletal pain. *Archives of Physical Medicine and Rehabilitation* [Electronic] 92(12):2041–56. (accessed April 29, 2014).

McPartland, J. M. 2002. *Strain-Counterstrain Technique.* Middlebury, VT: AMRITA Press.

McPartland, J. M. 2008. Expression of the endocannabinoid system in fibroblasts and myofascial tissues. *Journal of Bodywork and Movement Therapies* 12(2):169–82.

McPartland, J., and B. Miller. 1999. Bodywork therapy systems. *Medicine and Rehabilitation Clinics of North America* 10(3):583–602.

McPartland, J. M., A. Giuffrida, J. King, E. Skinner, J. Scotter, and R. E. Musty. 2005. Cannabimimetic effects of osteopathic manipulative treatment. *The Journal of the American Osteopathic Association* [Electronic] 105(6):283–91. http://www.ncbi.nlm.nih.gov/pubmed/16118355.

Martyn, C., and R. Hughes. 1997. Epidemiology of peripheral neuropathy. *Journal of Neurology, Neurosurgery, and Psychiatry* [Electronic] 310–18. http://www.ncbi.nlm.nih.gov/pmc/articles/PMC1074084/ (accessed August 13, 2014).

Mehdikhani, R., and F. Okhovatian. 2012. Immediate effect of muscle energy technique on latent trigger point of upper trapezius muscle. *Clinical Chiropractic* [Electronic] 15(3):112–20.

Meseguer, A., C. Fernandez-de-las-Penas, J. L. Navarro-Poza, C. Rodriguez-Blanco, and J. J. BoscaGandia. 2006. Immediate effects of the strain-counterstrain technique in local pain evoked by tender points in the upper trapezius muscle. *Clinical Chiropractic* [Electronic] 9:112e8.

Modi, R. G., and N. A. Shah. 2006. *COMLEX Review: Clinical Anatomy and Osteopathic Manipulative Medicine, Board Review Series.* Philadelphia: Blackwell /Lippincott Williams & Wilkins.

Moore, S. D., K. G. Laudner, T. A. McLoda, and M. A. Shaffer. 2011. The immediate effects of muscle energy technique on posterior shoulder tightness: a randomized controlled trial. The *Journal of Orthopaedic and Sports Physical Therapy* 41:400–7.

Murray, C. J., T. Vos, R. Lozano, M. Naghavi, A. D. Flaxman, C. Michaud, M. Ezzati, K. Shibuya, J. A. Salomon, S. Abdalla, et al. 2013. Disability-adjusted life years (DALYs) for 291 diseases and injuries in 21 regions, 1990–2010: a systematic analysis for the Global Burden of Disease Study 2010. *Lancet* [Electronic] 380(9859):2197–223.doi:10.1016/S0140-6736(12)61689-4 (accessed April 16, 2014).

Orrock, P. 2009a. Profile of members of the Australian Osteopathic Association: Part 1 – The practitioners. *International Journal of Osteopathic Medicine* [Electronic] 12(1):14–24. http://www.sciencedirect.com/science/article/pii/S174606890800059X (accessed February 18, 2014).

Orrock, P. J. 2009b. Profile of members of the Australian Osteopathic Association: Part 2 – The patients. *International Journal of Osteopathic Medicine* [Electronic] 12(4):128–39. http://www.sciencedirect.com/science/article/pii/S1746068909000492 (accessed February 18, 2014).

Osteopathic International Alliance (OIA). 2013. Osteopathy and osteopathic medicine: A global view of practice, patients, education and the contribution to healthcare delivery. [Electronic] Chicago, IL: OIA. http://wp.oialliance.org/wp-content/uploads/2014/01/OIA-Stage-2-Report.pdf (accessed April 27, 2014).

Osteopathy Australia. 2014. Osteo-what-athy? *Osteo Life* Summer: 3.

Pareyson, D., and C. Marchesi. 2009. Diagnosis, natural history, and management of Charcot-Marie-Tooth disease. *Lancet Neurology* [Electronic] 8(7):654–67. http://www.ncbi.nlm.nih.gov/pubmed/19539237.

Parmar, S., A. Shyam, S. Sabnis, and P. Sancheti. 2011. The effect of isolytic contraction and passive manual stretching on pain and knee range of motion after hip surgery: A prospective, double-blinded, randomized study. *Hong Kong Physiotherapy Journal* [Electronic] 29:25–30.

Peachey, T. 2011. *Marketing in the osteopathic practice*. Unpublished Masters thesis. Unitec Institute of Technology.

Peterson, B. E. 2011. Major events in osteopathic history.In *Foundations of Osteopathic Medicine*, ed. A. G. Chila, 3rd edn. Philadelphia: Lippincott, Williams & Wilkins.

Reddy, B. C., and S. Metgud. 2014. A randomized controlled trial to compare the effect of muscle energy technique with conventional therapy in stage II adhesive capsulitis. *International Journal of Physiotherapy and Research* [Electronic] 2(3):549–54. doi: http://dx.doi.org/10.16965/ijpr

Seffinger, M. A., H. H. King, R. C. Ward, J. M. Jones, F. J. Rodgers, and M. M. Patterson. 2011. Osteopathy philosophy. In *Foundations of osteopathic medicine*, ed. A. G. Chila, 3rd edn. Philadelphia: Lippincott Williams & Wilkins.

Selkow, N. M., T. L. Grindstaff, K. M. Cross, K. Pugh, J.Hertel, and S. Saliba. 2009. Short-term effect of Muscle Energy Technique on pain in individuals with non-specific lumbopelvic pain: A pilot study. *The Journal of Manual & Manipulative Therapy* [Electronic] 17(1):E14–E18.

Still, A. T. 1899. *Philosophy of osteopathy*. Kirksville, MO: self-published.

Tehan, P., and P. Gibbons. 2010. *Manipulation of the spine, thorax and pelvis: An osteopathic perspective*. Edinburgh: Churchill Livingstone/Elsevier.

Vernon, H. and S. Mior. 1991. The Neck Disability Index. *Journal of Manipulative and Physiological Therapeutics* 14, 409–415.

Wells, M. R. 2011. Biomechanics. In *Foundations of Osteopathic Medicine*, ed. A. G. Chila, 3rd edn. Philadelphia: Lippincott Williams & Wilkins.

Wong, C. K. 2012. Strain counterstrain: current concepts and clinical evidence. *Manual Therapy* [Electronic] 17(1):2–8. http://www.sciencedirect.com/science/article/pii/S1356689X1100186X (accessed January 28, 2014).

Wong, C. K., T. Abraham, P. Karimi, and C. Ow-Wing. 2014. Strain-counterstrain technique to decrease tender point palpation pain compared to control conditions: A systematic review with meta-analysis. *Journal of Bodywork and Movement Therapies* [Electronic] 18(2):165–73.

Woolf, A. D. and B. Pfleger. 2003. Burden of major musculoskeletal conditions. *Bulletin of the World Health Organization* 81:646–56.

Additional Resources

Finding an Osteopathic Practitioner

American Academy of Osteopathy https://netforum.avectra.com/eweb/StartPage.aspx?Site=AAO&WebCode=HomePage

British Osteopathic Association http://www.osteopathy.org/

Osteopaths New Zealand http://osteopathsnz.co.nz/

Osteopathy Australia http://www.osteopathy.org.au/

Further Reading

History of osteopathy

Lewis, J. 2012. *A. T. Still: From the Dry Bone to the Living Man*. Gwynedd, Wales: Dry Bone Press.

Osteopathic assessment, technique and basic sciences

Chila, A. G., ed. 2010. *Foundations of Osteopathic Medicine*. Philadelphia: Lippincott Williams & Wilkins.

Lederman, E. 2005. *The Science and Practice of Manual Therapy*. Edinburgh: Elsevier/Churchill Livingstone.

Osteopathic technique

DeStefano, L. A. 2011. *Greenman's Principles of Manual Medicine*. Philadelphia: Lippincott Williams & Wilkins.

Hartman, L. 2001. *Handbook of Osteopathic Technique*, 3rd edn. Cheltenham: Nelson Thornes.

Chapter 9

Functional taping

Introduction

In today's society, people seeking relief from pain have many options from which to choose. In the allopathic tradition, a customary first option is to seek care from their primary healthcare provider (PCP) who may, after initial evaluation, refer to a specialist for further assessment, prescribe a pharmacotherapy (prescription or over-the-counter), recommend a course of physical therapy, or may just suggest rest. Some may consider a referral to practitioners of alternative or integrative therapies including manual bodywork (for example, massage or structural bodywork), acupuncture, body–mind therapy, exercise therapy, or movement therapy.

In many cases, the complex nature of pain makes diagnosis, or even understanding a cause of the pain, extremely difficult. This presents challenges not only to the PCP or specialist, but also to any practitioner offering care to the client. With a confirmed diagnosis, integrative health practitioners may rely on established clinical guidelines and standards of care to treat pain. If a diagnosis is unclear or unconfirmed, selecting an appropriate referral and/or intervention can be daunting.

As a massage therapist, people come into my practice with and without a clear, confirmed diagnosis. They present with pain that is acute or chronic; nociceptive or neuropathic; caused by physical trauma, repetitive stress activity, or somatic dysfunction or disease; of a physical or emotional nature. In all circumstances, I am left with assessing how to address both the pain of the client and their presenting symptoms. I rely on the extent of my training and the legal scope of practice in my jurisdiction. My approach is to use the systematic manipulation of affected soft tissues with a variety of approaches—searching for the most effective pain and/or symptom reduction. In the past 8 years of my practice, I began supplementing my treatment options with functional taping in hopes to maximize the effect and duration of my treatment interventions.

History and Overview of Functional Taping

Functional taping involves the application of elastic or nonelastic tape to the skin to reduce pain, affect blood and lymphatic circulation, alter sensory input, support joint position, and to either limit or encourage movement patterns. The most common taping applications include traditional athletic taping, McConnell taping, and kinesiology taping.

Generally speaking, there are two different types of tape used in functional taping applications: elastic and nonelastic. The nonelastic taping applications (traditional athletic taping, McConnell taping) are most commonly used in athletic training rooms and physical therapy clinics. These applications are used to support joints and restrict movement. Elastic taping applications (kinesiology taping) are used to support both joints and soft tissues but do not restrict movement. Athletic trainers, physical therapists, chiropractors, and massage therapists increasingly use elastic taping applications.

Traditional Athletic Taping

Traditional **athletic taping** dates to 1893 with an article published in *The New York Polyclinic* by G. Virgil Gibney, MD, Professor of Orthopedic Surgery and Surgeon-in-Chief to the Hospital for the Ruptured and Crippled, based on his readings in the British medical literature that recommended strapping injured ankles with a cloth with a rubber adhesive placed on it. His technique, the "Gibney Basketweave," had success and would become the basis of taping applications not only to the ankle but also to other parts of the body. However, this rubber adhesive cloth was irritating. Johnson & Johnson began to experiment and develop different, less irritating adhesives and eventually developed the modern athletic tape used today.

Now embraced by athletic trainers worldwide, nonelastic athletic taping protocols are used to prevent injury or to facilitate an athlete's return to activity. The tapings limit the abnormal or excessive movements of injured joints and support the soft tissues compromised by the injury. Most trainers believe that the value of such restrictive taping protocols is an enhanced proprioceptive feedback loop provided by the tape during movement. It is thought this feedback supports ligaments and capsules of unstable joints, and support injuries to the musculotendinous units by limiting movement (Perrin 2012).

Athletic trainers also use elastic tape and wraps. Unlike the rigid athletic tapes, these tapes and wraps support body parts that require freedom of movement. They are also useful to apply compression to an area of acute injury. Frequently combined with ice, this helps to control swelling. Also, elastic wraps are used when protective pads need to be secured to the body (Lowry, Cleland and Dyke 2008; Holtzman and Harris-Hayse 2012; Paoloni et al. 2012).

McConnell Taping

In the mid-1980s, Australian physiotherapist Jenny McConnell, while working with a patient doing a step-down exercise and experiencing significant knee pain, experimented with manually gliding the patella medially and her patient immediately realized a reduction in pain. She then wrapped the knee with a nonelastic tape to hold the patella in this medial position and her patient remained pain free. After using this taping protocol on other patients with success, McConnell introduced her patellofemoral program to physical therapists in the United States. The success of her method was in controlling movements of the patella combined with strengthening the quadriceps muscles, and addressing internal rotation of the femur, monitoring pronation of the foot, and addressing shortening and excessive contraction of the iliotibial band.

Sidebar 9.1 Research
Warden and colleagues' 2008 meta-analysis looked at patellar taping for chronic knee pain (thirteen studies) and pain associated with osteoarthritis (three studies). The reviewers noted that the taping studies were of high quality, compared to the studies that were included in the meta-analysis for bracing to reduce knee pain. The taping was applied to exert a medially directed force on the patella and produced clinically meaningful reductions in pain, both immediately and during the follow-up periods reported.

McConnell Taping (MT) is rigid and supportive, usually worn for up to 18 hours. While evidence identifying the underlying mechanisms of action is not available, recent studies have shown that MT reduces pain and improves mechanical function in people suffering from patellofemoral pain syndrome (Campolo et al. 2013). Additionally, recent studies report significant effects on proprioception. MT over the skin stimulates cutaneous **mechanoreceptors** and more central nervous system integration, allowing for modulation of activity in many sections of the brain that enhances proprioception during knee movements (Callaghan et al. 2012).

The McConnell Institute website (www.mcconnell-institute.com) states that their principle concepts are based on the premise that causative factors for musculoskeletal symptoms are understanding how posture influences dynamic activities and that unloading soft tissues, usually with rigid, nonelastic tape, reduce pain and optimize effects of many treatment modalities. Today, these taping protocols are used not only at the knee joint, but also at the shoulder joint complex, on the elbow, hip, and the lumbar region of the spine.

Kinesiology Taping

Kenzo Kase, DC, originally developed a use of therapeutic elastic taping in 1973 in hopes that it would afford patients an extended benefit from the chiropractic and soft tissue interventions used in his practice. He theorized that applying a thin tape directly to the skin would work with the body's natural healing processes, enhance vascular and lymphatic circulation, encourage (rather than restrict) movement and mobility, and shorten therapeutic recovery time. Over a period of 20 years, he continuously researched and developed Kinesio® Tex Tape—a nonlatex, elastic tape about the thickness of the human skin and a heat-activated adhesive that could be safely applied and worn for an extended period of time with minimal discomfort and side effect.

Now called Kinesio® Taping, Kase introduced his taping method to clinical rehabilitation settings in Japan and achieved his first international exposure at the 1988 Seoul Olympic Games. Kase introduced Kinesio® Taping Method to the United States in 1995 and to Europe in 2001. The concept and use of Kinesio® Tape was soon endorsed by athletic trainers, physical therapists, and massage therapists, as well as many professional athletes and teams, including the Japanese volleyball team (2000 Olympic Games), US Postal Servicle Pro-Cycling Team (2001 Tour de France), Korean National Soccer Team (2002 FIFA World Cup), Alfred Nijhuis (Dutch soccer player during the 2002 FIFA World Cup), and the Women's Beach Volleyball Gold Medal match in the 2008 Olympic Games in Beijing. More recently, Kinesio® Taping has been used in many competitions during the 2012 Olympic Games in London and the 2014 FIFA World Cup Soccer Championships.

Since the development, visibility, and popularity of the Kinesio® Tex Taping and the Kinesio® Taping applications developed, promoted, and taught by Kase, three additional methods of elastic **kinesiology taping** have also become popular: Fascial Movement Taping (Capobianco and van den Dries 2009); NeuroStructural Taping, a series of pre-cut taping applications developed by Kevin Jardine (www.spidertech.com); Acupressure Taping (Hecker and Liebchen 2005). Additionally, many brands of elastic kinesiology tapes have entered the marketplace including Rock Tape, Mueller Kinesiology Tape, 3B Scientific Kinesiology Tape, and TheraBand™ Kinesiology Tape, to name a few. While each brand of tape is slightly different, they all have the same basic properties—they are nonlatex, mostly cotton, have an adhesive backing, and have the ability to stretch. They are all advertised as hypoallergenic and can be worn for an extended period of time (1–5 days).

> **Sidebar 9.2 Functional Taping**
> In this chapter, I refer to any use of elastic or nonelastic tape applied to the body as a therapeutic intervention.
> The term kinesiology taping is used in the scientific and healthcare literature and refers to the use of an elastic tape applied to the body as a therapeutic application. Kinesiology taping is not synonymous with Kinesio® Taping.
> Kinesio® Taping, Kinesio® Tex Tape, Kinesio®, Taping Method, and Kinesio® are registered trademarks of the Kinesio® Taping Association International (KTAI). Kinesio® refers to the holding company Kinesio® IP, LLC of Albuquerque, NM.
> Kinesio® Taping and the Kinesio® Taping Method refer to a definitive rehabilitative technique exclusively using Kinesio® Tex Tape. This tape and the related taping techniques were founded and developed by Kenzo Kase, DC.
> A Certified Kinesio® Taping Practitioner (CKTP®) belongs to a select group of practitioners that have completed a series of training workshops and have successfully passed a certification examination administered by the Kinesio® Taping Association International.

Theoretical Approaches to Pain Management

Today, practitioners have three mechanistic approaches when using the wide range of kinesiology taping applications: *Neurosensory*—to improve the afferent/**efferent** communications to the central nervous system to normalize tissue tone and to restore motor pathways and minimize pain; *Structural*—to minimize injurious range of movement, assist stability of joints, and minimize postural dysfunction; and *Circulatory*—to promote the movement of superficial fluids, reduce bruising, and to improve oxygenation to injured tissues. Each of these contributes to the management of pain directly or indirectly.

Neurosensory Effects

One premise of the mechanisms of action of kinesiology taping is the ability of the tape to lift the skin away from underlying tissues (Kase, Wallis, and Kase 2003; Hecker 2007; Capobianco et al. 2009) when applied to stretched skin. Recent pilot studies have begun to verify this basic assumption (Lang and Takakura 2013; Wong 2013) and perhaps be disputed by Parreira et al. (2014a, 2014b). The benefits associated with this mechanism have neurosensory and circulatory effects.

Because the skin and superficial fascia are rich in sensory neurons, it is reasonable to expect the application of tape to the skin to provide a sensory stimulus. When applied to stretched skin, the elasticity of the tape will cause a recoiling and develop undulations on the skin and in underlying tissues. These undulations create gradients of pressure differentials in interstitial spaces. In areas of lower pressures, the forces placed on sensory nerve endings and baroreceptors will be reduced, and consequently noxious stimuli detected from A-delta and **c-fibers** interpreted as pain will also be reduced. The sensory input provided by the tape will activate Merkel cells and A-beta fibers that, according to Gate Control Theory, will disrupt the noxious input from A-delta and c-fibers as well. This results in a reduction of pain sensations (Melzack and Wall 1965).

There are two other possible neurosensory mechanisms that may contribute to the ability of taping applications to reduce pain symptoms.

Firstly, we can consider counter-irritation. The relief from pain and the promotion of healing by irritating areas of the skin causes increased nerve signals traveling to the brain, making it more difficult for nociceptive signals to reach the brain (Calvino 1990; Schweinhardt 2011; Carlton 2014). These sensations can come from myriad sources including physical, thermal, and/or chemical, and have been reported in medical literature as early as Mackenzie (1909) and Williams (1923). It is reasonable to infer, then, that the application of an elastic tape to the skin, and the sensory interpretation that results, could, in fact, create enough irritation (or perhaps stimulation) to override nociceptive signals to the brain as well.

Secondly, a readily accepted mechanism of pain perception is the theory of central sensitization—that causes of pain may not only be from nociceptive signals that arise from injury or trauma in tissues, but may also result from changes in the brain as a result of repeated nerve stimulation (Gudin 2004; Perl 2007; Woolf 2011; McAllister 2012). Additionally, Flor (2003) postulates that pre-cortical processing of both painful and nonpainful input can provide feedback to the brain areas that were altered by somatosensory pain signals. Since elastic taping applications remain on the skin for several days, this repeated, nonpainful sensory information may be relayed to the brain similarly to any nociceptive pain signals at the pain application site. While it does seem unlikely that a taping application will completely override painful signals, perhaps the addition of nonpainful input may contribute to mitigating pain perception.

Microcirculatory Effects

The pressure gradients caused by the undulations created by tape recoiling also have circulatory effects (see Figure 9.1). The lifting of the skin reduces pressures on vascular and lymphatic vessels created by compressive stressors and/or inflammation. As compression on these vessels decreases, it becomes easier for fluids to flow through them. At the greater

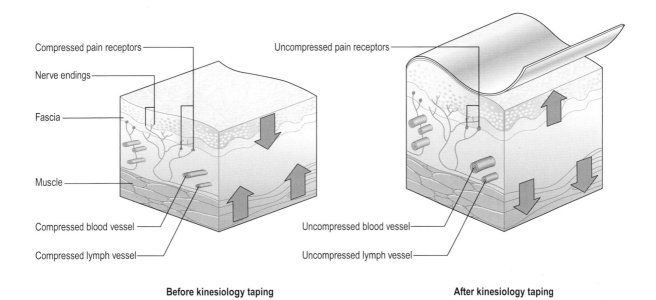

Before kinesiology taping   After kinesiology taping

Figure 9.1
This diagram demonstrates the recoiling of the elastic tape on the skin causing undulations and resulting additional space in the skin layers.
(Image adapted from an image provided courtesy fo the KTAI.)

amplitudes of undulation, interstitial pressures are less; fluids will move along these gradients in the direction of tape recoiling. This reduces fluid stasis and reduces swelling, edema, and bruising. The movement of interstitial fluids also reduces the fluid-induced pressures exerted on sensory receptors in the skin and underlying tissues and reduces pain sensations.

Structural Effects
One of the quintessential conundrums in manual therapies and bodywork is deciding if form dictates function or if function dictates form. The mutually influential elements of human anatomy (form) and physiology (function) continuously challenge practitioners in treatment planning and intervention selection, especially when dealing with pain. At times, misalignment of human structures

exhibits undue stress on both additional structures and physiological processes; at other times, physiological processes of the body exhibit undue stress on the body's structures. In both instances, pain can result. Manual therapists will often combine both structural interventions and methods that alter physiological processes to mitigate or

---

Sidebar 9.3 Patient Interviews
In response to the question, "Have your condition or symptoms or ability to function changed since receiving care?" a 28-year-old man with hip and leg pain replied: "Muscles tension/soreness that typically progresses to performance-limiting levels does not progress to those same levels with massage. Taping has changed movement habits, posture habits, and improved awareness of movement."

treat pain. Kinesio® Taping is a wonderful example of a complementary intervention that can affect both form and function.

Joint-centered structural Kinesio® Taping applications involve manually placing a joint (or joints) into a physiological efficient position within a pain-free range of motion. Tape is applied with significant stretch to support the joint in this new position. The recoil properties of the tape provide a continuous feedback to the central nervous system and to proprioceptors—muscle spindle and Golgi tendon receptors in muscle fibers, Pacini's corpuscles and Ruffini's endings in fascia and joint capsules—encouraging the joint to be held into this new position as long as the tape is applied and maintains its recoil ability. The ability to stimulate these deeper proprioceptors is based on the fact that similar proprioceptors are located in the deeper layers of the skin and that compressing and/or stretching the superficial proprioceptors in the skin will create a parallel reaction in the proprioceptors in the deeper fascia, muscle fibers, and soft tissues of the joints. Structural corrections, then, can help break pain cycles that may be caused by postural distortion or hypermobility of an unstable or misaligned joint.

The treatment of patellofemoral syndrome exhibits this nicely. The improper tracking of the patella over the femoral condyles often causes pain. Kinesio® Taping applications to support correct tracking of the patella have been documented to reduce pain and restore normal function of the patellofemoral joint mechanics (Callaghan 2012; Holtzman and Harris-Hayes 2012; Kuru, Yalman, and Dereil 2012; Campolo 2013).

Pain-causing postural distortions or joint misalignment may be the result of an imbalance in the gamma motor system in the muscles that stabilize joints. If the tone of muscle spindles is high, the muscle is "facilitated;" if the tone is low, the muscle is "inhibited." Kinesio® Taping applied from the insertion to the origin of a muscle (an inhibiting application), recoiling in the direction of muscle fiber lengthening, sends a sensory impulse to the spinal cord that the muscle is shortened and pulling on its tendon. This impulse initiates a reflex that causes muscle fibers to lengthen, thus mitigating a pulling force that may injure a tendon. KT applied from the origin of a muscle to the insertion of the muscle (a facilitating application), recoiling in the direction of muscular contraction, has the opposite effect. The stimulus from recoil gives the proprioceptors a signal to engage muscle fibers (Kase et al. 2003; Freedman 2014).

Some Kinesio® Taping practitioners and instructors (Capobianco and van den Dries 2009) support using the Applied Kinesiology Challenge/Therapy Localization Test (Pollard, Bablis, and Bonello 2006) to determine the direction of tape application. This test involves placing a directional drag on the skin and observing a change in pain symptom and/or range of motion and to apply the tape in the direction of a favorable or desired outcome. Langendoen and Sertel (2011) suggest taping from the origin of a muscle to the insertion of a muscle and that the amount of tension of the taping application will dictate facilitation or inhibition (more tension or less tension, respectively). Further study is needed to support these theories. My clinical experience, however, supports that, in many instances, a resulting joint repositioning or postural change will establish a new balance in the musculature, affecting joint positioning or posture, and clients report a resulting decrease in pain symptoms (see Figure 9.2).

Sidebar 9.4 Patient Interviews

In response to the question, "Have your condition or symptoms or ability to function changed since receiving care?" a 44-year-old man with knee pain for 5 years replied: "Prior to seeing John, I couldn't stand for short periods of time or walk even short distances without severe knee pain and swelling. After 2 years, I can walk and cycle for exercise and engage in daily PT. I can work without limitations and I feel like an active member of my household. Words can't describe how much my life has changed for the better."

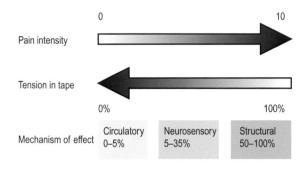

Figure 9.2

This graphic demonstrates: (a) the inversely proportional relationship between pain intensity and the tension of Kinesio® Taping application, and (b) the relationship between mechanisms of effect and the tension of Kinesio® Taping applications.

Kinesiology Taping and Current Pain Theories

The neuromatrix theory (Melzack 1999, 2005) acknowledges that pain is produced by an output of a widely distributed neural network in the brain rather than by a sensory, nociceptive input evoked by pathology. Loesser's Onion Skin Theory of Pain similarly incorporates the multidimensional aspect of pain—starting from a physical stressor, to how pain is perceived, to suffering caused by pain, one's behavior in reaction to pain and finally the interaction of the person in pain with their environment.

Kinesio® Taping applications can mitigate nociceptive pain sensations. The applications provide a visible and/or a tactile reminder to the pain sufferer of their discomfort. Emotionally, they acknowledge their pain and are actively participating in their own care. My clients have shared that the application of Kinesio® Taping helps to encourage modifying any behaviors that reduce their symptoms. One client reported that helpers in his workplace were more respectful of his attempts to work and offered to help him more frequently when he wore a short-sleeved shirt displaying a forearm taping application. These instances indicate that the Kinesio® Taping application appears to work in more than just the physical realm—but also in psycho-emotional and environmental realms. This illustrates the onion skin model of pain as described by Loeser and also in realms described by Melzack (2005) in his neuromatrix theory of pain.

Methodology

In order to select and administer appropriate pain management interventions, healthcare providers must first assess their client's condition and presentation. **Functional taping** has many possible outcomes and affects many different tissues and/or structures, all of which need to be considered—the skin, superficial and deep fascia, muscles, joint structure and function, physiological pathologies such as edema, inflammation, postural deviations, and compromised movement patterns.

Assessment

Typically, my assessment starts with a detailed client history where I cover diagnoses, injuries, symptoms, treatments or interventions used currently or in the past, and the client's treatment goals. Sometimes there is a clearly identified or articulated diagnosis (e.g. arthritis, sprained ankle) that explains the pain symptoms; at other times, this is not the case (e.g. undiagnosed, nonspecific low back pain, lumbago). Questions I frequently ask to help understand my client's pain include (but are not limited to): How would you describe your pain? What is your level of discomfort? How does this affect your day-to-day functioning? Where do you feel your pain specifically? Does the pain remain in one area or does it travel? When did you first feel the pain? Are there activities that aggravate the pain? Does anything you do relieve your pain? Have you ever had this pain or a similar pain before? When? For how long? How did you relieve it? Have you seen any other healthcare professional such as a physician, chiropractor, osteopath, physical therapist, acupuncturist, etc?

During this interviewing and active listening period, visual assessment of the client includes observing posture and body language, display of restlessness, anxiety or other emotional states, breathing patterns, energy level, and facial expressions. I then assess the client's posture for asymmetry, contributing joints for pain-free ROM, and movement ability including gait analysis.

The client then moves to the therapy table for palpation assessments. The assessments include visual—to detect skin color and textural variations—and manual palpation to detect temperature variations and elasticity of the skin and superficial connective tissues, swelling or edema, tissue gliding or adhesions. Moving to deeper tissues, muscles, musculotendinous junctions, tendons, and ligaments are palpated similarly to detect anomalies in contractile fibers and/or to identify areas of adhesions. Additionally, I examine the tissue for hypertone or hypotone, often due to excessive or impaired neurological function, respectively.

The assessment findings will guide massage session plan development and execution. After the execution of the therapeutic massage, areas of pain and extensive soft tissue work will be re-evaluated and re-assessed. I will apply functional taping if additional physiological or structural change is desired or to extend the duration affect of the massage. Because I am formally trained by the Kinesio® Taping Association International and have achieved the Certified Kinesio® Taping Practitioner (CKTP®) designation, I will only speak of Kinesio® Taping applications. Other tapes and taping applications follow similar principles and have been reported to achieve similar results.

Kinesio® Tex Tape

The Kinesio® Taping method is based on the trilogy of assessment, tape application, then reassess and modify if necessary. The Kinesio® Tex Tape is a latex-free, polymer elastic strand wrapped by 100% cotton fibers, backed with an acrylic, heat-activated

adhesive patterned like the human fingerprint. It is applied to a paper substrate with approximately 10–15% longitudinal stretch in its fibers. The tape is not designed to stretch horizontally. The cotton allows for evaporation of body moisture and quick drying of the tape after getting wet. The tape is about the thickness of the epidermis and can longitudinally stretch approximately 60% of its resting length. Rubbing the tape gently after it is applied to the skin activates the adhesive.

To maximize wearing time, the fingerprint pattern of the adhesive assists with the lifting of the skin from deeper tissue layers and also allows for areas from which moisture can escape. The elasticity of Kinesio® Taping allows for free movement of the taped area and retains its therapeutic effectiveness for 3–5 days on average. The tape must be applied to oil- and moisture-free skin and at least 30 minutes prior to significant activity or rigorous exercise. It is also recommended to remove body hair by shaving or trimming prior to tape application.

The tape is stretched to desired tension levels over the therapeutic area only. Tape is usually applied to stretched tissue.

Kinesio® Taping applications are contraindicated over any open wounds; over any active malignancy sites; over cellulitis, skin infections, irritations or rashes; or over deep vein thromboses (or suspected DVTs). While not contraindicated, approval from a physician is recommended when a client has diabetes, any kidney disease, congestive heart failure, coronary artery disease, or peripheral artery disease. Tape should also never cross the axilla or groin. KTT should be removed immediately if the client feels itchy or if there is any increase in pain symptoms.

Kinesiology Taping Cuts

The desired outcome of a taping application dictates the cut or design of a taping application and the amount of tension with which the tape is applied to the skin. The simplest cut is called an "I" strip (see Figure 9.3). This application is applied directly over

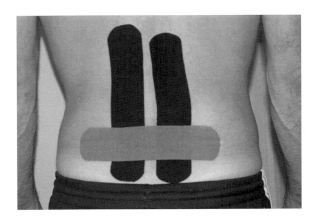

Figure 9.3
The application of I-strips along the paraspinal musculature and over painful spinal segments is effective in minimizing nonspecific low back pain.

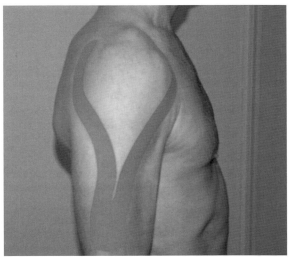

Figure 9.4
The application of a Y-strip surrounding the deltoid muscle group is a common application in the treatment of shoulder pain and dysfunction.

an area of injury or pain. The tension of the tape can be in the center of the "I", resulting in recoil towards the center of the application, or with no tension at one end of the application, resulting in recoil towards this base. This application is effective following acute injury to decompress tissues and reduce pain, over an area of myofascial adhesion to mobilize the underlying tissues, or when trying to stimulate proprioceptors to modify the position of a joint.

Another use of the "I" strip is called a functional correction application. Practitioners use this application when the desired outcome is sensory stimulation to either assist or limit motion. The tape is applied to the skin with no tension at its bases. Active movement created by the client creates the tension in the therapeutic zone of the tape. For example, to assist flexion at a joint, the joint is first placed into flexion. The tape is then applied 2 inches (5 cm) proximal and 2 inches (5 cm) distal to the joint. The practitioner secures the bases of tape with their hands and asks the client to actively move into extension. The practitioner then finishes the tape application by moving both hands towards the center of the tape. Theoretically, the client will

perceive stimuli that assist with flexion and resist extension. Current hypothesis is that mechanoreceptors will interpret this stimulus as normal joint position. Flexion will be assisted, as the perception of tension in extension will cause the joint to reposition into flexion to normalize the tension in the skin.

To treat areas of localized pain or tissue adhesion, a series of "I" strips may be applied to nonjoint areas including muscle bellies or fascial planes such as aponeuroses, retinacula, or areas of significant connective tissue convergence. These strips may be oriented in an "X" shape or in a "star" shape. Each strip will have a different angle of recoil and will create different areas of tissue decompression and/or fluid movements. This may contribute to greater symptom relief.

The most common application applied to muscle tissue is the "Y" strip (see Figure 9.4). This cut is created by simply cutting down the center of an "I" strip, creating an area that serves as an anchor or base and two "tails." It is designed to surround a muscle and the anchor is applied with no tension approximately 1–2 inches (2.5–5 cm) from an attachment. The tails of the "Y" are applied with equal tension and completely surround the muscle being taped. The direction of the application can be proximal (origin) to distal (insertion) to facilitate a muscle or distal to proximal to inhibit a muscle.

Over areas of inflammation, bruising or edema, a "fan" strip application is most appropriate to use (see Figure 9.5). The tails are placed, equally spaced and without tension, directly over the affected area. The anchor is placed proximal to an area of lesser congestion along a lymphatic pathway or proximal to a lymph node. The recoil of the fan strips changes the fluid pressures beneath the skin, resulting in a movement of fluids along the pathway of tape recoil. During active motion, the tape recoil also creates a massage-like action that may accelerate the draining of congested fluids. Anecdotally, I have also used "fan" strip applications over areas of localized pain to reduce symptoms with success. Perhaps, in addition

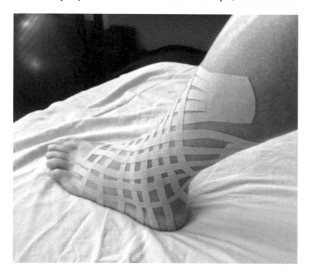

Figure 9.5
This fan-strip application is used to reduce swelling and pain after a lateral ankle sprain.

to creating pressure gradients to allow for movement of fluids, the recoiling of the strips of tape may also create gradients of decompression on sensory nerves, thus creating the symptom reduction.

There are several highly dissected cuts Kinesio® Taping applications similar to "fan" cuts. "Web" strip and "jellyfish" applications also contain several narrow strips of Kinesio® Tex Tape. These applications are most commonly used over a joint while at its extreme limit of motion, but can also be used over any tissue where there is edema or where pain is felt. These applications are most commonly used in acute pain presentations. There is minimal tension applied to the tape. The recoil of the strips causes significant rippling or undulations in the tape and creates a lifting of the skin from underlying tissues. This results in significant movement of inflammatory or edematous fluids. Additionally, the application also contributes

Sidebar 9.5 Research
Patients were asked to take no pain-relieving or anti-inflammatory medications 72 hours prior to the study by Gonzalez-Iglesias and colleagues (2009). Taping for acute pain from whiplash and range of motion were tested in this randomized clinical trial (RCT). Patients were allocated to the intervention group or sham taping group. The intervention group reported statistically significant decreases in pain and improved range of motion, compared to the sham taping group. These statistically significant findings were reported immediately following the intervention (or sham taping) and at 24 hours post taping (Gonzalez-Iglesias et al. 2009). These authors offer a hypothesis on mechanism of effect being tension in the tape applied to the intervention group, whereas no tension existed in the sham tape group. Thelan observed good functional outcomes for populations with shoulder pain; immediately following taping in the RCT, participants were able to move their shoulders, pain-free (Thelen, Dauber, and Stoneman 2008).

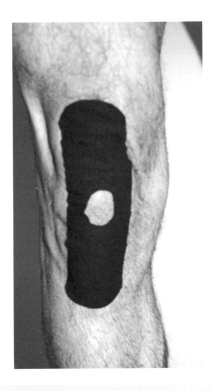

Figure 9.6
Donut applications are effective in reducing pain after trauma and in chronic situations such as osteoarthritis. Note the convolutions created by the recoiling of the tape.

to decompression in areas rich in sensory nerves, and significant relief of pain symptoms results.

A "donut" strip application is also created from the basic "I" strip. At the center of the strip, a circular opening is cut (see Figure 9.6). This opening is placed directly over a painful joint area, an area of localized inflammation, or an area of localized pain symptoms first. Then, the remaining tape is applied by applying tension in opposite directions away from the opening. The recoil of the tape draws tissue into the area of the opening and creates pressure and fluid gradients that will reduce edema, swelling from inflammation, and pain symptoms. It is also possible to create multiple angles of tissue

pressure and fluid gradients by layering "donut" strips in an "X" pattern or a "star" pattern. This may result in greater symptom relief.

Tension of Kinesio® Taping in Kinesio® Taping Applications

The desired outcome dictates the cut or design of a taping application and the amount of tension in the therapeutic zone. Because the tape is capable of stretching an additional 40% of its length, the variation of tension of taping applications can vary from 0% tension (tape simply applied to the skin without any added stretch or tension) to 100% tension (tape is stretched to its maximum length).

The Kinesio® Taping training seminars promote the theory that different tension applications yield different outcomes and results (see Figure 9.7). To create space and pressure gradients by lifting the skin from its underlying layers, zero to light tension is recommended. Applications with minimal tension yield best results when pain is acute. In subacute situations or when inhibiting muscle or fascia tissue is desired, light tension (15–25%) is the preferred application. To facilitate muscle or fascia tissue, moderate tension (25–35%) is suggested. During rehabilitation after painful injury or for the stimulation of proprioceptors to encourage repositioning of a joint or to alter postural and movement habits, heavy or severe tension (50–75%) should be applied. Full tension (75–100%) is applied when the suggestion of joint support is indicated (e.g. taping applied to ligaments when treating a sprained ankle).

Reassessment

Once a practitioner has the requisite client history and subjective information, completes their objective assessments, selects and applies an appropriate manual therapy intervention and Kinesio® Taping application, it is critically important to enter a period of reassessment. At the conclusion of the therapeutic session, I always recheck the taping application to ensure that the therapeutic zone is where I had originally

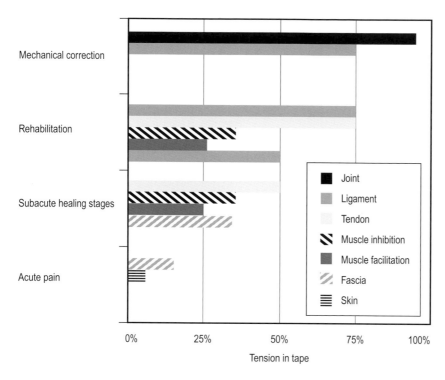

Figure 9.7
This figure compares the amount of tension applied to the therapeutic zone of Kinesio® Tex Tape to the tissues targeted and the type of taping application used.

intended, the application surrounds target tissues if needed, that edges of the anchors are not curling or pulling away from the skin, and the client is comfortable with the taping application. I also ask the client to walk or move around to be certain the tape is not pulling excessively on hair or skin and that movement is not impeded. If any of the aforementioned proves to be true, or raises any concern or uncertainty, I will remove the faulty Kinesio® Taping application and reapply.

To check the success of a taping application, I will reassess to understand if there has been any change in the client's pain symptoms by the end of their session. After the visit, I call the client and ask if they are experiencing any reduction in pain or other symptoms, if there is an increase in pain-free range of movement and performance of normal activities of daily living. This will give me an indication of the success of the therapeutic intervention and Kinesio® Taping application, or lack of it.

Sidebar 9.6 Patient Interviews
When asked, "What have you learned about this treatment approach or self-care that you would like healthcare providers to know about?", replies included:

- "Primary care doctors must understand that these resources are available and that this is a real and tangible way that they can help their patients."

- "Most importantly, I'd like them to know about the change in perspective on body function that can be gained from massage, such as the interaction between emotional/mental states and physical states, how to look at each "injury" as a unique situation that is not only affecting the area of pain instead of a preconceived diagnosis. I'd like people to know that this type of treatment is beneficial for overall health as well as specific injuries."

At the client's next visit, I will update with the client's history and subjective report of symptoms and activities. For an objective analysis, I will repeat each assessment originally performed and chart any change. If the outcomes were achieved, the manual therapy intervention and Kinesio® Taping application will be repeated. If the outcomes are less than what we desired, modifications will be made in either the tension used to apply the tape, the therapeutic zone, and the cut of the taping application, or the body part(s) taped.

Self-care Applications

Some Kinesio® Taping applications afford practitioners the possibility of instructing the clients on applying Kinesio® Tex Tape themselves. Practitioners must teach how to measure and cut tape, the appropriate body positioning and stretch of the tissues to which the tape will be applied, and the amount of tension applied to the tape in the therapeutic zone. Clients can then actively participate in their own pain management or recovery to ensure continuity of care with Kinesio® Taping applications between therapeutic sessions. Practitioners can sell the Kinesio® Tex Tape to clients directly, or clients can purchase the tape directly from a wide range of suppliers.

Several elastic, kinesiology tape brands sell individually packaged, pre-cut, standardized taping applications specific to a body region or to address a common complaint or symptom. The pre-cut tape can be slightly modified, mostly by shortening, to accommodate different body types. These individual packages include printed suggestions on appropriate application including body positioning, stretching the tissue to which the tape is applied, and amount of tension applied to the therapeutic zone.

Because the tape is available for purchase by the general public, and because "how-to" application videos are found on the worldwide web, many people will do their own personal research and make taping applications without the benefit of instruction from a trained or trusted practitioner. Usually, individuals will self-diagnose or self-assess and apply tape in the area

Sidebar 9.7 Patient Interviews

When asked, "Do you feel differently about yourself or your pain since receiving care?", replies included:

- "I understand my body much better and have a better understanding of factors that trigger pain/discomfort. I have learned to adapt my lifestyle to accommodate my condition and I'm getting closer to accepting this. I understand that I now have a chronic condition that needs regular care and maintenance but I'm optimistic that I'll continue to improve."

- "I have become more sensitive to small changes in feelings in muscles that are frequently worked on, and more confident that my body is functioning as it should. Anxiety about proper muscle function and performance has decreased."

of their symptoms or will accept a recommendation or instruction from a coach, training partner, or friend.

Self-applications, without the benefit of professional assessment, might present challenges that could interfere with achieving maximum benefit from Kinesio® Taping applications from a trained professional. Individuals might apply tape to an area of pain and not to the area causing the symptoms. The individual may not have a joint appropriately positioned for a support application; muscle and connective tissues may not be stretched sufficiently or at all, or the tension over the therapeutic zone may be insufficient or excessive. Additionally, individuals may not reassess properly after a self-taping application to monitor results and make modifications to the application if necessary.

Case Study

One of my clients is a 63-year-old professional oboist with a diagnosis of rheumatoid arthritis (RA). She originally came for massage 8 years ago for hip pain and continued to use massage prior to and after bilateral hip arthroplasty in 2008. In addition to massage therapy, she also received regular chiropractic care. A short time after surgery, she began to realize a generalized, warm, throbbing type of pain and a generalized sense of muscular weakness in her wrist, elbow, and shoulder. She explored several options with her rheumatologist and orthopedic surgeon including experimental stem-cell transplant therapy and elbow replacement surgery. Symptoms became severe and her ability to practice and perform decreased, affecting her ability to work. While there was no support in the literature or training materials available at the time for Kinesio® Taping applications as an intervention for RA, both the client and I agreed to try. Since beginning Kinesio® Taping applications with this client, Szczegielniak et al. (2012) have reported Kinesio® Taping as an effective intervention in physical therapy of RA in the hand.

The client's subjective history and resisted muscle testing indicated weakness in the flexors and extensors of the wrist and fingers and biceps brachii of her right upper extremity. Passive range-of-motion testing and reports from her orthopedic surgeon indicated ligamentous weakness in the right elbow and wrist. Postural analysis

revealed a slightly forward head posture and right shoulder positioning. Based on this information, the first Kinesio® Taping applications we opted to try included ligamentous support of the wrist with 50% tension and facilitation of the flexors and extensors of the wrist with 50% tension.

The client reported significant increases in pain and decreased mobility within the first hours of the tape application. She was instructed to remove all applications. On her next visit, the assessment tests were repeated and yielded the same results. The Kinesio® Taping applications were repeated with 25% tension, yielding similar results to the first application. I began to think that the facilitation applications were too stimulating. On the third visit, I eliminated the ligamentous application on the wrist and changed the forearm application to inhibit the flexors and extensors of the wrist and fingers. The client reported significant reduction of pain almost immediately and the relief lasted for about 4 days but she reported increasing fatigue in her arm.

On the fourth visit, I continued the inhibition tapings of the extensors and flexors and added an inhibition of the biceps brachii and triceps

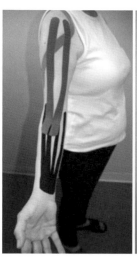 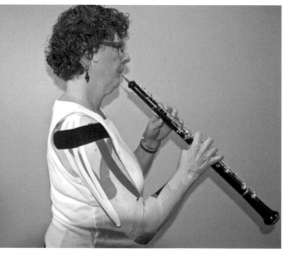

Figure 9.8
These photographs demonstrate the Kinesio® Taping application used to assist this musician maintain her practice and performance schedules.

brachii. At the suggestion of her chiropractor, I also added an inhibition of the deltoid group. After this application, the client reported both significant pain reduction and less fatigue than previously experienced.

On her fifth visit, she reported less pain and fatigue in her arm, but more fatigue in the shoulders. Repeating the postural analysis revealed an increase in the protraction of the right scapula and anterior rounding of the right shoulder. Tapings to reduce anterior gliding and depression of the humerus in the glenohumeral joint were introduced. The client reported significant relief (see Figure 9.8).

Without regular assessment, modification, and reassessment, the Kinesio® Taping applications would not have been successful. To date, 7 years later, we continue this application weekly. The client is mostly pain free and able to keep full practice and performance schedules.

Conclusion

Support for the use of elastic taping interventions is scant in the literature. What resources can be found are oftentimes of questionable quality (Beutel and Cardone 2014). However, while more research is needed to understand the mechanisms of action, we cannot ignore the fact that practitioners and individuals alike have been using kinesiology taping applications to relieve pain symptoms safely and effectively. Using interventions involving structural, circulatory, and neurosensory approaches, practitioners have been taping clients and patients of all ages and levels of activity. With few known and understood contraindications and concerns, applications have been used to treat myriad pain conditions that are localized, referred, or systemic, caused by specific pathologies, complex syndromes and even when etiology is unknown. Kinesiology taping is noninvasive, well tolerated, and inexpensive—making it difficult to overlook as a viable method of pain management.

References

Beutel, B., and D. Cardone. 2014. Kinesiology taping. Kinesiology Taping and the world wide web: A quality and content analysis of internet-based information. *The International Journal of Sports Physical Therapy* 9(5):665–72.

Callaghan, M. J., S. McKie, P. Richardson, and J. A. Oldham. 2012. Effects of patellar taping on brain activity during knee joint proprioception tests using functional magnetic resonance imaging. *Physical Therapy* 92(6):821–30.

Calvino, B. 1990. Is spinal cord dorsolateral funiculus involved in hypoalgesia induced by counter-irritation? *Behavioral Brain Research* 39(2):97–111.

Campolo, M., J. Babu, K. Dmochowska, S. Scariah, and J Varughese. 2013. A comparison of two taping techniques (Kinesio and McConnell) and their effect on anterior knee pain during functional activities. *International Journal of Sports Physical Therapy* 8(2):105–10.

Carlton, S. M. 2014. Nociceptive primary afferents: they have a mind of their own. *Journal of Physiology* 592:3404–11.

Capobianco, S., and G. van den Dries. 2009. *Power taping—theories and practical applications of fascial movement taping,* version 3.2. Los Gatos, CA: RockTape Inc.

Flor, H. 2003. Cortical reorganisation and chronic pain: implications for rehabilitation. *Journal of Rehabilitative Medicine* Supplement, 41:66–72.

Freedman, D. 2014. Kinesiology taping theory and application. Webinar, April 2, 2014.

Freedman, S., L. T. Brody, M. Rosenthal, and J. Wise. 2014. Short-term effects of patellar kinesio taping on pain and hop function in patients with patellofemoral pain syndrome. *Sport Health* 6(4):294–300.

Gibney, V. P. 1893. The modern treatment of sprained ankle. *The New York Polyclinic.*

Gonzalez-Iglesias, J., C. Fernandez-De-Las Penas, J. Cleland, P. Huijbregts, M. Del Rosario Gutierrze-Vega. 2009. Short-term effects of cervical kinesio taping on pain and cervical range of motion in patients with acute whiplash injury: a randomized clinical trial. *Journal of Orthopaedic & Sports Physical Therapy* 39(7):515–21.

Gudin, J. 2004. Expanding our understanding of central sensitization. http://www.medscape.org/viewarticle/481798 (accessed November 2, 2014).

Hecker, H., and K. Liebchen, K. 2005. *Acupressure taping.* Rochester, VT: Healing Arts Press.

Holtzman, G. W., and M. Harris-Hayes. 2012. Treatment of patella alta with taping, exercise, mobilization, and functional activity modification: a case report. *Physiotherapy Theory and Practice* 28(1):71–83.

Kase, K., J. Wallis, and T. Kase. 2003. *Clinical therapeutic applications of the KinesioTaping method,* 3rd edn. Tokyo, Japan: Ken Ikai Co.

Kuru, T., A. Yalıman, and E. Dereil. 2012. Comparison of efficiency of Kinesio® taping and electrical stimulation in patients with patellofemoral pain syndrome. *Acta Orthopaedica et Traumatologica Turcica* 46(5):385–92.

Lang, P., and M. Takakura. 2013. Pilot study: The effect of recoil on the tissue layer measured by diagnostic ultrasound, presented at the 2013 Kinesio® Taping Association International Research Sympoisum, Stanford University, Palo Alto, CA, June 9.

Langendoen, J., and K. Sertel. 2011. *Kinesiology Taping the essential step-by-step guide.* Toronto, Ontario, Canada: Robert Rose Inc.

Lowry, C. D, J. A. Cleland, and K. Dyke. 2008. Management of patients with patellofemoral pain syndrome using a multimodal approach: a case series. *The Journal of Orthopaedic and Sports Physical Therapy* 38(11):691–702.

McAllister, M. 2012. What is central sensitization? http://www.instituteforchronicpain.org/understanding-chronic-pain/what-is-chronic-pain/central-sensitization (accessed November 2, 2014).

Mackenzie, J. 1909. Counter-irritation. *Proc R Soc Med* 2 (Therapeutical and Pharmacological Section):75–80.

Melzack, R. 1999. From the gate to the neuromatrix. *Pain* Suppl 6:S121–6.

Melzack, R. 2005. Evolution of the neuromatrix theory of pain. The Prithvi Raj Lecture, presented at the Third World Congress of World Institute of Pain, Barcelona 2004. *Pain Practice: The Official Journal of World Institute of Pain* 5(2):85–94.

Melzack, R., and P. D. Wall. 1965. Pain mechanisms: a new theory. *Science* 19; 150(3699):971–9.

Paoloni, M., G. Fratocchi, M. Mangone, M. Murgia, V. Santilli, and A. Cacchio. 2012. Long-term efficacy of a short period of taping followed by an exercise program in a cohort of patients with patellofemoral pain syndrome. *Clinical Rheumatology* 31(3):535–39.

Parreira, Pdo C. C. Costa Lda, L. C. Hespanhol Jr., A. D. Lopes, and L. O. Costa. 2014a. Current evidence does not support the use of kinesiotaping in clinical practice: a systematic review. *Journal of Physiotherapy* 60(1):31–39. doi: 10.1016/j.jphys.2013.12.008. Epub 2014 Apr 24.

Parreira, Pdo C. C. Costa Lda, R. Takahashi, L. C. Hespanhol Jr., M. A. Luz Jr., T. M. Silva, and L. O. Costa. 2014b. KinesioTaping to generate skin convolutions is not better than sham taping for

people with chronic non-specific low back pain: a randomised trial. *Journal of Physiotherapy* 60(2):90–6. DOI:10.1016/j.jphys.2014.05.003. Epub2014 Jun 10.

Perl, E. R. 2007. Perspectives: Ideas about pain, a historical view. *Neuroscience* 8:71–80.

Perrin, D. H. 2012. *Athletic Taping and Bracing,* 3rd edn. Champaign, IL: Human Kinetics.

Pollard, H. P., P. Bablis, and R. Bonello. 2006. The ileo-cecal valve point and muscle testing: a possible mechanism of action. *Chiropractic Journal of Australia.* 36(4):122–6.

Schweinhardt, P. 2011. Commentary: The many faces of counter-irritation. *Pain* 152:1445–6.

Szczegielniak, J., J. Luniewski, K. Bogacz, and Z. Sliwiński. 2012. The use of KinesiologyTaping method in patients with rheumatoid hand—pilot study. *Ortopedia, Traumatologia, Rehabilitacja* 14(1):23–30.

Thelen, M.D., J. A. Dauber, and P. D. Stoneman. 2008. The clinical efficacy of kinesio tape for shoulder pain: a randomized, double-blinded, clinical trial. *J. Orthop. Sports Phys. Ther.* 38(7):389–95.

Warden, S. J., R. S. Hinman, M. A. Watson, Jr., K. G. Avin, A. E. Bialocerkowski, and K. M. Crossley. 2008. Patellar taping and bracing for the treatment of chronic knee pain: a systematic review and meta-analysis. *Arthritis & Rheumatism (Arthritis Care & Research)* 59(1):73– 83. doi 10.1002/art.23242.

Williams, H. F. 1923. Therapeutic value of counter irritation. *Transactions of the American Climatological and Clinical Association* XXXIX:74–9.

Woolf, C. J. 2011. Central Sensitization: Implications for the diagnosis and treatment of pain. *Pain* 152(3 Supplement): S2–S15.

Wong, V. 2013. MRI of the soft tissues before and after Kinesio® Taping, presented at the 2013 Kinesio® Taping International Research Symposium. Stanford University, Palo Alto, CA.

Additional Resources

Gibbons, J. 2014. *A Practical Guide to Kinesio® Taping,* 1st edn. Nutbourne, Chichester: Lotus Publishing.

Kase, K. 2003. *Illustrated Kinesio® Taping,* 4th edn. Albuquerque, NM: Ken Ikai Co.

Kase, K. 2006. *Kinesio® Taping in Pediatrics,* 2nd edn. Albuquerque, NM: Kinesio USA, LLC.

Kase, K., and K. R. Stockheimer. 2006. *Kinesio® Taping for Lymphoedema and Chronic Swelling,* 1st edn. Albuquerque, NM: Kinesio USA, LLC.

Kinesio® Taping Association International. 2009. *KT 1 Workbook*. Albuquerque, NM: Kinesio Taping Association International.

Kinesio® Taping Association International. 2009. *KT 2 Workbook*. Albuquerque, NM: Kinesio Taping Association International.

Kinesio® Taping Association International. 2009. *KT 3 Workbook*. Albuquerque, NM: Kinesio Taping Association International.

Kinesio® Taping Association International. 2014. *KT 4 Workbook*. Albuquerque, NM: Kinesio Taping Association International.

www.kinesiotaping.com

www.kttape.com

www.rocktape.com

www.spidertech.com

www.strengthtape.com

www.youtube.com

There are many instructional YouTube videos demonstrating kinesiology taping applications for myriad conditions and client presentations.

Traditional Chinese medicine bodywork: Tui Na

Introduction
The Art of Tui Na

A modality within **traditional Chinese medicine (TCM)**, **Tui Na** is the application of hands-on techniques, either directly to the affected injury region or on the related acupuncture meridians, acupuncture points, or Tui Na pressure points. Acupuncture requires complicated equipment such as needles for penetrating the skin, **moxa** to burn the needles, cups to pull the skin, a seven-star hammer for dermal stimulation, alcohol, and cotton balls to light a fire for the cups and sterilize the skin. Unlike acupuncture, Tui Na requires no equipment, and addresses pain mainly through the application of hands-on techniques: Tui Na practitioners apply their own body as a tool to heal the patient's pain. The techniques do not penetrate the skin so there is no possibility of infection, and acupuncture needle fainting is avoided. Tui Na is a welcomed treatment for all ages, from infants to the elderly, because patients are not afraid of it.

Tui Na includes what is well known as acupressure, manipulation of soft tissues and bone setting.

Acupressure is where the practitioner uses their fingers, fists, elbows, knees, and feet to stimulate acupuncture points instead of using needles.

Soft tissue manipulation is used to regain the size of the tissue and reset its original position. Practitioners use the manipulation techniques to reduce the swollen tissues, i.e. rehabilitate the disused or neurogenic atrophic soft tissues.

Bone-setting therapy, a key component in Tui Na, is an orthopedic treatment for motor system diseases such as bone fracture and joint dislocation from sports injury or trauma. Unique to Tui Na, bone setting does not require imaging testing, surgery, or anesthesia; instead, the practitioner applies traction to the long axis of the injured limb and reverses the mechanism of fracture. After the reduction, several small splints are used to cast the affected bone or joint with a topical plaster. The closed reduction is faster and less expensive than open reduction and internal fixation (ORIF), because it is less surgically time-consuming, does not need to be done at a surgical facility, can be done at the injury scene, does not require radiology testing or application of anesthesia medication; closed reduction also decreases the risk of complications due to foreign bodies (Knotts 2012).

Tui Na has no site limit: it can be applied at the scene of injury, and does not require a special treatment table or a chair, nor does it require diagnostic equipment. A Tui Na practitioner usually makes an initial diagnosis through palpation and can immediately provide treatments on site. For instance, in the case of a patient who suffers from a sprained ankle while hiking on a forest trail, a Tui Na practitioner is able to palpate the injured ankle and provide treatment to ease the pain on site.

Tui Na is a great hands-on tool to release stagnation of wind, damp, cold, **Qi**, and blood, and Tui Na produces few negative side effects, unlike herbal or pharmaceutical medicine that might cause chemical-based side effects. Tui Na treatments may result in slight short-term bruising if the purpose of the treatment is to release a blockage due to blood stagnation. For example, with an acute lower back pain, a Tui Na practitioner may press the popliteal fossa forcefully with the tip of the thumb, which may leave a bruising mark for a time. In TCM, side effects such as bruising are considered part of the treatment: the bruise is intended to release blood stasis, and inflammation is part of the healing process (McCarthy 2003).

The Function of Tui Na

Tui Na is well known in the treatment of pain management, not only as a quick way to stop pain, but also as a self-care tool that patients

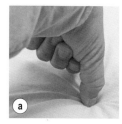
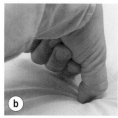
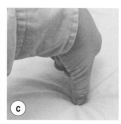
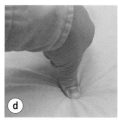
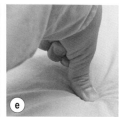

Figure 10.1

Yi Zhi Chan Tui Fa: One Finger Meditation Pushing Method. Photos a-e show a serious of thumb positions that demonstrate the full spectrum of the one-finger meditation method.

Meaning of the name:
Yi - one
Zhi - finger
Chan - meditation
Tui - pushing
Fa - method

Clinical purpose:
This method can be used to treat channel problems and is an excellent technique to help move chronically stagnant Qi and blood.

Application location:
This technique can be used on practically all parts of the body, especially on acupuncture points and Ah-shi points.

Application methods:
The method is one where the radial side of the thumb is held against the skin at the point selected and shaken and simultaneously kneaded for approximately 250 repetitions per minute.

can easily learn and apply to manage their own pain. Another application of Tui Na is to warm the affected area, and this is called balancing Yin and Yang. For example, applying Tui Na techniques on the Yang meridians, such as on the head or the back, increases Yang energy, which will warm the body, i.e. help the patient to fight cold; Yang energy also increases antibodies, helps the patient's immunity, and can aid fatigue by increasing energy (Ying Xia 2013).

In addition, Tui Na is also used to accelerate blood flow, which is intended to release spasms within muscles, tight tendons, and ligaments. This is called opening meridians, regulating Qi and blood, and is useful when treating chronic lower back pain (McCarthy 2003). Yi Zhi Chan Tui Fu, or One Finger Meditation Pushing Method, is commonly used to move chronically stagnant Qi and blood (see Figure 10.1).

With chronic joint pain or stiffness, Tui Na applies a treatment protocol called releasing adhesion, which lubricates joints to reduce or eliminate pain, and increases the joint range of motion. When a patient with a frozen shoulder receives Tui Na treatment, the shoulder's range of motion is limited. Tui Na's treatment principle on this is to return the shoulder range of motion to 180 degrees in abduction, 180 degrees in flexion, and 45 degrees in hyperextension and in internal rotation. Results of this treatment application typically find that female patients are able to touch T7 and male patients are able to touch T9 (thoracic vertebrae 7/9).

Tui Na is also useful for acute pain conditions. For example, it is the only Chinese medicine used for joint subluxation and dislocation. This treatment principle is called relocating joint. Tui Na can quickly resolve the issues of joint displacement, and it releases tension on the soft tissues in the joint and surrounding area (Yao-chi 2009), regaining normal joint movement and function. Unlike some joint manipulation techniques, Tui Na first releases the pressure and tension of the surrounding soft tissues, and then addresses the joint. Because the soft tissues are loosened, the joint can stay more firmly at the normal position for a longer period, and circulation is also improved because the loosened soft tissues are more able to supply blood to the area.

History and Related Modalities
The Names – "Tui Na" and "An Mo"

The name Tui Na (which literally means "pushing and grasping") was not presented in medical texts until *The Treasure of Tui Na for Kids* (小兒推拿秘訣), which was written during the Ming dynasty (AD 1368–1644). Prior to this, Tui Na was called **An Mo** (按摩) (which literally means "pressing and rubbing"). However, both terms exist in China, as explained below.

An Mo is believed to be the oldest tool to heal pain. The *Yellow Emperor's Internal Classic* (黃帝內經), the oldest medical text in China, written during the Warring States period (475–221 BC), includes nine chapters documenting the use of An Mo.

In China, the term Tui Na indicates a medical practice; it is the bodywork therapy based on the theories of TCM. The term An Mo is a relaxing massage that does not require any medical diagnosis. Thus, if one is looking for a relaxing massage, then a session from any spa will be appropriate; on the other hand, if one suffers from back pain and is looking for treatment, one should be admitted to a Tui Na department in a hospital (http://www.trhos.com/tcm/zhyamk/kpzs1.html).

The practitioners in Tui Na departments, who receive at least 5 years of medical school education, perform treatments based on the foundations of TCM, pathology, physiology, and diagnosis. In modern China, Western medical anatomy, physiology, and pathology are also applied in Tui Na practice to distinguish a disease; chemistry and radiology tests are also added to make further accuracy on the Western medical diagnosis.

The Modern History of Tui Na

Like other TCM modalities since the Ming dynasty, Tui Na was originally practiced and taught within families, and passed down through generations. After the Communist Revolution in 1949 in China, the new government made medicine standardized and systematized into a series of 5-year medical education programs. In 1956, a government-sponsored national Tui Na school was set up in Shanghai (上海). Two years later, in 1958, the nationwide Tui Na clinics were set up.

In 1979, the Department of Tui Na Therapy was established in the Shanghai Institute of Traditional Medicine College and, in July of that year, the first national Tui Na therapy conference was held in Shanghai (上海). Attending the conference were 108 famous experts from twenty-seven provinces, and ninety-eight Tui Na therapy theses were published.

Currently, Tui Na is widely practiced in Asian countries, including China, Hong Kong, Macao, Singapore, Tai Wan, Japan, and Korea, but it is less well known in the USA. Tui Na is taught as a separate but equal field of study in the major traditional Chinese medical colleges. Tui Na practitioners receive the same core training as acupuncturists and herbalists and enjoy the same level of professional respect.

Theoretical Approaches to Pain Management
Tui Na and Blood Circulation

Tui Na influences blood circulation locally, increasing circulation where Tui Na is being applied. Rolling Technique is used to promote circulation and relieve pain (see Figure 10.2) (McCarthy, 2003). Hyperthermia is achieved through increased blood

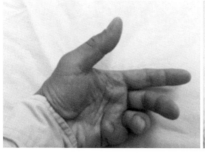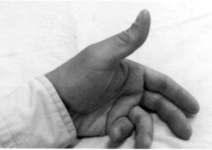

Figure 10.2
Gun Fa: Rolling Technique.

Meaning of the name:
Gun - rolling
Fa - technique

Clinical purpose:
This is a signature technique for Tui Na. Patients have a sensation of an object rolling above the application location. Through the vibration from the practitioner's hands, rolling technique promotes the circulation of the blood to the muscles and tendons and fascia and thereby helps to relieve pain.

Application location:
This technique can be used on all parts of the body except the head, face, chest, and abdomen.

Application methods:
Begin with your fifth finger edge on the treatment area, palm and fingers naturally flexed. Then, by extending your wrist, roll onto the back of your hand. Keep rolling until your arm is open and facing upwards with your fingers and wrist naturally extended, then roll your hand back to the starting position. The speed is about 300–360 times/minute.

circulation, promoting local blood capillary circulation and red blood cell production. In addition, the release of white blood cells is accelerated, which increases the oxygen within the local tissues, promotes the release of endorphins and plays an important role in the analgesic mechanism and repairing of injured tissues.

Tui Na and Endorphins

Endorphins come from endogenous morphine. They are a group of hormones produced and released by the pituitary gland in the brain and the hypothalamus in vertebrates when pain occurs or during recreational exercise, excitement, consumption of spicy food, or orgasm (Saravana Kumar and Gandhimathi 2012). Their function is to work as neurotransmitters: they have an ability to produce analgesia and a feeling of happiness and relaxation. Endorphins are simply understood as natural painkillers. Through acupressure techniques, pressing on the Tui Na blood points, acupuncture points, and tender spots, Tui Na encourages the body to release more endorphins.

The rotating technique is a very popular Tui Na technique to encourage endorphin release, one of many Tui Na maneuvers that works like a "runner's high." This is done by passively rotating the affected region on the axis of the joints. The maneuver can be applied on the neck, shoulder joints, elbow, wrist, fingers, lumbar joints, hip joints, knee joints, ankle joints, and toes. The force is gentle, the speed is steady, and the amplitude is increased gradually from the small to the limited range or to the physiological range, i.e. the physiological range refers to the total active range of motion in a joint. The purpose is to loosen the soft tissues surrounding the joint, promote joint flexibility, and encourage the body to secret endorphins to lower the pain level. Patients often say, "I am doing a lazy exercise," because the passive movement is done by the practitioner.

Tui Na and Muscular Hypotonia

Muscles are supposed to support the movements of the skeleton and prevent certain types of movement. In **hypotonia**, or low muscle tone, the muscle's initial state, speed, and stamina become weak, leading the patient to potentially suffer from many different diseases and disorders.

Tui Na enhances muscle tone and flexibility, helps the muscle functional enhancements, and increases muscle contraction (Yang 2011). It is also commonly used in the treatment of muscular atrophy and poliomyelitis hypotonia. Tui Na can not only increase the flexibility of muscles and tendons, but can also loosen the adhesion between the muscles and tendons and their surrounding tissues.

Tui Na and Joints

The best treatment period for any joint injury is the acute or subacute stage. Otherwise joint injury will continue into the chronic stage. Soft tissue adhesion in joints occurs if there is lymphatic stasis, synovial hypertrophy, tissue edema, or poor blood circulation.

According to the literature, 30–40% of patients with different degrees of joint injury will leave varying degrees of sequelae, such as a decrease in joint range of motion, joint disability, and muscle disuse atrophy (Zhi-Qiang 2007).

Sidebar 10.1 Patient Interviews

In response to the question, "What information do you wish your primary healthcare provider had given you to help make a better-informed decision to go to these treatment sessions or classes?" a 68-year-old female with knee and ankle arthritis replied: "My primary care provider does recommend acupuncture for musculoskeletal issues. It would have been nice if she had specifically mentioned Tui Na, referred me to some websites that discussed it and told me something about efficacy and outcomes for arthritis pain. It would also be nice to have a referral from the primary care provider or guidance on how to choose a qualified practitioner … [Tui Na and acupuncture] should be mentioned early on rather than as a last resort."

Tui Na promotes blood circulation and mobilizes and accelerates lymphatic fluid circulation, eliminates edema, releases soft tissue adhesion, and regains joint range of motion. It can increase the number of capillaries and their diameter, and therefore can greatly improve blood circulation. Tui Na also promotes reconstruction of the damaged capillary network, restoring elasticity of the vessel wall, making this treatment one of the best options for acute and chronic joint injury recovery. In China, it is my understanding that Tui Na treatment is most often selected by patients for rehabilitation, and the Tui Na department is the first to receive referrals from other Chinese and Western medicine departments.

Tui Na and Stomach Pain

In TCM, digestive system diseases are often considered to be directly related to the patient's emotional status. Emotional factors can stress the digestive system, e.g. you worry about the mortgage payment, your daughter is moving away to college, you feel anxiety regarding your performance because you are going to meet your senior manager, the swimming team you coach is preparing for the biggest meet of the season, or you are excited about planning a vacation. With such stress, anxiety, or overexcitement, your heart rate increases, adrenaline flows, blood pressure rises, and the result is gastrointestinal distress: pain and stomach cramps.

Tui Na therapy works on these neuroendocrine responses by increasing the release of endorphins, lowering blood pressure, and improving the gastrointestinal peristalsis. Tui Na can reduce the secretion of gastrin and enhance the intestinal absorption function, which has a better therapeutic effect on digestive system disease.

Tui Na and Children

Pediatric Tui Na has been used in TCM for over a thousand years. Even though Tui Na is not a relaxing massage, children enjoy it and do not find it painful, and it is very effective.

Unlike adults' pain, which is more chronic and associated with the constitution, i.e. either deficiency or stasis in Qi and/or blood of the internal **Zangfu** organs, children's pain is usually an acute state. Pediatric Tui Na uses a system of acupuncture **meridians** and acupuncture points that are different from adult ones. Children's Qi and their meridian systems are not fully developed, their Zangfu organs—especially their lungs and spleen—are not fully functioning yet.

Adults' joint pain is usually caused by emotional stress and, because stress causes tight tendons, tendons are more likely to be injured. Children's pain is usually sourced from an injury, which often means a local stagnation of meridians. When children cry, it directly helps to release the stagnation. When more treatment is necessary, Tui Na works very well for local soft tissue circulation. In addition, Tui Na practitioners may also apply a topical herbal plaster to the painful area: herbs to ease the pain, promote blood circulation, and expel wind, damp, and cold.

Congenital torticollis is a condition commonly treated with Tui Na in traditional Chinese hospitals. Among all TCM modalities, Tui Na is well known as the best treatment for this neck condition. Tui Na treatment loosens the spasms of the sternocleidomastoid muscle, and the procedure is effective, painless, and without side effects. After the treatment, the parents are instructed on specific Tui Na techniques and additional self-care to use at home to further assist in maintaining the results. Each treatment is only 15 minutes, once every other day, and usually the muscle will be loosen after 5–10 visits (Feng 2002).

Methodology
The Types of Medical Services in China

China has two types of medical service: the first type is hospitals where Western medical services are the primary care provided, with a small department of Chinese medicine, and even though small, it has all services that are provided in Chinese medicine hospitals including Chinese herbal medicine (中藥科), acupuncture (針灸科), and Tui Na (推拿科). The second type is hospitals where Chinese medicine is the only service provided. Chinese herbal medicine is widely used for internal medical diseases and is good for endocrine/hormonal disorders; genitourinary, urinary tract, and bladder infections; and digestive, respiratory, gynecological, and dermatology conditions. Acupuncture is often used as a preventive medicine and is good for promoting health and energy, and is very helpful for sleep disorders and drug and alcohol addictions, and smoking cessation. Many people find that acupuncture and **moxibustion** only 3–4 times a year is very beneficial for many chronic illnesses such as asthma. This procedure is usually done in July, because TCM believes that the herbal property of the moxibustion enters more meridians and Zangfu organs during the hottest season of the year.

Tui Na is well known in the treatment of pain management, not only as a quick way to stop pain, but also as a self-care tool that patients can easily learn and apply to manage their own pain.

In China, Tui Na departments have inpatient and outpatient clinics. Tui Na practitioners in the outpatient clinics will treat their patients with Xiao Tui Na, and refer the patients in certain conditions to the inpatient department for Da Tui Na.

Da Tui Na is performed simultaneously by more than five practitioners while the patient is under local anesthesia. Conditions suitable for Da Tui Na are herniated disc sciatica and dislocation of joints.

Xiao Tui Na is usually a one-on-one practice, but at times requires two or three practitioners to perform the procedures. Outpatient clinics perform this type of Tui Na treatment.

The pain conditions usually treated with Xiao Tui Na can be both acute and chronic, and commonly include (but are not limited to) the following:

- headache and migraine; soft tissue related neck, back, and hip pain

- shoulder pain including frozen shoulder, shoulder impingement, pain from traumatic injuries such as dislocation, displacement, or sports related

- sciatica from a slipped disc, spinal stenosis, piriformis syndrome and pelvic injury

- wrist pain including carpal tunnel syndrome, Blackberry thumb (DeQuervain's disease), and sports injury

- ankle pain including sprains

- knee pain including pain from the medial collateral ligament (MCL), the lateral collateral ligament (LCL), or other ligaments and tendons, and pain from conditions affecting cartilages such as the patella and meniscus.

Sidebar 10.2 Patient Interviews

When asked, "Do you feel different about yourself or your pain?", a 68-year-old patient with arthritis replied: "The difference in my ankle since treatment with Tui Na and acupuncture borders on magical. I didn't expect to have improvement in its range of motion, but it happened. I haven't needed a Synvisc injection in my knee for several years because there is so much less pain. Tui na and acupuncture have helped postpone the need for a knee replacement. If I have another musculoskeletal issue, Tui Na and acupuncture are now my first choice of treatment."

The Four Diagnostic Methods in TCM

When a patient presents for Tui Na pain treatment, I go through a TCM diagnostic procedure consisting of observation, auscultation and olfaction, interrogation, and pulse taking and palpation.

Observation

Under natural daylight, I use my sense of sight to carry out a systematic and purposeful inspection of a patient's body parts, secretions, and excretions, because the outer changes actually reflect the inner constitution.

The observation establishes the patient's physiology and pathology. First, I focus on the patient's face to study the eyes, manners, complexion of the body constitution, face color, and vitality. Second, I look at the patient's tongue to learn the deeper sight of the constitution of the pain that is either from a deficiency or an excess condition; and then I inspect the pain region to learn whether it is swollen or depressed, and the color and vessel condition of the area.

In the Tui Na department, practitioners focus on the source and duration of the pain, as these dictate the treatment plan and outcome. For example, when the painful site shows edema, the tongue shows signs of bruising and distended vessels; these provide a sense of the source of a repetitive injury and the duration of the disease.

Orthopedic tests are also part of the main observations in Tui Na clinics. I perform the full range of joint motion evaluations and special orthopedic tests, such as Cozen's test for lateral epicondylitis and the straight leg test for sciatica. Neurological examinations are also part of the diagnostic procedure for pain treatment, and imaging tests play an important role in treatment decision-making.

Auscultation and olfaction

Auscultation is a method of listening. In Chinese medicine, listening is to "listen to learn the whole body." I listen to the patient's voice, breath, and cough.

Voice

- A loud and coarse voice indicates an acute condition with a high level of pain.

- A weak and low voice indicates a chronic condition, and the pain might be related to the pathogenic change of internal organs, for example, a chronic low back pain where the pain is constantly sore and is worse after exertion. This indicates that the pain is from kidney Qi deficiency.

- A lack of desire to speak indicates a chronic condition and functional dysfunction. These patients often show edema, have a cold sensation, and are sluggish and fatigued; male patients might show erectile dysfunction and female patients might show amenorrhea.

- Incessant talking indicates a condition of pain related to inflammation.

Breathing

- Loud and coarse breathing indicates an acute condition with a high level of pain.

- Weakness, shortness of breath, and difficulty breathing indicates a chronic condition. The pain occurs from pathogenic change of the internal organs.

- Sighing indicates the origin of pain is from tendons.

Coughing

- Wheezing indicates the pain is related to edema.

- Coughing with sticky sputum indicates the pain is related to a condition of inflammation.

- Loud coughing indicates the pain is acute.

- Weak coughing indicates the pain is chronic and of a low degree.

Olfaction is an important aspect of diagnosis and is used to identify the patient's abnormal odors from the oral cavity, body secretions, and excreta:

- Rancid odor indicates the pain is tendon related and the patient is emotional.

- Burned odor indicates the pain is inflammation related.

- Sweet, fragrant odor indicates the pain is muscle related.

- Rotten odor indicates the pain is related to stiffness. There is lack of range of motion, and the patient lacks cardio exercise.

- Putrid odor indicates the pain is related to joints and edema.

Interrogation

I interview the patient to learn about the pain's onset and development, past treatment, present symptoms, other past medical history and family history:

- origin of the current pain to know the cause of the onset, development, treatments, present symptoms, and other information of diseases

- past medical history relevant to the chief complaint, for example, inquiry of neck pain history and imaging test results that might be relevant to the current hand and finger numbness

- living and occupational environmental conditions to help identify the patient's posture at work, and when sleeping and standing; the temperature of the environment such as windy, cold, and moist; handedness (right or left); family, for example, a female patient suffers from right shoulder and elbow pain because her 1-year-old daughter always needs to be held; and social history, for example, a patient with long-term disturbed rest at night might more commonly suffer from joint pain

- pain after edema indicates the source is on the surface

- pain before edema indicates the source is on the deep side

- pain and edema occurring at the same time indicates the source is from the fluid

- pain stays but the edema spreads indicates the prognosis is good

- pain spreads but the edema stays indicates the prognosis is bad

- pain in the joint is less but the edema is worse, indicating infection or bone tuberculosis (TB)

- pain is very minimal but the edema is hard to touch, and edema and pain are progressively worse indicates cancer

- pain is related to emotional stress if the taste in the mouth is bitter

- pain is related to digestive disorders if the taste in the mouth is sweet

- pain is related to gastritis if the taste in the mouth is sour

- pain is related to hypertension if the taste in the mouth is spicy

- pain is related to chronic nephritis if the taste in the mouth is salty

- pain is related to endocrine diseases if the taste in the mouth is light

- pain is related to the presence of a tumor if the taste in the mouth is astringent or dry

- pain is related to diabetes if the taste in the mouth is fragrant

- pain is related to nasopharyngeal disease if the patient has halitosis.

Pulse taking and palpation

Pulse taking is done through the second, third, and fourth fingers and touching over the patient's radial artery on the wrist to feel the pulse rate, depth, and length, and the quality or type of pulse. When taking the pulse, I am able to receive abundant information about the patient's entire body,

the source of the pain and its development, and the prognosis:

- Tight pulse indicates pain with a cold sensation; the patient is sluggish and fatigued.

- Wiry pulse indicates pain with a tendon-related condition; the patient is emotional and stressful.

- Irregular pulse indicates pain related to poor blood circulation.

- Hidden pulse indicates the pain is severe.

- Rapid pulse indicates the pain is inflammation related.

- Slow pulse indicates the pain is musculoskeletal related.

Palpation in Chinese medicine is used to make the first-hand diagnosis; as well as touching the area of pain, the affected region will also be palpated to make a further and more accurate diagnosis, for example:

- I palpate the low back region from L4 to S3 for sciatica patients.

- I palpate the L5 to S1 region for heel pain or plantar fasciitis.

- I palpate the related iliotibial (IT) band for patella displacement.

- I palpate the neck to learn its condition in relation to cervical spondylosis.

Hands-on Techniques

Traditional Chinese Medicine (TCM) includes Tui Na treatment as well as other modalities, such as acupuncture needling and Chinese herbal remedy prescriptions. Listed below are some of the typical procedures I would use for a patient in pain.

Diagnosis

Tui Na medical facilities can be found in both out-patient clinics and inpatient hospital settings. For example, a patient, Michael, is suffering from sciatic pain or a "prolapse of the lumbar intervertebral disc" on L4 and L5. Typically, the Tui Na practitioner starts with a comprehensive interview. In this situation, I would ask Michael a series of questions, then make an initial diagnosis based on Western medicine (prolapsed lumbar vertebrae) and traditional Chinese medicine (Bi syndrome). Further, I would perform the necessary orthopedic test (e.g. straight leg) and neurological assessment (e.g. foot plantar flexion), as well as ordering radiology tests as needed.

Sidebar 10.3 Research

In this meta-analysis, Kong and colleagues (2012) examine twenty-eight randomized controlled trials (RTCs) for Tui Na and other Traditional Chinese Medicine (TCM) treatment's effect on low back pain in an inpatient context. Despite searching English language databases, all the studies were conducted in China between 2005 and 2012. The Tui Na treatments ranged from 20 to 30 minutes, and the study duration ranged from 3 days to 8 weeks. These studies used the visual analogue scale (VAS) for pain and the Oswestry disability index (ODI) or Japanese orthopedic association (JOA) score for low back pain to measure functional status. Two studies maintained that inpatients in the Tui Na plus acupuncture group experienced more obvious improvements on functional status. Six trials in the meta-analysis showed favorable effects of Tui Na plus Chinese herbal medicine on pain. Combined with acupuncture, the meta-analysis also showed significant effects on pain. One study reported a long-term effect on functional status when compared with acupuncture. Although the methodological quality varied, these authors found statistically significant changes for pain and function, mostly when Tui Na was combined with other aspects of TCM. These findings suggest that Tui Na has promising therapeutic value in treating low back pain in an inpatient setting.

Sidebar 10.4 Research

McCarthy, a Tui Na practitioner from Ireland, suggests certain Tui Na techniques when treating neck and shoulder-related pain. These are described in the text and include applications of Tui Na for pain associated with rheumatoid arthritis of the upper back, hands and fingers, frozen shoulder, whiplash, and neck rotation dysfunctions (McCarthy 2003).

Acupuncture treatment

In some cases, a practitioner will apply acupuncture needling before a Tui Na treatment. In this situation, Michael would be asked to lie on his side on a treatment table; usually, lying on the unaffected side is recommended. I might also use an electro-acupuncture machine, long-wave infrared lamp, moxibustion, laser acupuncture, ear seed embedding, and cupping techniques.

Tui Na treatment

For this treatment, I would ask Michael to lie prone so that I could start a series of Tui Na techniques, such as palpation, on the affected region. In Michael's case, I would palpate the spine, lumbar soft tissues, iliac bones, and joints, and compare the skin temperature on both legs. Next I would open acupuncture meridians, warming the affected regions, and start with mild techniques such as dragon rolling, phoenix rolling, kneading, pressing, pushing, and chafing on Michael's lumbar region, hamstring, popliteal fossa, calf, and ankle.

When the affected regions are warm, I would begin the main period of treatment to address the chief complaints. During this stage, I would focus on loosening the soft tissues around the lumbar spine and sciatic nerve, using techniques such as grasping on the low back muscles, elbow pressing on the buttocks, and rotation of the lumbar hip, knee, and ankle joints.

Outcome Measures

Typically, and in Michael's case, I would recommend weekly treatments. Each visit would start with an interview including the common questions for pain management:

- How was the last treatment?

- Within a pain scale of 0–10, how would you rate your pain after your last visit?

- How is your pain today?

The treatment outcomes from the last visit must also be discussed. From my twenty-plus years of clinical experience, I have found that treatment outcomes are the best tool for determining the next treatment approach/principles, Tui Na techniques for the current treatment, and self-care remedy post treatment. If the prior treatment proved effective in decreasing pain, then I either do not change the plan or introduce a slight change according to the patient's recent health status and symptom severity.

I not only track pain but use palpation on the affected region to measure the treatment progress and outcomes. For example, low back pain and cold skin temperature in this region are symptoms of kidney Yang deficiency; therefore, if Michael's skin appears warm, then Tui Na treatments on this back area may have improved his kidney Yang deficiency and pain. If the intended outcome from the prior treatment is not reached, I review my diagnosis, treatment principles, Tui Na treatments, and the patient's self-care "homework," and make necessary adjustments.

Self-care Education

I love to tell my patients that self-care education is a series of "self-care homework" tasks that are quite crucial for the success of the treatment. I have found this to be true because the homework not only maintains the treatment outcome but also helps my next treatment. For example, I had a female patient with pain in her left knee due to degeneration, and the homework I recommended involved practicing an exercise while lying on a bed, and avoiding long-distance walking. When she came for her second visit, her knee pain was worse because she

had been hiking for 5 miles on a trail with a heavy backpack. After she understood that the hike had contributed to her knee pain, and agreed to stop long-distance walking, her condition improved significantly by the fifth visit.

If a patient attends weekly appointments, then "homework" will be prescribed for the rest of that week. Some homework recommendations consist of daily exercises, herbal prescriptions, dietary suggestion, posture recommendations, and lifestyle suggestions. For example, as Michael has sciatic pain, I would prescribe a Chinese herbal formula and teach him an exercise, to be practiced daily, to strengthen his low back muscles. In addition, dietary and posture recommendations would be included as well as recommending sleeping in a supine position, on a harder bed, with legs bent at 90 degrees at the hips and knees.

Sidebar 10.5 Patient Interviews

When asked, "Do you do any regular self-care to relieve or prevent ongoing pain?", replies included:

- "Aside from massage therapy, I receive acupuncture treatments twice each month. I have a structured PT routine designed by a personal trainer that I perform on a daily basis. I take medications to help with depression and chronic pain and I see a therapist twice each month."

- "I swim, stretch, walk, have massages bi-monthly. I have had surgery on knees and thumbs."

- "I use ice and/or heat, as needed. I also do some stretches for ankle and knee and exercises to strengthen the muscles around my knee."

Case Study

A 54-year-old patient was a successful import–export businessman complaining of right shoulder pain. When he phoned my clinic to make an appointment, I briefly interviewed him to learn about his chief complaint. The shoulder pain started about 20 years previously from a martial arts practice, and has been "on" and "off" since then, with aggravation in the past couple of weeks.

He reported that he was injured in a martial arts practice about 20 years ago while living in Hong Kong: he fell hard, hitting his right shoulder on the floor. The patient received initial medical care: just shoulder immobilization and oral pain relief.

After he immigrated to Seattle, he could not find a Chinese medicine provider who was specialized in traumatology. The shoulder became worse, and the range of motion progressively became worse.

When I met him in the initial visit, he was a slim, well-nourished patient whose job required overseas travel and heavy goods lifting. Observation found that the right deltoid, supraspinatus, infraspinatus, and teres major muscles showed atrophy, possibly due to disuse. Shoulder range of motion in abduction was at 65 degrees, flexion was at 95 degrees, and hyperextension was at 30 degrees. The acromion process was very prominent. The pain location was at the lesser tuberosity of the humerus, the greater tuberosity of the humerus, and, the most painful area, the supraspinatus tendon. The pain usually only occurred during shoulder movements.

In my Tui Na treatment for his right shoulder pain, I often started with dragon rolling around the shoulder from the front to the back and stayed at the top for a long period of time until the whole shoulder was warm. Next, I used a technique called "grasping" on the deltoid muscle. With this technique, I used my fingertips to dig into the muscles to separate the adhesions and to promote blood circulation. I put my thumb at the rear side of the deltoid and the rest of my fingers on the front side, while I held his right wrist. I grasped his deltoid at the same time and raised his right arm gradually and gently, I then applied a Tui Na technique called "holding a globe" on the shoulder. With this technique, I forcefully

kneaded the front and back of his shoulder with my palms until they were warm and red.

The patient received these treatments once a week for about 3 months. I measured and evaluated the pain scale and the shoulder range of motion: his pain level decreased and the range of motion increased with each visit. Three months later, the pain was very mild and the shoulder abduction was at 165 degrees. The atrophic muscles came back to the same size as those of the left shoulder, except for the supraspinatus muscle.

Conclusion

Tui Na is one of the three main TCM modalities in Chinese medicine hospitals, and it is practiced to the same degree as acupuncture and herbal medicine.

Tui Na treatment combines the world's oldest medicine with modern Western medical anatomy, physiology, pathology, and diagnosis. The manual techniques are widely used in other therapies worldwide and the treatment results are remarkable. In addition, the therapy has been considered safe for patients of all ages from infants to the elderly, and even for correcting fetal position.

The greatest advantage of Tui Na is that it focuses on the specific pain, no matter whether it is an acute or a chronic pain associated with the joints, muscles, or the skeletal system. Tui Na enhances muscle tone and increases soft tissue flexibility, loosens the adhesions between soft tissues, and resets dislocated joints.

Tui Na treatment is not only very effective for soft-tissue trauma as it quickly softens the spasms, promotes blood flow, helps the body promote better circulation of the lymphatic system to drain edema, promotes new cell production, and accelerates injury healing, but it also quickly resets dislocated or displaced joints. Hence, it is the first choice of treatment for patients when they suffer from musculoskeletal issues.

References

Feng, X. U. 2002. Pediatric massage therapy in children with congenital muscular torticollis 52 cases. *Chinese Manipulation & Qi Gong Therapy,* 18(2):48–9.

Knotts, C. 2012. http://www.ncbi.nlm.nih.gov, /pmc/articles/PMC3348749/ http://www.ncbi.nlm.nih.gov/pmc/articles/PMC3348749/ (accessed December 23, 2014).

Kong, L. J., M. Fang, H. S. Zhan, W. A. Yuan, J. H. Pu, Y. W. Cheng, and B. Chen, B. 2012. Tuina-focused integrative Chinese medical therapies for inpatients with low back pain: a systematic review and meta-analysis. *Evidence-Based Complementary and Alternative Medicine* Volume 2012, Article ID 578305, 14 pages. doi:10.1155/2012/578305.

McCarthy, M. 2003. Palpatory literacy, Chinese therapeutic bodywork (Tui Na) and the remediation of head, neck and shoulder pain. *Journal of Bodywork and Movement Therapies* October: 262–77.

Saravana Kumar A., and R. Gandhimathi. 2012. *International Journal of Pharmacology Research* http://www.ijprjournal.org/File_Folder/88-108.pdf (accessed December 23, 2014).

Yang, L. I, 2011. Effects of Tuina on muscular tension of flexor and extensor in patients with knee osteoarthritis. *China Journal Of Orthopaedics And Traumatology* 24(7):575–7.

Ying Xia, G. D. G.-C. W. 2013. *Current research in acupuncture.* Houston, New York, Heidelberg, Dordrecht, London: Springer.

Yao-chi, W. U. 2009. Clinical study of tuina for stiff neck. *Journal Of Acupuncture And Tuina Science* 7(4):225–7.

Zhi-Qiang, L. 2007. Lateral calcaneal "V" shaped incision treatment for calcaneocuboid joint calcaneal fracture. *Chinese Journal of Trauma* 23(10):734–5.

Introduction

The *Feldenkrais Method*® of somatic education offers a student-centered approach to learning movement that enhances posture and balance, and reduces pain of both physical and emotional origin. While people of all ages and abilities come to the *Feldenkrais Method* to improve a variety of functions, pain is the primary motivator (Buchanan, Nelsen and Geletta 2014). *Guild Certified Feldenkrais Practitioners*CM (also known as *Guild Certified Feldenkrais Teachers*®) provide a supported, safe, and secure environment for students (or clients) to learn patterns of postural support and mobility. Once students feel comfortable, change in acute and chronic pain patterns become possible. *Feldenkrais* practitioners believe that small, slow, gentle movements bypass habitual pain patterns and re-establish or improve functional abilities that enhance students' participation in personal and professional activities of daily living.

Overview of the Feldenkrais Method

The *Feldenkrais Method* assists people to connect with their natural ability to move, think, sense, and feel. The method incorporates elements of developmental, organic learning to facilitate organization of a whole, integrated self-image. Central to successful outcomes for *Feldenkrais* students is their active participation during lessons, with application into daily life. *Feldenkrais* practitioners assist students to experience postural clarity and discover their innate capacity to improve balance (Feldenkrais 1985, 1996).

Posture and balance include how one orients and organizes within the current environment and in relationship to the field of gravity for potent action. Feldenkrais stated: "posture relates to action, and not the maintenance of a given position. Acture would perhaps be a better word for it" (Feldenkrais 1985, 108). Balanced posture or acture

is foundational to the *Feldenkrais Method* and is relevant in all orientations, including standing, sitting, and lying. Part of the *Feldenkrais* process is learning to continually find clarity in acture, recognize the absence of effort and resistance, and discover the ability to reverse action and breathe easily. Inefficient acture reflects demands on the person that interfere with moving effortlessly in any direction at any time.

Feldenkrais practitioners guide students through movement experiences that invite attention to, and sharpen awareness of, their present and potential actions. Students investigate habitual and familiar behaviors that are used, for example, to walk their neighborhood streets. They examine nonhabitual yet available behaviors that allow them to walk a new trail at a favorite park. They explore unfamiliar and undiscovered behaviors from which new skills emerge, such as walking on stilts through the park.

Feldenkrais practitioners teach the method in two complementary group and individual formats. They typically present *Awareness Through Movement*® (ATM) lessons to groups and provide **Functional Integration**® **(FI)** lessons to individuals.

Awareness Through Movement

Awareness Through Movement (ATM) lessons (see Figure 11.1) typically last 30–60 minutes, with a practitioner verbally guiding a group or individual through a movement exploration sequence. ATM utilizes a variety of positions including lying, sitting, or standing. Practitioners consider the current capabilities and pain levels of students and make accommodations so that seemingly impossible or difficult movements become possible and easy. They remind students to avoid pain and to perform movements within comfortable ranges. Movement sequences develop from simple to complex as students evolve their ability and awareness (Feldenkrais 1977, 1981).

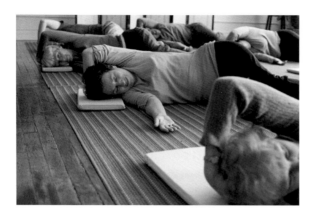

Figure 11.1
Example from an *Awareness Through Movement* lesson.
(Copyright 2007, Rosalie O'Connor. Used with permission of the Feldenkrais Guild® of North America.)

Students expand their movement patterns as they explore new pathways for easier function. Movement sequences arise from human development, such as: rolling over, standing up from the floor or a chair, turning to look over one's shoulder, and reaching overhead (Feldenkrais 1977, 1981).

Typical exercise often focuses on stretching, moving quickly, strengthening, and pushing through pain. In contrast, ATMs offer slow, attentive explorations that encourage awareness of physical, mental, and emotional states. As students expand their repertoire of healthful movements, their self-efficacy evolves along with their understanding of efficient and resilient function. This self-knowledge grows through intimate, direct experience with their physicality that concurrently clarifies the self-image. A practitioner can draw from hundreds of ATM lessons that vary in function, difficulty, and complexity to provide a student-centered approach to learning to act more effectively in the world with less or no pain (Feldenkrais 1977, 1981).

Functional integration

Feldenkrais practitioners use individually focused *Functional Integration* (FI) lessons (see Figure 11.2) to offer fully clothed students physically guided experiences that use gentle, educated touch to inform them about current behaviors and suggest movement alternatives. Feldenkrais stated:

> [Functional Integration] *turns to the oldest elements of our sensory system—touch, the feelings of pull and pressure; the warmth of the hand, its caressing stroke. The person becomes absorbed in sensing the diminishing muscular tonus, the deepening and the regularity of breathing, abdominal ease, and improved circulation in the expanding skin. The person senses his most primitive, consciously forgotten patterns and recalls the well-being of a growing young child (Feldenkrais 1981, 121).*

Practitioners use bolsters and padding to support, enhance, and facilitate movement while the student is lying on a table, seated, or standing. Each lesson is tailored to meet individual needs for comfort,

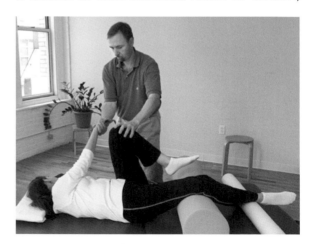

Figure 11.2
Example from a *Functional Integration* lesson.
(Copyright 2007, Rosalie O'Connor. Used with permission of the Feldenkrais Guild® of North America.)

safety, and ability to achieve goals of relieving pain, expanding flexibility, and improving coordination (Feldenkrais 1981).

The intentions of FI lessons are similar to ATM, but often the trajectory of learning is more rapid. Through the integration of touch, this mode affords more customized guidance, enriched communication between practitioner and student, and enhanced self-awareness.

History

In this section, we provide a biography of Moshe Feldenkrais, DSc, originator of the *Feldenkrais Method*. We then present variations that are closely based on Feldenkrais's teachings.

Moshe Feldenkrais, DSc

Moshe Feldenkrais, DSc (1904–1984; see Figure 11.3) lived a nonconventional life that began in an Hassidic Jewish community in Eastern Europe. He survived the pogroms of World War I and immigrated as a teenager to Palestine where he worked as a laborer, tutor, and cartographer. He was athletic, studied jujitsu, and devised his own self-defense techniques (Feldenkrais 2010; Kaetz 2007).

While in Palestine, he injured his knee playing soccer. A physician advised him that he had a 50% chance of a permanently extended knee if he underwent surgery (Elinor Silverstein 2015, personal communication). Another physician suggested Feldenkrais could retrain his nervous system to regain function and reduce pain (Elinor Silverstein, 2015, personal communication). Feldenkrais seriously studied the literature, including Coué's writings on autosuggestion, and was able to restore his function (Feldenkrais 2014; Elinor Silverstein 2015, personal communication). In retrospect, these events mark his method's beginning.

In the 1930s, Feldenkrais studied engineering at the Sorbonne in Paris and worked in the Joliot-Curie laboratories. While there, he met the originator of judo and earned a black belt. When the Nazis occupied Paris during World War II, Feldenkrais left for Great

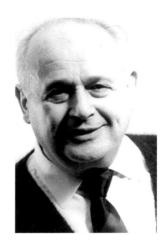

Figure 11.3
Moshe Feldenkrais.
(Courtesy of Feldenkrais Institute, Tel Aviv, Israel.)

Britain (Feldenkrais 2010). He worked with preeminent exiled scientists doing anti-submarine research for the Royal Navy. His knee pain, aggravated by recurring slips (Elinor Silverstein 2015, personal communication), became a renewed focus of attention. While continuing to work on defense systems, he resumed his studies of biology, evolution, psychology, human development, and learning for interdisciplinary insights into healing, and explored the effects of small movements and mental imagery to improve his function. He delivered a series of lectures to his colleagues about his scholarship and direct experience that became the foundation of his method (Feldenkrais 1996).

After World War II, Feldenkrais returned to the newly created Israel and worked for the military. He began offering lessons in his nascent method, which soon took all of his attention. He taught three groups to become teachers of his method, first in Tel Aviv, Israel (1969–1971), then San Francisco, CA (1975–1978), and Amherst, MA (1980–1981) (Feldenkrais 2010). He suffered a traumatic brain injury in a motor vehicle accident while teaching in Switzerland and was unable complete the

Amherst training (Elinor Silverstein 2015, personal communication).

He returned to Israel for treatment, including the then novel surgery to reduce intracranial pressure. While convalescing, Feldenkrais used his own method to restore his speech and other functions (Elinor Silverstein 2015, personal communication). Many years before neuroscientists could document **neuroplasticity's** existence, Feldenkrais had incorporated it into his method and demonstrated it personally and with his students (Elbert et al. 1995; Feldenkrais 1977). He died in 1984 from the effects of his brain injury.

Models Based on the Teachings of Moshe Feldenkrais

Several individuals have developed somatic education approaches that are substantially grounded in Feldenkrais's teachings. The first was Thomas Hanna, who learned about the work of Feldenkrais in the early 1970s and integrated his studies with Feldenkrais into Hanna Somatic Education®.

A recent survey of US *Feldenkrais* practitioners revealed that 28.9% of responders held additional certification in one or more of these approaches (Buchanan et al. 2014). The top four approaches, beginning with the most frequent, were: Bones For Life® developed by Ruthy Alon, the Anat Baniel Method®, Sounder Sleep System® designed by Michael Krugman, and Child'Space® Chava Shelhav Method (Buchanan, Nelsen and Geletta 2014, unpublished data).

Theoretical Approaches to Pain Management

Feldenkrais wrote this overview of his approach. Although Feldenkrais wrote this over 30 years ago, it is highly relevant today. The major reason students pursue *Feldenkrais* lessons is to relieve pain, with back pain being the most common complaint (Buchanan et al. 2014). Feldenkrais succinctly outlined the distinctive features of his method and illustrated the observed effects of lessons on students.

> For many years I have been involved in working with people who have turned to me for help. Some complain of physical pain, others of mental anguish, and only a few ever speak of emotional troubles. I have some difficulty in explaining to my followers that I am not a therapist and that my touching a person with my hands has no therapeutic or healing value, though people improve through it. I think that what happens to them is **learning,** but few agree with this. What I am doing does not resemble teaching as understood at present. The accent is on the learning process, rather than on the teaching technique. After each session my pupils have a new sense of well-being: they feel taller, lighter, and breathe more freely. They often rub their eyes as if they have just woken from a sound and refreshing sleep. More often than not they say that they have become relaxed. The pain is always abated and often it is gone altogether. In addition, face wrinkles nearly always disappear, the eyes become brighter and larger, and the voice deeper and more resonant. The pupil becomes youthful again (Feldenkrais 1981, 7).

He emphasized that his method to alleviate painful conditions is a learning approach to changing interrelated physical, mental and emotional components of an individual's behavior.

While collaborating with top scientists who were applying early general systems theory to develop defense systems, Feldenkrais utilized similar integrative thinking to synthesize his perspective on how maladaptive behaviors, including chronic pain, arose in humans. He argued that people often ignored pain and failed to adequately examine behaviors that contributed to their pain. He stated: "Normally, one learns from experience, by correcting earlier patterns of behaviour. When a person continues to use a stereotyped pattern of behaviour instead of one suitable to the present reality, the learning process has come to a standstill" (Feldenkrais 1996, 153). In essence, people learned to ignore and perfect their pain. From his perspective, individuals needed to pay close attention to the behavior that created the pain, and change that behavior in order to change their pain. This is a learning process in which students must engage their attention, curiosity, and awareness under conditions that are safe, secure, and supportive.

One major implication of this approach is that students need to avoid pain and stop reinforcing it. Instead, in the *Feldenkrais Method*, practitioners encourage students to look for comfort and ease while doing movements with less effort and without provoking pain. For example, *Feldenkrais* practitioners guide students to move slowly while engaging flexor muscles to lengthen instead of stretching tight or overactive extensor muscles. The concern with stretching is the potential for stimulating pain receptors that increase extensors contraction and cause more pain. Students learn to habitually seek, notice, and appreciate actions that feel good instead of searching out those that provoke pain (Feldenkrais 1996).

Feldenkrais explicitly emphasized the interrelationships among sensing, feeling, thinking, and moving for understanding the organization of behavior and how to improve it through learning (Feldenkrais 1977, 1985, 2010). He believed changing behavior, or learning, was possible throughout life and that learning resulted in changes in the nervous system, including the organization of the brain. For example, Feldenkrais proposed that the cortical sensorimotor maps of the ring finger of the left hand of musicians would differ significantly from those of non-musicians (Feldenkrais 1977). Decades later, neuroscientists confirmed the existence of such neuroplastic changes in string players (Elbert et al. 1995).

One theoretical framework that encompasses neuroplasticity and the emergence of behavior from the interactions among multiple components—including cognition, perception, emotion, and action—is dynamic systems theory. This theory evolved from general systems theory and influenced the work of several developmental psychologists

and movement scientists. Thelen and Smith's 1994 book on dynamic systems caught the attention of several *Feldenkrais* practitioners who considered their theoretical presentation to epitomize the foundations of the *Feldenkrais Method* (Ginsburg 2010; Buchanan 2012).

At this time, there is little research specifically assessing the appropriateness of dynamic systems theory as a suitable framework for the *Feldenkrais Method*. However, there is a growing body of peer-reviewed literature supporting the effectiveness of *Feldenkrais* lessons for people with painful conditions (Chinn et al. 1994; Bearman and Shafarman 1999; Lundblad, Elert, and Gerdle 1999; Malmgren-Olsson, Armelius, and Armelius 2001; Smith, Kolt, and McConville 2001; Malmgren-Olsson and Bränholm 2002; Malmgren-Olsson and Armelius 2003; Kemp, Ersek, and Turner 2005; Schön-Ohlsson, Willén, and Johnels 2005, 2006).

Early on, Feldenkrais noted that people with challenging issues impacting the neck and back "maintain the cervical and lumbar curves rigidly in the same form, even during sleep. They wake up with a sense of tiredness and stiffness of the neck and spine which are only to be expected" (Feldenkrais 1996, 121). Recent research indicates that people with pain often have impaired sleep (Baliki et al. 2008). Disturbed sleep is also problematic because sleep is necessary for the removal of neurotoxic wastes from the brain that accumulate during wakeful activity (Xie et al. 2013). Another concern is the impact of insufficient sleep on learning. Sleep is useful both in preparation for learning activities, as well as afterwards for the formation and consolidation of memory and in support of neuroplastic activity (Walker 2008). Feldenkrais experientially understood the role of sleep on learning: "Students attempting these lessons should do one every evening immediately before going to sleep. Within a few weeks they will find a considerable improvement in all functions essential to life" (Feldenkrais 1977, 55). Additionally, an informal survey of *Feldenkrais* practitioners and students indicated positive effects on sleep itself from *Feldenkrais* lessons (Buchanan 2014).

Recent neuroscience research has demonstrated that pain, besides interfering with sleep, has functional impacts on the brain beyond the perception of pain. For example, people with chronic back pain have changes in the prefrontal cortex that are associated with increased negative emotions (Baliki et al. 2006). They also develop altered cortical functional connectivity that decreases cognitive function and impairs attention. The longer the pain has been present, the greater the negative effects (Baliki et al. 2008).

In summary, the *Feldenkrais Method* is a distinctive, global learning approach that guides people

Sidebar 11.1 Research

In a recent rheumatology review of neck pain, the authors describe Feldenkrais as: "The core principle of Feldenkrais is to first improve one's kinesthetic and proprioceptive self-awareness via guided practice sessions, and ultimately to transform unhealthy habits, movements, and postures into movement patterns that offer the individual greater comfort and ease during performance of physical tasks" (Plastaras et al. 2013, 2). This review describes a small but promising study on patient–reported outcomes, pharmaceutical and medical costs. The researchers found that 100% of patients reported some level of improvement in their headaches or musculoskeletal pain after Feldenkrais treatments. In addition to patients feeling better, pharmaceutical and medical costs were reduced by 40%. These authors continue to summarize benefits from the Feldenkrais approach for fibromyalgia-related pain: patients reported reduced pain, fatigue, and improved sleep. The authors conclude this section with: "… the favorable risk-to-benefit ratio and long-term cost-effectiveness should give physicians reasons to encourage active participation [in Feldenkrais]" (Plastaras et al. 2013, 3).

to change behaviors that cause pain, alter their self-image, and impair their quality of life. *Feldenkrais* practitioners have suggested that dynamic systems theory is an appropriate framework for explaining and understanding this method. While recent research seems to support the proposals that Feldenkrais made decades earlier about the influence of pain on physical, mental, and emotional aspects of people's lives, more research is needed to clarify these connections.

Methodology

In this section, we present elements and techniques that are typically used in designing and providing *Feldenkrais* lessons. These components are applicable to the delivery of both ATM and FI lessons, and inform the behavior of both practitioners and students.

Assessment

A *Feldenkrais* lesson is as dynamic as the student, the day, and the pain complaint. For *Feldenkrais* practitioners, assessment begins with the initial communication with students and is continual throughout practitioner–student interactions. The initial session includes discussion of lifestyle activities, functional areas of limitation, and the effects of pain on activities. Practitioners learn why students seek lessons and what they desire to learn. These why and what questions are revisited every lesson.

As students share their story, we utilize all our senses to gather information to formulate learning opportunities. We notice how students are organized skeletally and how they move around the room. We consider their postural support and observe the dynamic relationships throughout their bodies. We observe the presence and location of restricted or excessive movements, which become focal points of learning. As a result of such movements, students may have formed compensatory movement patterns that interfere with efficient mobility and function; these, too, become themes for learning.

For example, we watch students walk, stand, or perform a task related to their professional or recreational activities. If a student presents with pain in the sacral area when standing, walking, and transitioning between these movements, we identify if the student bears more weight on one leg, and how she initiates and organizes movement through the foot, ankle, knee, and hip relative to the pelvis. While the student walks, we look at postural organization and the quantity and quality of movements including trunk rotation, head carriage, and arm swing. We repeat a similar process of observing students each time they change postures during a lesson.

We discuss *Feldenkrais* concepts of learning, self-image, and efficient movement. We create an initial plan at the start of a lesson or series, recognizing this plan is adaptive, flexible, and likely to change in response to the student's learning trajectory within and across lessons.

Strategy

Here we describe several major strategies that we commonly integrate into lessons. While not exhaustive, this listing presents essential and distinctive features of the *Feldenkrais Method*.

Creating a safe and supportive learning environment

First and foremost, from the *Feldenkrais* perspective, it is essential to provide students with a safe and secure environment that reduces the fight-or-flight response and sets appropriate conditions for learning. We are attentive to the space in which lessons occur, including being mindful of temperature, sound, lighting, flooring, color, décor, and potential distractions. Our commitment is to create an environment conducive to learning while recognizing when students are curious, grow weary, or become distracted. We clarify and support the students' goals and remain aware of their ever-changing self-image.

We use bolsters, padding, small balls, and other props to support students' body weight. This often increases comfort and allows students to relax and let go of excessive muscle tension. As the musculature reaches a more neutral state of tonus, there are increased possibilities to explore new movements and advance learning.

Communication

The success of *Feldenkrais* lessons is predicated on the clarity of communication that emerges from the relationship between the student and practitioner. Our quality of touch is paramount in exchanging information with the student. Relevant, gentle touch can initiate movement, engage the student's curiosity, and create a previously unimaginable sense of accomplishment without overwhelming the student. Each time we use touch to connect with the student, there is guiding communication indicating a direction, speed, depth, and pathway through the skeleton to produce more efficient movement. This type of touch embodies somatic empathy (Feldenkrais 1996; Cheever 2000; Cheever and Cohen 2003).

Touch may be as simple as one finger gently placed to indicate a point of reference marking the beginning or end of a movement. We can also imitate similar quality of touch through simple verbal communication that directs small, gentle movement exploration with the intent to discover pain-free movement. Our approach is to apply just enough pressure or verbal direction to facilitate reorganization of movement and associated anatomical structures without escalating pain.

Practitioners must organize their own posture and action in order to effectively communicate with students. This ensures students receive clear information that is uncomplicated by practitioners' disorganization. Our extensive direct experience with the *Feldenkrais* repertoire facilitates our ability to teach new patterns to students. Specifically during FI, we can couple with students to transmit forces through our skeletal structure to clarify direction of force, depth of pressure, and speed of movement. As a result, there is an intentional mirror image of action between students and ourselves. We use the least amount of force required to initiate change in order to avoid engaging the fight-or-flight response. It is important for practitioners to sense the difference between touch that is pushing or forcing versus guiding or suggesting. We use touch with students to guide movement, clarify the shape and texture of their bodies, and facilitate change in their behavior.

We quiet ourselves and focus on these intentions at the start of and as needed during lessons. We then assist students verbally and manually to explore their current movement abilities, and gently guide them to experience additional possibilities for more effective action.

Reference postures and movements

We use the baseline observations of students' postures and actions for contrast and comparison throughout and at the end of lessons. We also direct students' attention to these details so they can refine their abilities to detect changes in their organization, make choices that create ease and comfort in daily activities, and facilitate their learning.

Within the lesson

Feldenkrais practitioners use distinctive strategies within lessons. We identify a selection of them here.

Repetition

We direct students to repeat movements, but without counting repetitions as is common with therapeutic exercise. Instead, repeating movements with slight variations, changes in postural orientation, and with shifts of attention are part of a process of layered learning. We incorporate pauses and brief rests to allow students time to notice changes that enhance learning.

Small movements

We structure lessons and guide students to produce small, differentiated movements. These small motions help students experience comfort that reduces co-contraction that can inhibit movement and aggravate pain. They learn to refine coordination, and become familiar with perceptual and kinesthetic qualities that accompany such movement. Later during lessons, we incorporate these smaller movements into larger, functional activities.

Imagination

Feldenkrais practitioners routinely incorporate mental imagery into lessons. We invite students to imagine movements if they cannot act without provoking pain, and we encourage mental rehearsal to stimulate learning. Nearly every lesson involves at least brief periods of mental imagery, while there are entire lessons that use the imagination.

Reversibility

We teach students to initiate and complete a movement, and also to reverse path and return to their starting position. In this process, we include opportunities to interrupt, pause, and reverse direction at various points along the movement trajectory. These variations create a richer image of the action that deepens students' understanding of its coordination and control, and open up options for adapting movement when contexts and circumstances change.

Rest

Feldenkrais practitioners incorporate pauses and rests in lessons to allow students time to notice changes that promote integration and learning of refined movement. We frequently alert students to notice changes in their sleep patterns, as students may improve the quality of sleep or recognize the need for more sleep associated with learning. Additionally, we often suggest that students review selected movements before going to sleep and upon waking to aid their learning.

Constraints

Feldenkrais practitioners often constrain areas that move easily to create conditions that invite areas with restricted motion to increase their engagement. An example is instructing students to rest in prone with their foreheads on the backs of the hands. This limits movement of the neck and shoulders. We then guide students through actions of the pelvis and legs that encourage thoracic movement.

Education for self-care

The end of the lesson is as important as the beginning. As we guide students to sit or stand and repeat reference movements, we invite them to notice changes. We verbally review themes and offer reminders of organizing principles from the lessons. This is an important transition time that integrates the lessons learned on the floor or table into students' daily activities.

Monitoring Outcomes

Monitoring outcomes is an ongoing process in the *Feldenkrais Method* that practitioners use to adjust lessons to students' needs. We continually attend to comfort and pain levels and often use scales and body diagrams to track these levels within and across lessons. One commonly used tool to track pain levels is the visual analog scale (Carlsson 1983). The practitioner gives the student a paper with the 10-cm line and asks her to place a mark representing her current level of pain. Afterwards, the

practitioner presents another paper and asks the student to rate her pain again. By presenting the scales on separate papers, the practitioner minimizes biasing the student's response due to visual referencing of her prior response. Figure 11.4 is an example from Buchanan's students.

Throughout lessons, we observe students' behavioral states including: relaxation and alertness, quantity and content of speech, facial expressions, emotions, breathing characteristics, muscle tonus, skin color, and movement characteristics including smoothness, transmission of forces through the skeleton, and changes in range.

Our Personal Practices

Many *Feldenkrais* practitioners use the method in traditional practice settings and others integrate into numerous, innovative approaches (Buchanan et al. 2014). Here, we offer synopses of how we have used the *Feldenkrais Method* during our careers.

Patricia Buchanan

My practice has evolved through three phases. Initially, through my *Feldenkrais* Professional Training Program, I integrated new skills and perspectives as the core of my work as a physical therapist with a

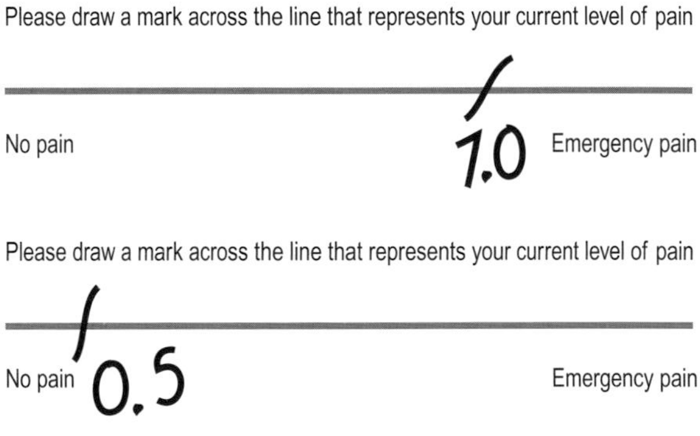

Please draw a mark across the line that represents your current level of pain

No pain — 7.0 — Emergency pain

Please draw a mark across the line that represents your current level of pain

No pain 0.5 — Emergency pain

Figure 11.4
Visual Analog Pain Scale. The line is 10 cm long; scoring is simply a matter of measuring the placement of the mark.

Sidebar 11.2 Research
Lundquist and colleagues used the visual analogue scale (VAS) and other pain assessment tools when comparing the effects of Feldenkrais on neck or shoulder pain for patients with visual impairment. This randomized controlled trial reported significantly less pain from the VAS and Visual, Musculoskeletal, and Balance Complaints questionnaire than controls, post treatment and at the 1-year follow-up. These authors conclude that Feldenkrais is an effective treatment option for this population (Lundquist, Zetterlund, and Richter 2014).

small private practice, and later with home health and hospice care. While training, I began learning about dynamic systems theory. I realized that I wanted to meld my interests as a new *Feldenkrais* teacher and an athletic trainer, my original healthcare profession, with the study of motor development from a dynamic systems perspective.

Soon, I entered my second, academic-centered phase. My personal practice was small while completing my doctoral studies and focused on research and teaching. I was grateful for the opportunity to introduce students in athletic training and physical therapy educational programs to the *Feldenkrais Method*. I believe this is an important way to guide healthcare providers to enhance their understanding of movement while refining their skills of observation, assessment, and intervention. I offered my *Feldenkrais* services to a modest number, but wide range, of people struggling with pain and dysfunction including musicians, athletes, adults, and young children with neurological conditions.

Now, I am in my third, solo practice phase. I offer an integrative learning approach to improving movement outside of academia and health care. My primary focus is on guiding female athletes and active women who have been struggling with pain or underperforming to resolve their pain and enhance their performance.

Nancy Haller

I have maintained a full-time healthcare-related practice as a solo *Feldenkrais* practitioner since completing my certification. I see a wide variety of clients with complaints of pain including the cervical area, headaches, shoulders, thoracic and lumbar regions, sciatic pain, motor vehicle collisions, and labor and industries injuries. Here are some of the other ways that I apply the *Feldenkrais Method*.

Equine focus: in the arena with equestrians and horses, there is a delicate balance between human posture and the carriage of the horse. When the two are synchronized, there is ease for both in all gaits.

This ease continues by meeting the equestrian's expectations for functional activities of the horse, whether trail riding, reining cattle for round-up, or performance of dressage patterns. My work began with equestrians and evolved to add horses; both have an active nervous system ready to learn how posture, balance, and movement are changeable and can improve. Linda Tellington-Jones created **Tellington Touch**®, a method for animals, partially based on the teaching of Moshe Feldenkrais.

Working with dancers or other athletes to improve their posture enhances the length and depth of extensions, the speed and articulation of the feet, height and accuracy of jumps, lifts, and balance. Grace in movement from the integration of delicate awareness of where the point of balance is, through the toes, ankle, knee, hip, and support of the head carriage during spins, runs, pulls, throws, swings, and leaps is developed in the lesson.

Stage presences, vocal acumen, breathe control, embouchure, tone, or finger skills necessary to speak, sing, or play an instrument can become the center of the lesson. I focus on postural support and balance to allow the musician, speaker, actor, or teacher to perform with greater potential for controlled sound at chosen volumes and tempos.

Children develop individualized patterns formulated during infancy that continue to be repeated through the decades of their lives. Injuries and misuse of the body can lead to residual posture and movement patterns which create pain and restrict mobility. These symptoms may be present without resolve until new optional patterns are introduced. I address chronic pain or old injuries with the discovery of alternate posture and movement patterns.

People affected by brain injury, trauma, physical or emotional abuse, or symptoms of post-traumatic stress disorder often find the *Feldenkrais Method* a resource to restore a sense of calm and internal support by creation of additional awareness of safety within their personal posture and balance. My focus and intention is to develop a safe and secure environment for the client to move slowly through the positions of psychological memory to restore clarity of human dignity and ease in well-being.

I work with those who feel restricted by their pain, mobility, personal trauma, injuries, or illnesses and desire to learn skills to improve their posture, balance, and movement. My clients want to take control of possibilities and engage in strategies with potential for change. I like to teach someone to fish rather than cook dinner.

Sidebar 11.3 Patient Interviews

When asked, "What have you learned about this treatment approach or self-care that you would like healthcare providers to know about?", replies included:

- "Healthcare providers need to provide all avenues of healing to their patients; it's a collaborative effort, many avenues to help relieve pain and encourage healing."

- "That it is important to encourage and be open to alternative treatments and to listen to those providers' recommendations or diagnoses. They should support any efforts that a patient makes to be proactive in preventative care."

- "Clients should be encouraged to participate and share responsibility for own health outcomes. Providing information and support encourages this. It is the responsibility of healthcare providers to equip themselves with a broader approach to health management."

Case Study

"Make the impossible possible, then easy, comfortable, pleasurable and finally aesthetically pleasing" (Feldenkrais 1981, 92).

In January 2007, Gordon, then 57 years old, experienced a left-sided cerebrovascular accident. Gordon suffered right-side body paralysis that reduced his ability to work as an engineer and participate in activities of daily living and he had cognitive and memory difficulties. After 10 months of physical therapy, he regained approximately 15% use of his right upper extremity. He had limited grip and could only lift four pounds. He complained of constant, intense pain bilaterally in the cervical and scapulothoracic areas. He developed sleep apnea and began using a continuous positive airway pressure machine.

After discharge from physical therapy, Gordon's primary care physician referred him to me [Haller] for a series of ten *Feldenkrais* lessons beginning in July 2008. He was unable to lie or sleep on his back due to pain. Gordon spoke of his inability to work effectively because of pain, limited right upper extremity function, memory problems, and difficulty staying awake. His self-image as a father and virile man suffered due to these physical and cognitive difficulties.

During Gordon's first lesson, he had poor control of his right lower extremity that presented with decreased weight bearing, increased tone and stiffness, and difficulty bending his hip and knee. He had limited trunk rotation with little differentiation. As a result, he walked with a side-to-side sway, had difficulty changing directions while walking, and fatigued quickly. He struggled with transitioning between standing, sitting, and lying. He had poor postural control and tended to have most of his weight on his left leg while leaning his upper body to the right and forward. He had difficulty balancing on one leg, the right worse than the left, which made activities requiring balance and weight transfer very difficult.

Gordon's right forearm was habitually supinated with his fingers flexed. He had swelling and increased flexor tonus in the right hand with little active extension. The right index finger was particularly flexed and difficult to open. Gordon used his left hand to peel open his right hand and was unable to grasp and pick up small objects. His right shoulder and arm hung anterior to his body, which made raising his arm overhead difficult.

Throughout the assessment, I verbally guided Gordon through movement patterns of weight distribution and helped him explore skeletal support when standing and sitting. In standing, I had him use the wall for support to allow for more stability and perceptual information during movement explorations.

During our lessons, I verbally and manually guided Gordon through numerous balance-related explorations. I encouraged him to practice these movements between sessions as part of his self-care and learning.

I often had Gordon in side lying with a large bolster under the top leg, and foam pads supporting his head and thoracic area. I focused on pelvic movements, including anterior and posterior tilts. The roller provided a weight-supporting tool while I rotated the femurs in conjunction with pelvic movements. I used many slow, small pelvic movements and integrated them with alternating spinal flexion and extension to engage each vertebra and expand movement possibilities in more differentiated directions.

Gordon had a postural habit that included a depressed sternum and forward head and shoulders. I supported this pattern with light compression in the thoracic region to reduce muscular tension. As the muscles lengthened, thoracic mobility improved, scapulae slid more easily, clavicles could move upward, and upper extremity and neck mobility improved.

These changes in core posture made it easier to focus on upper extremity function. I manually guided Gordon to support and reduce flexor tone and progressed to sensorimotor activities with the fingers in extension. I had him use both hands so that the left hand could assist the right hand and enhance perception. We did movements with palms together or with fingers interlaced.

Gradually, Gordon could squeeze a ball that fitted in his hand. He slowly progressed to smaller items. He practiced crumpling paper, tossing it on the floor, and picking it up. With each functional accomplishment, we added another challenge.

We practiced sitting and finding locations on the floor where Gordon could place his feet for skeletal support so he could improve his trunk and head carriage. We did similar experiments to clarify skeletal support during standing and walking. At times, we used a roller under each foot while sitting to mobilize and provide sensory information to the foot and ankle to increase balance and function when walking and standing. I had Gordon practice walking under varying conditions, including forwards and backwards.

Gordon's progression was at times easy and difficult, rapid and slow. Despite this variability, he displayed tenacity and constantly played with the ideas and movements during the ten sessions. His motivation was key to his improvement. By the end of our sessions in October 2008, Gordon's pain was intermittent and decreased in intensity by 50%. He could sleep on his back and woke rested. He could elevate his right arm, extend his fingers, and turn a doorknob. He had a clearer sense of balance when walking and standing. He reduced the sway in his gait, increased counter-rotation, and improved his arm swing. With reduced co-contraction in his right lower extremity and trunk, he had greater ease and quality of transitional movements. Perhaps most meaningful to Gordon, he recovered sufficient function to resume wearing pants with a zipper.

Conclusion

Certified practitioners of the *Feldenkrais Method* of somatic education verbally and physically guide students to learn and improve function through self-exploration. Students engage and play with movements during *Functional Integration* and *Awareness Through Movement* classes. Each lesson is student-focused, in a safe, secure, and supported learning environment. This maximizes possibilities for students to examine current behaviors, explore alternative movements, and add new patterns to their repertoire. By improving their abilities to sense, feel, think, and move, students create greater ease and efficiency in posture, balance, and activities of daily living, and thereby reduce pain of both physical and emotional origin.

References

Baliki, M., D. Chialvo, P. Geha, R. Levy, R. Harden, T. Parrish, and A. Apkarian. 2006. Chronic pain and the emotional brain: Specific brain activity associated with spontaneous fluctuations of intensity of chronic back pain. *The Journal of Neuroscience* 26(47):12165–73.

Baliki, M., P. Geha, A. Apkarian, and D. Chialvo. 2008. Beyond feeling: Chronic pain hurts the brain, disrupting the default-mode network dynamics. *The Journal of Neuroscience* 28(6):1398–1403.

Bearman, D., and S. Shafarman. 1999. The Feldenkrais Method in the treatment of chronic pain: A study of efficacy and cost effectiveness. *American Journal of Pain Management* 9(1): 22–7.

Buchanan, P. A. 2012. The Feldenkrais Method® of somatic education. In: *A Compendium of Essays on Alternative Therapy*, ed. A. Bhattacharya, 147–172. Rijeka, Croatia: InTech.

Buchanan, P. A. 2014. Spring. Seriously, for a moment: Unwired and soft-wired. *SenseAbility* 66(63):9–11.

Buchanan, P. A., N. Nelsen, and S. Geletta. 2014. United States *Guild Certified Feldenkrais Teachers®:* A survey of characteristics and practice patterns. *BMC Complementary and Alternative Medicine* 14:217.

Carlsson, A. M. 1983. Assessment of chronic pain. I. Aspects of the reliability and validity of the visual analogue scale. *Pain* 16(1):87–101.

Cheever, O. 2000. Connected knowing and "somatic empathy" among somatic educators and clients of somatic education. *ReVision Journal* 22(4):15–23.

Cheever, O., and L. Cohen. 2003. The Feldenkrais Method. In: *Complementary and Alternative Medicine in Rehabilitation*, ed. E. Leskowitz, 39–50. St. Louis: Churchill Livingstone.

Chinn, J., D. Trujillo, S. Kegerreis, and T. Worrell. 1994. Effect of a Feldenkrais intervention on symptomatic subjects performing a functional reach. *Isokinetics and Exercise Science* 4(4):131–6.

Elbert, T., C. Pantev, C. Wienbruch, B. Rockstroh, and E. Taub. 1995. Increased cortical representation of the fingers of the left hand in string players. *Science* 270:305–7.

Feldenkrais, M. 1977. *Awareness Through Movement*. New York: Harper & Row.

Feldenkrais, M. 1981. *Elusive Obvious*. California: Meta Publications.

Feldenkrais, M. 1985. *The Potent Self: A Guide to Spontaneity*. San Francisco: Harper San Francisco.

Feldenkrais, M. 1996. *Body and Mature Behavior: A Study of Anxiety, Sex, Gravitation and Learning*. Madison, CT: International Universities Press.

Feldenkrais, M. 2010. *Embodied Wisdom: The Collected Papers of Moshe Feldenkrais*. San Diego, CA: Somatic Resources.

Feldenkrais, M. 2014. *Thinking and Doing*, trans. R. Ofir. Longmont, CO: Genesis II Publishing.

Ginsburg, C. 2010. *The Intelligence of Moving Bodies: A Somatic View of Life and its Consequences*. Santa Fe, NM: AWAREing Press.

Kaetz, D. 2007. *Making Connections: Hasidic Roots and Resonance in the Teachings of Moshe Feldenkrais*. Metchosin, British Columbia: River Centre Publishing.

Kemp, C., M. Ersek, and J. Turner. 2005. A descriptive study of older adults with persistent pain: use and perceived effectiveness of pain management strategies. *BMC Geriatrics* 5:12.

Lundblad, I., J. Elert, and B. Gerdle. 1999. Randomized controlled trial of physiotherapy and Feldenkrais interventions in female workers with neck-shoulder complaints. *Journal of Occupational Rehabilitation* 9(3):179–4.

Lundqvist, L. O., C. Zetterlund, and H. Richter. 2014. Effects of Feldenkrais method on chronic neck/scapular pain in people with visual impairment: a randomized controlled trial with one-year follow-up. *Arch Phys Med Rehabil* 95(9):1656–61. doi: 10.1016/j.apmr.2014.05.013. Epub 2014 Jun 4.

Malmgren-Olsson, E., and B. Armelius. 2003. Non-specific musculoskeletal disorders in patients in primary care: subgroups with different outcome patterns. *Physiotherapy Theory & Practice* 19(3):161–73.

Malmgren-Olsson, E., and I. Bränholm. 2002. A comparison between three physiotherapy approaches with regard to health-related factors in patients with non-specific musculoskeletal disorders. *Disability And Rehabilitation* 24(6):308–17.

Malmgren-Olsson, E., B. Armelius, and K. Armelius. 2001. A comparative outcome study of body awareness therapy, Feldenkrais, and conventional physiotherapy for patients with nonspecific musculoskeletal disorders: Changes in psychological symptoms, pain, and self-image. *Physiotherapy Theory & Practice* 17(2); 77–95.

Plastaras, C., S. Schran, N. Kim, D. Darr, and M. S. Chen. 2013. Manipulative therapy (Feldenkrais, massage, chiropractic manipulation) for neck pain. *Curr Reumatol Rep* 15(7):339. doi: 10.1007/s11926-013-0339-x. file:///C:/Users/Marissa/Downloads/

Manipulative%20Therapy%20for%20Neck%20Pain.pdf (accessed July 8, 2015).

Schön-Ohlsson, C., J. Willén, and B. Johnels. 2005. Sensory motor learning in patients with chronic low back pain: A prospective pilot study using optoelectronic movement analysis. *Spine* 30(17):E509–16.

Schön-Ohlsson, C., J. Willén, and B. E. Johnels. 2006. Optoelectronic movement analysis to measure motor performance in patients with chronic low back pain: Test of reliability. *Journal of Rehabilitation Medicine* 38(6):360–7.

Smith, A., G. Kolt, and J. McConville. 2001. The effect of the Feldenkrais method on pain and anxiety in people experiencing chronic low back pain. *New Zealand Journal of Physiotherapy* 29(1): 6–14.

Thelen, E., and L. B. Smith. 1994. *A Dynamic Systems Approach to the Development of Cognition and Action*. Cambridge, MA: MIT Press.

Walker, M. P. 2008. Sleep-dependent memory processing. *Harvard Review of Psychiatry* 16(5):287–98.

Xie, L., H. Kang, Q. Xu, M. J. Chen, Y. Liao, M. Thiyagarajan, J. O'Donnell, D. J. Christensen, C. Nicholson, J. J. Iliff, et al., 2013. Sleep drives metabolite clearance from the adult brain. *Science* 342:373–7.

Additional Resources

Feldenkrais Guild of North America http://www.feldenkrais.com

International Feldenkrais Federation http://feldenkrais-method.org/en

Interactive movement practices: Trager®

Introduction

I was introduced to Trager® as a bodywork modality in 1985. My work at the time was managing a *vipassana* meditation retreat center on San Juan Island in Washington State, for Thai Buddhist monk Dhiravamsa. He told me that he had experienced bodywork all over the world and he felt that *Trager* was the closest form to the practices we were learning at the center (Dhiravamsa 1990). Shortly afterwards, I received my first *Trager* session in Seattle. I felt very comfortable on the massage table and my body was moving very freely. I had never felt my body move with such ease and comfort. After the session I went for a walk and noticed remarkable feelings in my body. It was as if I was floating; my body felt so light and fluid. Every step felt effortless as if my feet were barely touching the ground. The nature around me was intensely alive, reflecting the feelings I was having in my body. Now, 30 years later, I can still feel those effects, and see in the nature around me what I had seen on that walk.

Essence of Trager®

In the Trager Approach®, the body is treated as a communications medium between the client and the practitioner. The first part is the table work, in which the client is a passive recipient of rhythmic movement of her body. The movement is attuned to the tonicity of the client's body and gently challenges the pains and limitations that have accumulated in the client's body-mind. The practitioner intends to underwhelm instead of overwhelm: pain-free movement through approximation of connective tissue, through "weighing" the tissue, and through creating joint movement, and entrainment between the practitioner's and client's body movement.

The second part involves active movements off the table, called **Mentastics®** on the part of the client. Dr. Milton Trager developed these movements to recreate the experience of the table work, first to bring relief to his own body, second as self-relief and homework for the client. Once again the principle of underwhelm applies so as not to take the client into pain by challenging her bodily resistance. These movements are based on two basic guidelines: no effort, no pain. In using these methods—table work and Mentastics®—Trager was intent on teaching the unconscious mind to let go of conditioning. He believed that injury is often held in the mind and autonomic nervous system long after injured tissue has been repaired (Blackburn 2015).

During my first *Trager* class I realized why Dhiravamsa had suggested that I pursue that form of bodywork. What was emphasized the most was the inner state of mind of the practitioner, presence, or what Trager called "hook-up." This mind-state practice of the practitioner is the third and most unique feature of the *Trager* approach. The body-centered awareness that Trager was emphasizing was very similar to the continuous body-centered sensory scanning in *vipassana*. Two important factors are helpful in understanding this connection: first, the living body essence exists continually in the present moment (Wilber 1981). Second, every sensation, including pain, we experience in our body is always occurring now. The ability to feel these presencing sensations is called sentience (Hart 1987; Hanna 1995).

Trager emphasized that we are always working on the unconscious mind of the client. By creating pleasurable sensations—such as floating, passive stretching, elastic rebounds in the joints—practitioners could help clients change their mental conditioning. This is an interactive process, resulting from a sharing of practitioner and client presence (Blackburn 2015).

History

Milton Trager was born in 1910. As he matured, he was highly influenced by the Physical Culture movement started by Bernarr Macfadden in the late 1800s. The proponents emphasized clean living, healthy thoughts, good diet, lots of exercise, exposure to the elements, and living in places that had easy access to sun, outside activities, and nature (Lisken1996).

President Teddy Roosevelt (1858–1919) was probably the most famous exponent of another movement of the time: changing one's life through positive thinking and physical challenge (Burns 2014). Many persons, especially younger ones, were drawn to these examples. Many of the proponents of Physical Culture were individuals like Theodore Roosevelt and Milton Trager who were weak and sickly as children. They inspired many in the United States to take charge of their life and become productive, healthy citizens. The phrase "mind over matter" was very much the slogan of the day.

Trager followed those examples. He became very active physically: as a professional dancer, vaudeville performer, acrobat, bodybuilder, and boxer. In telling his own story, Trager states his discovery that he could treat people with his hands came spontaneously when he worked on his overly tired boxing coach. Both he and the coach were surprised by the results. He started experimenting with treating persons with physical problems. Trager believed, like Physical Culturalist Jack Lalane 20 years later, that healthy persons could influence the sick and weak to revamp their connection with their bodies and their lives. In the 1930s, he started developing his own forms of bodywork as a lay practitioner, focusing on back injuries and post-polio sufferers. Though Trager never clearly described how he derived all the facets of his work, it is clear that rhythmic movement, light touch, self-conscious interactions with gravity, and muscle fluttering were influenced by his own physical activities as well as his experiments in treating disabled clients. He was able to relieve many of their symptoms by applying his own hands as well as the "can do" attitude of Physical Culture (Blackburn 2003).

Trager served in the navy during WWII as a pharmacist's mate and refined his own techniques by working with soldiers returning from battlefields with mental and physical injuries. After the war, he set up shop in southern California where he resumed his practice treating many different conditions. In 1952, Trager decided to go to medical school to legitimize his methods. Upon finishing his courses in medicine, he was accepted for an internship in psychiatry on the island of Oahu, Hawaii. He was granted a variance to practice medicine in Hawaii. He worked in the mornings and on-call as an MD, and in the afternoons using his own hands-on bodywork approaches (Liskin 1996).

In 1975, he was invited by the Esalen Institute in California to demonstrate his hands-on work. After that demonstration, his star began to rise. Many persons wanted to learn his methods. The *Trager* Association was formed in 1980 and a teaching protocol was established. As the Association grew, Trager was assisted in classes by his early students in developing the specific principles, applications, and the characteristics of his work. The *Trager* Association developed an in-depth training program and ongoing certification requirements independent of the few existing massage schools (Liskin 1996).

Theoretical Approaches for Pain Management from a Trager Perspective

The ongoing challenge in Trager's approach that underlies each of the theoretical aspects below was to discover procedures in which the client experiences pleasure even while letting go of limits, and producing new freedoms of movement and coordination that normally would cause discomfort.

The elements of this section derive from Trager's interactions with clients and students over the years (see Figure 12.1). Trager himself never developed a handbook for *Trager*. In classes, he would demonstrate on a client and then come by and correct students as they tried to apply what they had observed. It was left to his assistants and fledgling

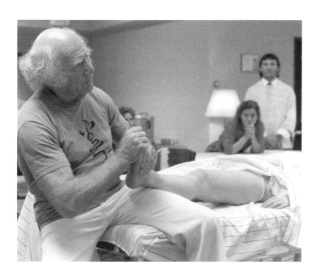

Figure 12.1
Milton Trager at the table.
(Used with permission Trager Institute.)

teachers to compile and keep updating a student training handbook for learning his approach. In classes, Trager placed great emphasis on students being in "hook-up" while they were working on one another. He also would take the class through *Mentastics* movements, so that students could capture the essence of pain-free non-efforting, and presencing sentience. During the table work, Trager would rarely answer technical questions or describe what he was doing in anatomical language. He would have students put their hands on his hands so they could feel what he was doing (Liskin1996; Juhan 1989).

No Pain

Trager often explained that, if you are causing pain, you are not doing *Trager* (Trager 1982). In trainings, he stressed that we should not use pressure to remove pain. Even though *Trager* practitioners work on places where the client has been experiencing pain, there is no attempt to push against resistance. The client receives very

pleasurable effects from resonant movement. The movement rhythm matches the elasticity in the client's body and sends a very powerful signal to the brain (Foster et al. 2004). The muscles, nerves, and joints that would be required for the client to create the same movement by herself become passive receivers. Hence the unique rhythmic movements send signals to the brain that do not trigger guarding reflexes (Juhan 1989; Blackburn 2004b).

Sidebar 12.1 Research
Foster and colleagues applied the Trager approach to treating headaches in a small clinical trial with three arms: medication only (control group), medication and attention (attention control group), and Trager and medication (intervention group) (2004). The findings were that the Trager group experienced a decrease in both medication use and headache frequency. These authors further found that Trager and physician attention improved headaches and quality of life (Foster et al. 2004). These promising results suggest that the provider–patient relationship and a patient-centered approach are essential components to effectively caring for patients with pain conditions.

Self-care

"You cannot give anything you haven't got" (Trager 1986a, Trager 1986b videos). By this statement Trager meant that practitioners have the responsibility to release their own bodily guarding patterns, including painful restrictions. Trager insisted that practitioners receive sessions themselves: pause, step back, and practice *Mentastics* when they feel overloaded; maintain a state of presence (hook up); attend to their own body mechanics; never overwhelm client's resistance; and work from a place of comfort. These self-care guidelines foster sensitivity in the practitioner, enhancing their ability to read whether or not the client is experiencing pain (Blackburn 2004c).

Finding Resonance

Practitioners move from their *whole* body as they match the client's body rhythm. This allows their hands to remain soft and sensitive, and allows the client to feel more securely held. Moving and feeling from her whole body brings the practitioner more information about the clients' amplitude of movement and vectors of free movement. The client's feeling of trust and safety grows because she can feel the motion being generated from the practitioner's whole body. Thus, entrainment and mutual assurance can take place, as with a mother rocking a baby from her whole body. The client feels the practitioner's whole body sensing and matching the rhythm of her intrinsic body movement. Modalities that overwhelm bodily defenses require more strength on the part of the practitioner, and produce more pain and guarding in the client (Blackburn 2004b).

Less is More

Here are two approaches to not producing pain. One is to assist the connective tissue in doing what it is already doing by using variations of positional release. The other is to underwhelm the bodily defenses by combining movements that follow lines of least resistance, so that the client receives quite pleasurable signals to the brain. When practitioners are working with tremendous client pain and guarding in the body, the less they do, the more effective they are. Milton Trager: "When you feel resistance, do less" (Trager1986b video). Reducing the pressure, allows the practitioner to *feel* more, allows the client to feel safer, reduces client anxiety, and can inspire client's somatic curiosity. This is the underwhelm approach, i.e. one that does not challenge resistance directly. Using micromovements, "weighing" and supporting body parts bring presence, trust, no pain, and new information to the client. The state of presence (hook-up) (Blackburn 2004a) allows practitioners to discern movement restrictions *before* they take the client

into pain. Practitioners deal with the subtle reflexes of guarding by backing off, trying a new direction of movement, or new hand support placement. *Trager* clients become less fearful as they realize that their sessions are not increasing their pain. This allows the practitioner to connect through the client's present bodily sensations rather than through the client's fear-ridden memories.

Establishing Trust

One way of bringing the client into feeling safe with body movement is to ensure that he feels continually supported. This support is easily supplied when the practitioner "weighs" parts of the client's body. The practitioner positions her hands and body so that she can comfortably support the weight of the body part in motion. The client feels supported because in weighing, the mass of the body part being moved is directly transferred through the practitioner's center of gravity to the ground. Weighing reduces guarding reactions and builds confidence in the client as he entrusts the movements of her body parts to the practitioner. After childhood, it is rare for a part of our body to be supported and moved through gravity by another person. This can create therapeutically pleasurable sensations of trust for the client. As the client surrenders into being weighed, the practitioner can easily feel the changes in the client's muscles, joints, and other connective tissue. Practitioners can also feel changes in quality of movement, tissue temperature and tonus, and bodily cues, like reflexive releases. Surprisingly, the amount of client somatic awareness can also be felt by the practitioner who is in weighing mode. To follow cues from the client's body, such as subtle guarding and reflexive releases, practitioners work with soft hands that shape themselves to, rather than imposing themselves on, the client's body (see Figure 12.2). This allows practitioners to follow the changes that are implicit in the client's body as the client lets go (Blackburn 2004b).

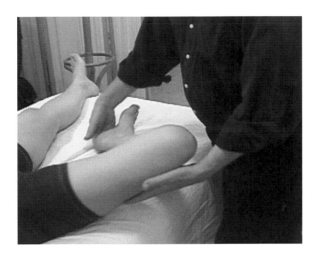

Figure 12.2
Weighing the leg. Chie Muranaka model.
(Reproduced with kind permission from Chie Muranaka.)

Mentastics®

Practitioners teach *Mentastics* (mental gymnastics) so that clients can recreate the feelings and releases that occurred during the table work. The guidelines for Mentastics include: Don't try, don't effort; you will accomplish more release and relaxation if you keep your self-created movements in the range that are pleasurable to you. Keep checking in between movements to feel the changes in your body. Ask yourself: "How little can I do? What is even less than that?" Weigh your arm and then let it drop and feel the effortlessness and elasticity at the end of the drop. Trager's quote on *Mentastics*: "I do these movements because they pleasure me." (Trager 1989 video). *Mentastics* are composed of proprioceptive interactions with gravity, dynamic positional releases, and somatic awareness guided by attention to pain-free and effort-free movement (Blackburn 2004c). *Mentastics* are designed to move the body using momentum, centrifugal and centripetal force, gravity, and tissue elasticity. Using these elements to create movements allows injured connective tissue and nerves to experience

the movements in a receptive non-engaged state. The signals that go from them to the brain are not reinforcing the limits that have been imposed by the gamma sensory motor system. That is why it is very important to find ways to create painless movement to change mental guarding (Trager and Guadagno 1988; Juhan 2003, 2014).

Changing the Mind

Pleasure is a stronger impulse for changing fear-based mental conditioning than the imposition of pain. In neuroplasticity research, the transformative phase in creating new brain synapses occurs when we can replace painful signals with pleasurable ones (Hansen 2006; Newberg 2013). With the gentle rocking of *Trager*, the client experiences parasympathetic effects rather than sympathetic reactions. Much of our mental conditioning comes from traumatic events in our past. Long after the body has healed itself, the mind is still holding on to certain memories and injuries from the past. Mentally holding on to the past creates fear of repeating the past. The combination of pain and fear creates much of our suffering.

Presence

Trager believed that presence, or **hook-up** (Blackburn 2004a; Blackburn and Price 2007), on

> **Sidebar 12.2 Research**
> Fear conditioning is well-established in research on emotions (Moseley and Vlaeyen 2015). The **fear-avoidance model** has been widely attributed to pain-related disability (Lethem et al. 1983; Rose et al. 1992; Vlaeyen and Linton 2000, 2012). Trager might have been ahead of his time, combining movement and addressing fear avoidance in the same practice. Promising research from Vlaeyen and colleagues addresses dysfunction and chronic pain in the hope of understanding the magnitude of the full effect fear has on functional ability, or disability for people suffering from chronic pain.

the part of the practitioner could directly transfer to the client. As the client experienced presence from the practitioner, the client's relationship with her body and her life would also be changed. Trager repeatedly said: "Hook-up is like measles; you catch it from someone who's got it" (Liskin 1996, 131).

There are various ways that the practitioner can create presencing interactions with the client other than Trager's. One way is to use words to trigger somatic-proprioceptive awareness in the client so that she realizes that her participation is creating the bodily releases she is feeling. As she engages with her proprioceptive awareness into places where the practitioner is working, the client can feel herself having a direct role in changing the tissue. There are a variety of ways the *Trager* practitioner can extend Trager's approach (Blackburn 2013).

Turning Towards Pain

The sections above discuss theory as it relates to Trager's work. To better understand how to deal with clients' pain, I studied various meditative approaches that focus attention directly into the pain. My own practice of *vipassana* over the years provides helpful personal experience. The medium of the meditations are the sensations arising in the body, and a continual monitoring of what is occurring now at the mental, emotional, and physical levels. In my own learning of these processes, much of the experience was quite difficult because I was not used to focusing directly into pain.

I wanted a way to take clients into their pain without creating the effects I had experienced in *vipassana*. It became obvious to me that the thoughts, emotions, and physical sensations are continually reflecting one another. There is a direct connection between what is felt in the body and the activity in the mind. An aspect that occurs with all negative thoughts and emotions is that the body enters a sympathetic state; tissue tightens, breath shortens, body surfaces become cold, and

everything is preparing for fight or flight. As this happens, the memories and negative reactions of fear are also colliding with the normal thought processes of the mind. To reverse this process, I help clients create a proprioceptive interaction with areas of pain, quantifying and qualifying different aspects of the pain (Fehmi and Robbins 2010). I teach clients who would normally dissociate from their pains to realize that they can safely access them directly. Clients start to notice how their reactions to pain arise, based upon how they are paying attention inside. The more proprioceptive attention they bring into the pain, instead of trying to avoid it, or associate it with negative memories, the more they can feel the pure pain signal without fear or irritation (Young 2006).

In 1996, I had confirmation of my evolving approach when I interviewed a hand surgeon named Paul Brand, MD, who specialized in pain. He wrote *The Gift of Pain*. He had done much of the primary research with Hansen's disease and discovered that the biggest problem for patients with leprosy is that they do not feel pain. In his book, he presented many stories about patients, including himself, he had helped go directly into their pain (Brand and Yancy 1993). The stories were very inspiring. Not only did patients move beyond their reactive pain patterns by going directly into their pain, but their whole lives were transformed. He was not trying to take people out of pain, but used pain to bring them deeply into their own healing.

Sidebar 12.3 Patient Interviews

In response to the question, "Have your condition or symptoms or ability to function changed since receiving care?" replies included:

- "Less pain, more flexibility, better posture."

- "Pain is relieved and I have a lot of mobility."

- "It's energizing to not have pain."

Methodology
Interacting with the Client

After reviewing her intake form, I start my sessions by asking the client's sense of where she is at in her life, and how that relates to her body issues. While sitting, standing, and walking, I always ask clients: "What are you feeling in your body right now?" I compare that response with the postural and movement patterns I observe. In the body-work phase, I apply *Trager* in combination with the various methods I describe below. Because of my spiritual counseling training, I also help my clients discover inner obstacles such as, memories, emotional themes, and stressors that impede their bodily changes.

My work is client-centered, meaning that I depend on my client as an equal partner in the process. Their subjective bodily experiences are highly valuable, so I am continually eliciting and responding to client feedback. I can feel through a continual process of assessment, improvisation, and verbal cues how the hands-on work is affecting the client's mind, body, emotions, and spirit. For example, if the client reports feeling pain, I can adjust my approach so that there is no longer pain. We remain engaged dynamically, myself through palpation, the client through proprioception. Part of the process is to ask the client what he is feeling after I feel a release in that body part. Usually, the more that he is feeling, the more release has taken place. When my client realizes that his pain has changed because of his own somatic awareness, he emerges from the experience with tools he can practice on his own.

In my personal practice, there are a variety of ways I have adapted and expanded the underlying approaches Trager taught. Every session is unique, the number of sessions necessary is not predictable, and the tools I apply vary on the individual's needs, desires and treatment goals.

Emphasis on the Clients' Responses and Interactivity

From my beginnings as a *Trager* practitioner, I used words to guide clients into their body sensations at the onset and conclusion of every session. This approach stemmed from my training in *vipassana* meditation. This practice, which derives from Shakyamuni Buddha, is a strong tool for breaking habits and conditioning, and freeing minds and bodies from the past (Thera 1979; Heron 1992). At the beginning of my sessions, I ask clients to follow my hands as we work with different parts of their bodies. This addition to *Trager* applications produces a profound effect on the client as well as me. I remember an early session I gave an MD anesthesiologist in which I told him: "You take people out of pain by taking them out of their bodies; I intend to take you out of pain by bringing you directly into your body." He was totally surprised by what happened—he became totally pain free. At the end, he said, "I'm going to have to totally change my understanding of pain and conscious awareness" (Blackburn 2006).

Engaging in Shared Presence

Trager would actively engage the client in reciprocal proprioceptive interactions with the practitioner's touch: "Push against me lightly, even lighter than that! That's right; I can feel you coming in, now notice the direction I am moving your arm, and bring it further in that direction, or don't let me take it further" (Trager, 1989 video). In these interactions, he was stimulating tissue

---

Sidebar 12.4 Patient Interviews

When asked, "Do you do any regular self-care to relieve or prevent ongoing pain?", replies included:

- "Mild stretching each a.m."

- "Walking, Pilates, techniques my practitioner has suggested."

- "When tension or pain is present I will do small amounts of self massage and infrequent stretching."

response, somatic awareness, and active engagement in the body parts which were experiencing what Thomas Hanna called *sensory motor amnesia* (Hanna 1993). In my own forms of shared presence, I engage with clients' proprioceptive actions such as: "Push against me with your breath, touch my hands from inside your body, describe the pain, go right into where the pain is the strongest." Trager used hook-up as an interactive tool, limited by the proviso "no pain, no effort" (Juhan 1993, 2014).

Side-lying Somatics

Trager is normally done with the client in prone or supine positioning. Starting in 1987, I adapted some *Trager* applications to side-lying positioning, what I now call side-lying somatics (see Figure 12.3). There are tremendous advantages to side-lying work, especially in dealing with pain. As long as my client is bolstered in a way that leaves the upper arm and leg fully supported, I can move the torso in all three directions. I found that when clients have spinal fusing or scoliosis, I can find directions of movement that are not available when prone or supine. For lower lumbar pain, I apply torqueing

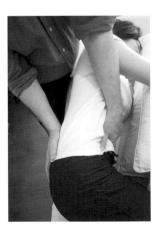

Figure 12.3
Side-lying somatics. Chie Muranaka model.
(Reproduced with kind permission from Chie Muranaka.)

movements between the lower abdomen and the lower back so that the client experiences abdominal shortening and low back lengthening while being moved in various directions. Probably the biggest advantage in side-lying with relationship to pain is that gravity is passing through the body in the direction that shortens connective tissue in the rotator cuffs as well as the hip joints, combined with less body surface on the table, which makes it easy to move the whole body while focusing specifically into those areas of shortened or decompressed connective tissue (Hanna 1995; Blackburn 2002a, 2002b).

Positional Release and Trager

I have found that positional release produces very welcome effects in the body and mind of clients. As I take over the work of a muscle or a joint, the clients enter a parasympathetic state, creating feelings of trust and curiosity rather than fear. For example, a client had a frozen shoulder. She could not raise her arm above horizontal. I noticed that she was anteriorly rotated. First I put her in side-lying position so that the affected shoulder was off the table. I placed a pillow in her armpit so that the head of the humerus and acromioclavicular joint had some extra space. By supporting and moving her forearm, I could reposition the whole arm, which could naturally retract. This felt very good to her. Then I gradually lifted her arm so that the weight came directly into her rotator cuff and by extension into the pectoral girdle. When her arm was in this position, she took deeper breaths and her shoulder joints (glenohumeral and sternoclavicular) naturally decompressed. From that point on, I could gradually bring her whole arm into neutral and bolster her in that position. I then used *Trager* movements to affirm that she was fully free.

I found that the sensitivity of soft hands and gentle movement I had learned in *Trager* became the means of assessing the directions of repositioning as well as confirming the therapeutic changes occurring. I studied *dynamic positional release* with

Denise Deig. Her approach mirrors many of the principles that Trager advocated in his work. She teaches what she calls *indirect method* (Deig 2006).

Noting the Difference between Pain and Suffering

Practitioners and clients tend to conflate pain and suffering. Pain signals come from our bodies much of the time without prompting suffering. Often, we adjust ourselves to turn off a pain signal and are unaware that we have repositioned ourselves unless the pain persists (Blackburn 2006). Pain only exists now, whereas memory of pain is in the past. Paradoxically, if we ask the client: "What are you feeling *now* in your body," often clients cannot tell us. I always ask this question at the beginning of every session to give me a sense of the client's degree of somatic awareness. We commonly use pain to recharge our past memories instead of embodying the present. To help the client release the overlay of past memories, I create tactile sensations which he can interact with right where the pain or tightness is located. As he breathes into (expanding with the in-breath, contracting with the out-breath) that place where my hands are, the tissue softens and he relaxes.

Suffering is quite different. Suffering usually has some elements of fear and negative emotions associated with the pain (Hinds 2003). When we experience a pairing of pain with negative fearful reactions such as guilt, danger, anger, hopelessness, failure, death, we then react to the pain with various degrees of suffering. Clients can feel weak, oppressed, cursed, and resigned to their fate. On the other hand, the pain can be used to create a pathway towards letting go of suffering. I have used this approach with dying patients in a cancer hospital in Japan. I was invited by the medical staff who were observing the sessions. I would place my hands directly on very painful tumors, and ask patients to fill my hands with their breath. I found ways to move their body parts without creating more pain. What then happens is a palpable shift away from their defensive reactions, which takes them not only out of fear but into a strong sense of aliveness (Ford 1992, 1999).

Focusing and Bodywork

Focusing is based on a process developed at the University of Chicago in the 1960s under the direction of Eugene Gendlin PhD (Gendlin 1982, 1996). His team discovered that clients who felt into their bodies in psychotherapy made much more rapid progress. In focusing, there is a direct correlation between the client's increased ability to describe pain verbally and increased ability to move physically and release pain. For example, my client felt suicidal because she was in extreme pain. After having hemorrhoid surgery, the sutures cut through her anal sphincter. As I worked with her, I asked her what the pain felt like. She told me that the pain in her anus felt like hot coals. I mirrored her words and ask her if she could increase the pain by blowing internally on the pain. She found that she could do that. I then asked her if she could cool the pain. Surprise, she found that she could also do that. Now she had a tool she could use on her own. She practiced this tool at home and when she came to her next session, she was visibly more relaxed. I pursued the same process with her each session. She found various ways of interacting with the pain: writing poetry, drawing it, enriching her feeling vocabulary, and bringing movement from our sessions into her whole body. The closer she came to describing what she felt in her body, the closer she came to pain-free movement in her body, and regaining enthusiasm for her life. Her wound responded directly to her willingness to probe the tissue somatically. So focusing is also helpful when I cannot put my hands directly on a part of the body, for example, the genitals, internal abdomen, open wounds, and inside the skull (Blackburn 2008).

What is called a *"felt shift"* in focusing means that the client's verbal and interactive processing has produced a dramatic change in the client's conscious awareness and physicality. This shift is usually in the direction of more ease and expansive awareness inside, outside, and in one's inner life. I find that these changes are parallel to the changes Trager was trying to produce with hook-up, except that they involve much more conscious participation on the part of the client, who is becoming the author of her own experience.

Decompression Somatics

Decompression is a specific form of positional release; using micro-movements, I shorten the connective tissue, joints, tendons, ligaments, and fascia in order to create relaxation while finding the direction of ease. The client is encouraged to interact with the sensations produced. Often, it feels as if the tissue is melting. It takes very little verbal support to guide them directly into a body part and have them interact with the compressions and tactile stimulation of my hands. For instance, a client's lungs in the upper chest and upper back are underused. This seems to happen often in aging, emotional withdrawal, and grieving. I encourage the client to breathe into her upper chest and back and to expand her breath laterally and then use my hands to help her contract medially with the out-breath. This creates a reduction of anterior rotation and an incredible rush of vital energy in the client.

In applying **decompression somatics,** I often follow the fascial connections in Tom Myer's *Anatomy Trains* (Myers 2001). Instead of applying a direct approach of deep pressure to overcome the resistance of various muscle and fascial links, I use indirect approaches, i.e. positional release and client somatic interactions. In a painful or hypertonic body part, I use *tapping* (tactile stimulation) to deepen client proprioception and interaction. This produces no additional pain and often releases the pain and hypertonicity. The purpose of the tapping is to help clients feel through the different layers of tight tissue so that they have a more three-dimensional experience.

As the client brings his awareness into what he can feel, I apply very gentle positional releases and start a process in which the client's somatic awareness is guiding my hands far away from where we are in contact (see Figure 12.4).

Case Study

A 70-year-old female psychoanalyst reported intolerable pain, left mid-thoracic, 7th–8th rib subluxation, and had suspended almost all of her activities because of back pain. Specifically, the pain was unrelenting while awake, intermittent while asleep. "The pain feels sharp, stabbing, and electrical. In the beginning I felt surprised and confused because it was so deep. As it continued, I felt fear and despair and hopeless that it would never go away." For 2 months she had managed her back pain by lying still on a heating pad much of the time except when working with clients. "Simple things like talking, looking to the side, laughing, or adjusting my position would increase the pain; it literally hurt to be with my friends."

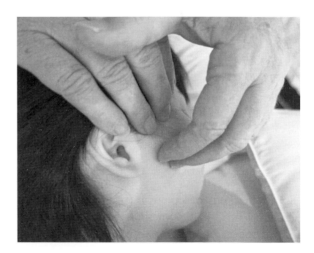

Figure 12.4
Decompression somatics for temporal mandibular joint pain—Noriko Baba model.
(Reproduced with kind permission from Noriko Baba.)

She had a history of polio as a child, Hashimoto syndrome as an adult, as well as broken right wrist and a severed tendon in her left foot. She could feel exactly where the pain was centered in the costovertebral joint.

Treatment

The patient was bolstered in a side-lying position, left-side up. She felt some pain in this position at first when she inhaled, but when her left arm and shoulder were retracted and supported she was able to take deeper breaths. The subluxation felt like the 8th rib was folded partly under the 7th. I placed my hands parallel to her ribs and asked her to focus her in-breath into my hands. As she exhaled, I compressed the ribs toward her vertebrae, which seemed to help her pain somewhat and soften the connective tissue between the ribs and her vertebrae. I could then gently bring some rocking motion to her torso while torqueing the intercostal muscles between her 7th and 8th ribs. Gradually I could feel the ribs repositioning, as she continued to breathe deeper and deeper into her lungs. She reported that her pain was greatly relieved. I said that I could feel her breathing into my hands, expanding her ribcage from inside her body. Later she said that this immediate relief was something she would never forget. I continued to treat the rest of her body in a side-lying position, on both sides so that she could feel the range of the change that had occurred.

As we continued to work together over a series of sessions, she discovered that her early childhood memories of polio had created unconscious assumptions that she would always suffer in her body; that her rib would remain inflexible and guarded. Once the rib felt more mobile and alive, we could work other body issues that stemmed from her past.

She later stated that the relief of the intense pain has shifted her experience of her body. She could then learn to:

> Follow the pain and be curious about it. Pain feels as though it occurs in the context of a larger body, rather than being the focus of the whole body. There is a subtle, but noticeable shift in my perception of my body in space, and some increased interest in taking care of it in a kindly way, as opposed to viewing it as something that only hurts me. Instead of viewing the pain as some sort of psychological or spiritual flaw of mine, [I learned] to simply be interested in it, to be curious about it. And that is a much gentler way to experience myself.

Conclusion

Dr. Milton Trager put the client's body into motion without stimulating pain, fear, or resistance. He used Mentastics for eliciting feeling responses in the client's self-generated movements that bypassed unconscious guarding. He taught clients and practitioners to share a state of presence by feeling weight, by measuring effort, and by giving up "trying." Hook-up, or presencing, became the cornerstone of Trager's approach. He was convinced that pain and inhibition were coming from the client's mind. The basic approaches to changing the mind of the client involve various kinds of somatic interactions between practitioner and client and within the client's own consciousness.

References

Blackburn, J. 2002a. *Why I work on the side: a quiet evolution in bodywork.* Washington State AMTA Newsletter, March Issue.

Blackburn, J. 2002b. *Why somatics, introduction to side-lying.* Somatics class manual.

Blackburn, J. 2003. Trager® psychophysical integration an overview. *Journal of Bodywork and Movement Therapies* 7(4):233–9.

Blackburn J. 2004a. Trager®-2: Hooking up: the power of presence in bodywork. *Journal of Bodywork and Movement Therapies* 8(2):114–21.

Blackburn, J. 2004b. Trager®-3: Trager® at the table. *Journal of Bodywork and Movement Therapies* 8(3):178–88.

Blackburn, J. 2004c. Trager®-4: Mentastics®- presence in motion. *Journal of Bodywork and Movement Therapies* 8(4):265–77.

Blackburn, J. 2006. *Presencing pain: doorways to healing.* Presencing Newsletter 2.

Blackburn, J. 2008. *A meeting of words and touch.* The Focusing Institute Newsletter vol. XIII (1).

Blackburn, J. 2013. *Teamwork and transformation: a presencing paradigm.* Presencing Newsletter 31.

Blackburn, J. 2015. Trager® – psychophysical integration. In *Modalities in massage and bodywork,* ed. E. Stillerman, 2nd edn, 402–19. New York: Mosby.

Blackburn, J., and C. Price. 2007. Further implications of presence in the manual therapies. *Journal of Bodywork and Movement Therapies* 11(1):68–77.

Brand, P., and P. Yancy. 1993. *Pain, the gift nobody wants.* New York: Harper Collins.

Burns, K. 2014. *The Roosevelts: an intimate history.* NPR video. ASIN: B00JKJ0XJU.

Deig, D. 2006. *Positional release technique, from a dynamic systems perspective.* Indianapolis, IN: Somatic Publications.

Dhiravamsa. 1990. *Dynamic way of meditation: the release and cure of pain and suffering through vipassana meditative techniques.* New York: Harper Collins.

Fehmi L., and J. Robbins. 2010. *Dissolving pain – simple brain training exercises for overcoming chronic pain.* Boston, MA: Trumpeter Books.

Ford, C. 1992. *Where healing waters meet: touching the mind and emotions through the body.* New York: Station Hill Press.

Ford, C. 1999. *Compassionate touch: the body's role in emotional healing and recovery.* Berkeley, CA: North Atlantic Books.

Foster, K. A., J. Liskin, S. Cen, A. Abbott, V. Armisen, D. Globe, L. Knox, M. Mitchell, C. Shtir, and S. Azen. 2004. The Trager® approach in the treatment of chronic headache: a pilot study. *Altern Ther Health Med* 10(5):40–6.

Gendlin, E. 1982. *Focusing,* 2nd edn. New York: Bantam.

Gendlin, E. 1996. *Focusing oriented psychotherapy.* New York: Guilford Press.

Hanna, T. 1993. *The body of life: creating new pathways for sensory awareness and fluid movement.* Rochester, VT: Healing Arts Press.

Hanna T. 1995. What is somatics? In *Bone, breath and gesture: practices of embodiment,* ed. D. Johnson, 341–52. Berkeley CA: North Atlantic Books.

Hansen, R. 2006. *Self-directed neuroplasticity.* San Rafael, CA: The Wellspring Institute for Neuroscience and Contemplative Wisdom.

Hart, W. 1987. *The art of living: vipassana meditation as taught by S. N. Goenka.* New York: Harper Collins.

Heron, J. 1992. *Feeling and personhood: psychology in another key.* London: Sage.

Hinds, E. 2003. *A life larger than pain: the pathway from resignation to renewal.* Albuquerque, NM: Health Press.

Juhan, D. 1989. *An introduction to Trager psychophysical integration and mentastics movement education.* Mill Valley, CA: The Trager Institute.

Juhan, D. 1993. *The physiology of hook-up: how Trager® works.* Mill Valley, CA: The Trager Institute.

Juhan, D. 2003. *Job's body,* 3rd edn. Barrytown, NY: Station Hill Press.

Juhan, D. 2014. *Resistance/release notes.* on-line article, http://www.jobsbody.com/pages/articles/

Lethem, J., P. D. Slade, J. D. Troup, and G. Bentley. 1983. Outline of a fear-avoidance model of exaggerated pain perception–I. *Behav Res Ther* 21(4):401–8.

Liskin, J. 1996. *Moving medicine: the life and work of Milton Trager.* Barrytown, NY: Station Hill Press.

Moseley, G. L., and J. W. Vlaeyen. 2015. Beyond nociception: the imprecision hypothesis of chronic pain. *Pain.* 156(1):35–8. doi: 10.1016/j.pain.0000000000000014.

Myers, T. 2001. *Anatomy trains.* New York: Churchill Livingstone.

Newberg, A. 2013. *The metaphysical mind: Probing the biology of philosophical thought.* Self published.

Rose, M. J., L. Klenerman, L. Atchison, and P. D. Slade. 1992. An application of the fear avoidance model to three chronic pain problems. *Behav Res Ther* 30(4):359–65.

Thera, N. 1979. *The heart of Buddhist meditation.* New York: Samuel Weiser.

Trager, M. 1982. Trager psychophysical integration and mentastics. *The Trager Journal* Vol. 1.

Trager, M. 1986a. *Trager addresses group with parkinsonism video.* Mill Valley, CA: Trager Institute.

Trager, M. 1986b. *Interview with Milton Trager video Part 1 and 2.* Mill Valley, CA: Trager Institute.

Trager, M. 1989. *Mentastics with Milton video.* Mill Valley, CA: Trager Institute.

Trager, M., and C. Guadagno. 1988. *Trager® mentastics: movement as a way to agelessness.* Barrytown, NY: Station Hill Press.

Vlaeyen, J. W., and S. J. Linton. 2000. Fear-avoidance and its consequences in chronic musculoskeletal pain: a state of the art. *Pain* 85(3):317–32.

Vlaeyen, J. W., and S. J. Linton. 2012. Fear-avoidance model of chronic musculoskeletal pain: 12 years on. *Pain* 153(6):1144–7.

Wilber, K. 1981. *No boundary: Eastern and Western approaches to personal growth.* Boulder, CO: Shambala.

Young, S. 2006. *Break through pain: a step-by-step mindfulness meditation program for transforming chronic and acute pain.* Boulder, CO: Sounds True Inc.

Additional Resources

Becker, A. 1973. Parameters of Resistance. *The Journal of the American Osteopathic Association* Sept: 75–87.

Blackburn, J. 1999. Trager® Movement. In *Therapeutic Exercise: Moving Toward Function*, ed. C. M. Hall and L. T. Brody. New York: Lippincott Williams & Wilkins.

Blackburn, J. 2007. *How I re-discovered the effectiveness of decompression, introduction to decompression.* Somatics class manual.

Blackburn, J. 2012. *Guiding the client into presence.* Presencing Newsletter 22.

Calais-Germain, B. 1993. *Anatomy of movement.* Seattle, WA: Eastland Press.

Feldenkrais, M. 1977. *Awareness through movement.* New York: Harper and Row Publishers.

Juhan, D. 1998. The Trager approach: the feeling that is healing, *Positive Health* March: 55–60.

Korr, M. 1986. Somatic dysfunction osteopathic manipulative treatment and the nervous system: a few facts, some theories and many questions. *The Journal of the American Osteopathic Association* 86(2):l09–l4.

NhatHanh, T. 2003. *No death, no fear: comforting wisdom for life.* New York: Riverhead Books.

Oschman, J. 2000. *Energy medicine: the scientific basis.* New York: Harcourt Publishers.

Rogers, C. 1989. Client-centered, person-centered, approach to therapy. In *A Carl Rogers Reader*, ed. I. Kutash and A. Wolfe. New York: Houghton Mifflin.

Rossi, E. 1993. *The psychobiology of mind-body healing.* New York: W. W. Norton.

Savage, F. 1990. *Osteoarthritis: a step by step success story to show others they can help themselves.* Barrytown, New York: Stanton Hill Press.

Selye, H. 1976. *The stress of life.* New York: McGraw-Hill.

Introduction

Yoga has earned substantial support in recent years as an intervention benefiting people with pain (Bussing et al. 2012; Cramer et al. 2013; Holtzman and Beggs 2013; Ward et al. 2013). With four meta-analyses since 2012 documenting decreased pain and function-specific benefits, this ancient holistic system has become an evidence-informed practice to address pain-related issues ranging from osteoarthritis to fibromyalgia and irritable bowel syndrome. Indeed, the American Pain Society now includes yoga in its guidelines for the treatment of people with chronic low back pain (Chou et al. 2007). This chapter seeks to offer health professionals an understanding of yoga as more than a trendy body-mind-spirit movement for personal health. Rather, applied therapeutically by trained practitioners, yoga is also an evidence-informed intervention highly effective for integrative pain care.

The complexity and diversity of yoga therapy is well matched to the complex and multifaceted nature of pain. Yoga therapy is an interactive process, allowing for individualized, humanistic interventions of the immensely personal experience of pain. These interventions incorporate

cornerstones of successful pain programs: awareness and self-regulation, acceptance, and restoring functional movement. Our current understanding suggests that integrating yoga techniques into pain management has the potential to provide favorable outcomes in many different populations with difficult-to-change pain conditions (Bussing et al. 2012; Cramer et al. 2013; Holtzman and Beggs 2013; Ward et al. 2013).

History of Yoga

Yoga is both a philosophy and a lifestyle, originally intending to decrease suffering and to foster the attainment of inner peace. Yoga techniques date back more than 5000 years (American Yoga Association 2006), pre-dating both written history and Hinduism, the Indian religion with which yoga is most often associated. Until the twentieth century, the tradition of yoga was passed from teacher to student. Thus, its techniques were based on lived experiences rather than controlled scientific studies.

During the past 100 years, yoga practices have become more popular outside India, especially in North America. While its spiritual intent seemed most important throughout the majority of yoga's history, the Western adaptation has shifted to emphasize the physical dimensions that require flexibility and agility. Less often, Western yoga studios combine the physical practice with aspects of spiritualism, chanting, and meditation. On the surface, it appears that the goal of most individuals attending yoga in North America is solely physical. A focus on gymnastic yoga postures makes it difficult to understand how yoga can be therapeutic for people in whom movement is limited and painful.

Historically, the most common yoga path was classic yoga, known in India as Raja yoga. This yoga includes eight distinct and interrelated activities

---

Sidebar 13.1 Patient Interviews

In response to the question, "Have your condition or symptoms or ability to function changed since receiving care?" a 68-year-old woman with multiple pain conditions for the past 15 years, replied: "I understand more about pain which is the first line of defense. I understand what I need to do and believe that when I do it, it does relieve my pain. I fully understand that to calm my central nervous system is the only way to deal with a number of the conditions I have as a result of central sensitization such as IBS and headaches."

that bring physical, mental, emotional, and spiritual well-being. It begins with *"yamas,"* which require introspection regarding how you act/live in the world, and *"niyamas,"* which provide guidance on how you treat yourself. The practice of *"pranayama"* introduces breath awareness and breathing exercises. The physical postures most widely associated with yoga in the West are known as *"asana"* and appear as the fourth branch of yoga (see Figure 13.1). *"Pratyahara"* seeks to develop awareness of self/withdrawal of external sense while *"dharana"* involves concentration, so that one can practice *"dhyana,"* or meditation. The eight-part system of yoga culminates with *"samadhi,"* the attainment of inner peace or enlightenment. Yoga also includes three lesser known paths towards *samadhi*: serving others through Karma yoga, fostering love and devotion through Bhakti yoga, and gaining wisdom through Jnana yoga. Although aspects of these are important for some with chronic pain, they will not be discussed here.

The physical postures of Raja yoga are important, though not only for the purposes of strength, flexibility, and calorie burn. Skilled teachers guide yoga students to practice deeper awareness of their body, breath, thoughts, emotions, and spirit during the postures of yoga. As a student of yoga brings attention to his or her body position and posture, to areas of increased muscle tension or poor muscle activation, and to breathing patterns, thinking patterns and emotions, the physical practice of yoga transforms into a process of self-discovery. Yoga not only enhances physical abilities; it integrates awareness and self-regulation of body position, muscle tension, breath, thoughts, and emotions.

All yoga is therapeutic. Yet yoga classes and yoga therapy are not the same. Yoga therapy is a process in which an individual, trained and experienced in the entire spectrum of yoga modalities and philosophy, guides individuals through yoga techniques and practices specific to the client's therapeutic needs. While yoga teachers can begin teaching students with 200-hour training

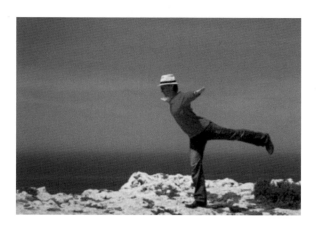

Figure 13.1
Asana: Yoga postures can be used for so many goals besides more flexibility and strength.
Use them to improve balance, confidence, contentment, energy, peacefulness, and even to have fun and find more joy in your life.
(Reprinted with permission, Life Is Now Pain Care Inc.)

Sidebar 13.2 Patient Interviews
In response to the question, "Have your condition or symptoms or ability to function changed since receiving care?" a 59-year-old woman with back and hip pain for 38 years, replied: "Neil's work has given me more control over, and insight into, my ability to lessen pain. I have been able to reduce pain medications substantially. The Pain Clinic agreed that after seeing Neil, I was now able to manage my own pain. I do exercises he taught me (body scans, body awareness, breathing awareness, calm breathing, yoga, etc.) every day. And I have now been teaching Gentle Yoga myself, in a Maintain Your Independence program for seniors, for more than a year. Students have commented that the classes have helped physically and mentally, including relieving pain.

programs, yoga therapists require 1,000 hours of training, practicum, and mentorship for certification before working with clients. The International Association of Yoga Therapists has standardized the training and curriculum requirements. The goal of this extensive training is to align yoga therapy within regulated health professions (International Association of Yoga Therapists 2014).

Theoretical Approaches to Pain Management

Yogic views on pain have both similarities to, and differences from, current Western pain theories. The similarities far outweigh the differences. Let's first look at the differences.

Pain and chronic pain have specific definitions according to the International Association for the Study of Pain (IASP 1986). These attempt to make pain real and measurable, and directly linked to tissue health. Yoga philosophy, on the other hand, views pain as an experience of life that is not limited to the physical body. *Dukkha* is interpreted as both suffering and pain, and the practice of yoga is to decrease suffering.

The prevailing understanding of chronic pain is that it is complex, individual, multifaceted, and

Sidebar 13.3 Research

Historical definitions of Pain: Aristotle (384–322 BCE) defined pain as an emotion, not as a mechanical sensation (Jackson 2002). Galen (AD 130–201) defined pain as a sensation, and not an emotion (Perl 2007). In Perl's conclusion, he writes: "Considering the evidence, it seems reasonable to propose pain to be both a specific sensation and an emotion, initiated by activity in particular peripheral and central neurons" (Perl 2007, 78).

The IASP's most recent definition of pain: An unpleasant sensory and emotional experience associated with actual or potential tissue damage, or described in terms of such damage (IASP 2014).

biopsychosocial (IASP 1986). Yoga is a system that views individuals as unique, complex, and multidimensional, including the body, mind, and spirit. Even more complex is the **Pancamaya** model that views individuals as having five aspects or layers (see Figure 13.2). The outermost layer of our being is what we can see, the physical body. Next comes the energetic aspect, in which breath is integral. Deeper still are the layers that correlate to intellect, emotion, and wisdom, where we regulate thoughts and emotion with meditation. At the center of our being is the higher self or spirit. It is here that we find meaning, and purpose, in life. These aspects, within yoga philosophy, are considered to be integrated,

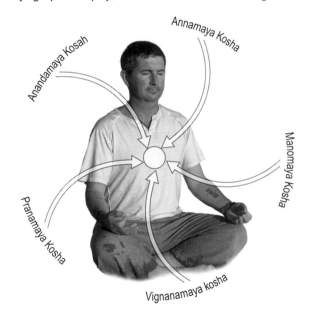

Annamaya Kosha

Anandamaya Kosah

Manomaya Kosha

Pranamaya Kosha

Vignanamaya kosha

Figure 13.2

Pancamaya model: This model describes humans as having five aspects of self and of existence. These are typically referred to as layers or sheaths, yet they are not truly separate or distinct. Similar to a biopsychosocial view of pain, it is impossible to affect one aspect of self without having effects on all.

(Reprinted with permission, Life Is Now Pain Care Inc.)

rather than separate aspects of an individual, similar to a biopsychosocial perspective.

Current pain science shows that, when pain persists, there are measurable changes in our lives, including breathing (Kolar et al. 2012; Mostoufi et al. 2012; Smith, Russell, and Hodges 2014), body awareness (Lotze and Moseley 2007; Wand et al. 2011), posture (Smith, O'Sullivan, and Straker 2008), muscle tension (Roland 1986; Wallwork et al. 2009), thoughts (Campbell and Edwards 2009), emotions (Sturgeon and Zaurta 2010; Crombez et al. 2012; Wideman et al. 2013), relationships (Snelling 1994; Smith and Osborn 2007), and sense of purpose in life (Plach, Heidrich, and Waite 2003; Schleicher et al. 2005), similar to Yogic views. Yoga philosophy suggests that pain and suffering are experiences that not only impact multiple aspects of self, but disconnect us from what is important in our life. The practice of yoga helps those in pain reconnect to what is important. Science also shows how persistent pain can create distortions in body image (Smith et al. 2014) and thoughts (Wideman et al. 2013). Yoga techniques provide an opportunity to practice awareness of body sensations and of our thoughts.

The body-self neuromatrix model, proposed by Melzack (1999) to deepen our understanding of pain, also shows similarities with these same yoga views. This model suggests that pain is an output of our brain, influenced by all inputs (cognitive, sensory, and affective) to the brain. This is a hopeful message: pain can be influenced by altering any and all inputs into the brain. Historically, yoga did not directly address the brain, yet it provided an equally hopeful message: suffering can be influenced by how we practice yoga, and by how we live.

Current science discusses this as "plasticity" (Siddall 2013): like plastic that can be reshaped through the application of force over sufficient duration, we can reshape our nervous system. These changes include chemical, functional, and structural shifts in neurons and our nervous systems, when pain persists, and when we recover (Seminowicz et al. 2011; Wand et al. 2011). Neuroplastic changes are promoted by repetition, by physical activity, by novel learning situations, and by focused attention (Marchand 2014; Silverman and Deuster 2014). The persistent practices of yoga include each of these important factors.

Over at least the last 100 years, prevailing pain theories have viewed pain arising from physical injuries as distinct from pain arising from life events, or psychological or spiritual trauma. Yoga philosophy, on the other hand, has not separated physical from emotional or spiritual suffering. Consistent with this view, recent brain scan research shows marked similarities in the brain changes associated with chronic pain and depression (Chou 2007). Yoga philosophy also differs from Western pain management based on yoga's core belief in impermanence (*anitya* in Sanskrit). Simply put, yoga posits that everything changes, even pain and suffering. Unfortunately, chronic pain is often considered unchangeable within an allopathic model when medications or surgery are ineffective. Here, yoga offers a view more consistent with neuroplasticity, and once again provides a more optimistic perspective. Life with no suffering may not be possible, but pain, like all things, changes.

Sidebar 13.4 Research

According to the National Institutes of Health (NIH) in the US, research into the therapeutic value of Yoga suggests that this approach, with carefully selected poses, can be beneficial for low back pain and associated functional improvements. This section, titled "What the Science Says about Yoga", includes promising results for improvements in quality of life, stress reduction, lower heart rate and blood pressure, help in relieving anxiety, depression, and insomnia, and improved overall physical fitness, strength, and flexibility (NIH 2015).

When asked, "Do you feel different about yourself or your pain?", the 59-year-old woman in pain for 38 years replied: "I can step outside myself mentally more now, and see the pain from a distance. This allows me more perspective, and gives me more control over the pain. Also I have become much more aware of how my breath, body and spirit affect each other, and how to better use my body and mind to calm and sometimes eliminate my pain. In a curious way I am grateful for having had the experience of pain, as Neil's work has connected me with a deeper, nourishing, spiritual thread. It may sound odd, especially from someone not religious, but I feel that I have found my soul, when I was not really consciously aware I had been losing it."

Similar to Western pain management programs, yoga classes include varied approaches to overcoming pain. Given the individual nature of pain, we should expect that approaches addressing the multifaceted nature of pain will be most effective, and those with a linear, mechanistic, or psychological view of pain will be less beneficial and to fewer individuals.

Clinical practice suggests that, for people in pain, the best outcomes from yoga will arise when pain management includes breathing in a more relaxed manner, attending to the pain and to the body in new ways, decreasing muscle tension, calming thoughts and emotions, and finding ways to move with more ease (see Figure 13.3). In other words, yoga is a complex system of self-management, appropriate for the complex, individual experiences of chronic pain, and is supported by recent pain models, theories, and neuroscience. The specific techniques of yoga therapy described in the next section offer safe opportunities to practice important pain management strategies.

Methodology

Yoga therapy is a complex and individualized process rather than a clearly definable singular technique. The techniques of yoga therapy include

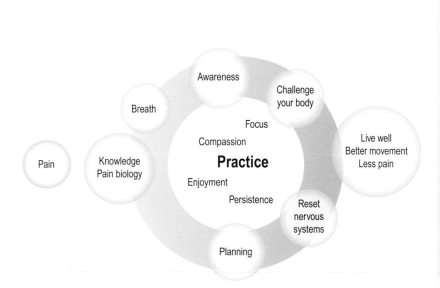

Figure 13.3
Pain Recovery Model: Self Care Complex pain problems require complex recovery strategies. This diagram shows the self care practices required to move from Pain (on the left) to Live Well, Better Movement and Less Pain (on the right). Self care is a nonlinear, individual process, requiring considerable practise of all pain care components in order to move towards mastery.
(Reprinted with permission, Life Is Now Pain Care Inc.)

assessment and treatment by a yoga therapist, combined with self-assessment and self-regulation. The yoga therapist's role in pain care is to create a supportive and interactive process with the client. Collaboratively, and based on the Pancamaya model, aspects of the body, mind, and spirit that have been impacted by the experience of pain are addressed. The yoga therapist considers the eight aspects of **Raja yoga** as guides, instructing the client in techniques that address the client's goals for recovery. In addition to functional and pain-control goals, the yoga therapist ensures that the client experiences techniques seeking to improve awareness, self-regulation, and a greater sense of peace.

Before describing specific techniques, it must be noted that between yoga therapists and yoga therapy training programs there are many different approaches. Some focus on the body and structural alignment, while others focus on the mind, on psychology, or on the spirit. Still others focus on the integration of each. All systems and techniques intend to decrease suffering, and promote inner peace, through individual processes based on the needs of the person in pain.

As both a physical therapist and yoga therapist, my approach includes integrating current pain science, the lived experience of an individual's persistent pain, and yoga practices. I am most interested in how we can use the insight gained from practicing yoga to make positive changes in our pain and in our lives. This chapter provides an opportunity to identify the key techniques of yoga therapy for people in pain, and to consider such questions as: "Why it is that yoga has been shown so effective for many complex and difficult pain conditions?"

What follows is a typical protocol employed within yoga therapy. It begins with a subjective and objective assessment, which will guide the therapeutic techniques and processes.

Assessment Techniques
Subjective assessment

The first, and most important, assessment process provides the time necessary for the client to tell their story, and for the practitioner to actively listen. This is therapeutic, builds trust, develops a caring relationship, and offers important guidance for the yoga therapist. Concurrent with listening for the following information, the breathing pattern, movement, posture, and body tension are visually assessed:

- The body-mind-spirit aspects of the individual's pain, and how it has impacted each aspect of their existence (biopsychosocial, body-mind-spirit, and Pancamaya views).

- Treatments or self-care techniques that have been helpful, and which ones have not.

- Information provided by other health professionals, including serious medical conditions, and contraindications to yoga and movement.

- The individual's interpretation of the condition, belief of how this might impact the future, what they believe is possible, and additional support needed. Most will also want to know my interpretation: what I think is wrong, how they can improve, how I can help, and how they can help themselves.

- Current and previous medications, and the effectiveness and dose of other treatments.

- Typical pain-related questions are asked to identify relationships of the pain to movement, work, sleep, stress, food, and medications.

- Questionnaires can be useful for baseline measurements of pain: life activities (Brief Pain Inventory), emotional aspects of pain (PHQ9 and GAD7). If the subjective assessment points to neuropathic pain, the DN4 form provides appropriate baseline data.

- The individual's previous experience with yoga, meditation, or other body-mind-spirit practices should be obtained.

- Ayurvedic constitution is assessed (Buhrman 1997).

- The individual's goals in relation to the pain and movement are discussed. What does the individual want from yoga therapy?

At the end of the initial patient interview, similar to Western medicine and physical therapy, I use clinical reasoning to generate possible explanations for individual's current pain and disability. Subsequently, the objective assessment includes evaluations to rule out or confirm these potential explanations.

Objective assessment components

- Posture: sitting and standing

- Muscle tension: supine, sitting, standing, and during movements and yoga postures

- Ease and smoothness of movement, including motor control

- Flexibility and muscular tightness

- Balance

- Ability to breathe calmly at rest, in different postures, with movement, and with movement towards pain

- Awareness of body position, muscle tension, and innocuous body sensations

- Responses to yoga postures, including sense of safety, emotional responses, and alterations in pain intensity

As a physical therapist and yoga therapist, my initial assessment concludes with developing a clinical (non-medical) diagnosis related to tissue pathology and nervous system sensitization. When a specific diagnosis is not possible, I collect a list of key problems related to the pain, noting interactions with the individual's ability to move with ease and engage in activities of daily living.

Although this initial assessment includes a focus on the physical body, during subsequent appointments my assessment expands to include interactions of pain with thoughts, emotions, and spirit. Techniques described below, such as body scans, meditation, and yoga nidra, assist me in assessing the individual's persistent pain experience.

Through a series of yoga therapy sessions, clients often become more and more aware of non-physical aspects of pain. Progressive efforts in self-exploration and self-regulation can lead to the discovery of deeper meaning to an individual's pain, or path of recovery. With each session, I modify therapeutic home practices, guided by, and supporting the new awareness and continued improvements.

Ongoing assessment is imperative to positive outcomes in yoga therapy. The client is instructed in a technique. Then, through collaborative interactions, the client and I evaluate progress toward the client's goals. I may request that the client persists with a technique, knowing that positive changes will take additional practice; when a technique increases agitation rather than calming it, I will turn to an alternate technique, and evaluate its effectiveness.

Yoga Therapy Techniques for People in Pain

The foundations of yoga therapy for people in pain are breathing techniques (pranayama) and physical postures (asana). Breath awareness, breath control techniques, and the postures of yoga can be used to address many of the issues related to persistent pain. Each addresses stress and pain, calming sensitized nervous systems, regaining a sense of control, strength, and function, improving confidence and flexibility, restoring body awareness and image.

Equally important in yoga therapy are the practices of greater self-awareness (pratyahara), concentration (dharana) and meditation (dhyana). Drawing

Sidebar 13.6 Research
In a 2005 study of yoga, exercise and self-care for chronic low back pain, Sherman and colleagues enrolled 101 participants. The researchers employed a viniyoga protocol, described as safe, easy to learn, and therapeutically oriented … "Although all the sessions emphasized use of postures and breathing for managing low back symptoms, each had a specific focus: relaxation; strength-building, flexibility, and large-muscle movement; asymmetric poses; strengthening the hip muscles; lateral bending; integration; and customizing a personal practice" (Sherman et al. 2005, 850). The results showed a sharp decrease in medication use for the yoga group. The yoga group had further positive results in functional status and decreases in pain (Sherman et al. 2005).

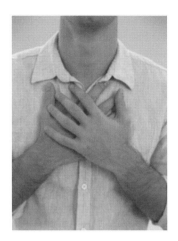

Figure 13.4
Supported breathing: Placing your hands on your rib cage, or on a client's rib cage, not only provides the biofeedback required to alter breathing patterns, but also calms fight–flight and heightened muscle tension.
(Reprinted with permission, Life Is Now Pain Care Inc.)

attention inward in order to restore or cultivate body awareness, learning how to focus on thoughts and experiences other than pain, and creating a greater sense of peace are established and effective pain management techniques (Marchand 2014).

Yoga therapy also employs less-studied techniques of pain management—hand positions (mudras), chanting, and repeated affirmations (**mantras**) are considered effective techniques to alter pain experiences within yoga therapy.

This section describes select yoga therapy techniques from a Western pain management perspective. Each technique has vastly greater uses, interactions, and effects than those described here. A comprehensive discussion of yoga therapy techniques is available at www.iayt.com.

Pranayama
Prana is life force, and pranayama is the practice of gaining greater control of breathing. Breathing techniques are foundational to yoga and to people in pain (see Figure 13.4). Pain changes breathing (Terekhin and Forster 2006). Breath can become more rapid, shallow, recruiting anterior neck and scapular muscles more related to protective responses than improving tidal volume. Vicious cycles develop between pain and these protective responses. I instruct people in pain to practice breathing techniques daily for 30 minutes or more to create long-lasting changes in the nervous system.

One of the most commonly used breathing techniques in yoga is ujjayi breath. This technique involves slowing and smoothing out both inhale and exhale, by tightening the vocal cords. This creates a soft sound (described as "like a wave gently rolling onto a beach"), bringing greater awareness to one's breath, and to its qualities. **Ujjayi breath**, translates as victorious breath, and is often used during more strenuous physical postures of yoga. The sound and sensations of ujjayi can increase one's ability to maintain attention to breathing, at the same time as learning or performing the physical postures of yoga. Given that painful movement is often associated with breath holding, and breath holding is associated with increased sympathetic nervous system arousal, maintaining awareness of breathing while we move with pain becomes an important aspect of pain management. Conditioned breath holding with difficult movements could be a major barrier to regaining ease of movement when pain persists.

Clinically, people in pain report variable success with breathing as an immediate pain control technique. To promote more lasting changes in the central, peripheral, and autonomic nervous systems, we should expect that consistent practice is required. As such, in yoga therapy, I instruct people in pain to practice breathing techniques daily, for 30 or more minutes, over a period of 4 to 6 weeks, before they decide if the breathing technique will provide sufficient pain relief.

There are many other breathing techniques within yoga. In addition to pain relief and improving ease of movement, these techniques can be used to assist with many of the problems associated with persistent pain: regaining self-efficacy, decreasing anxiety, feeling more energetic, and calming muscle tension, thoughts, and emotions (Busch et al. 2012).

I have the yoga therapy clients use specific hand positions with the intention to reinforce the effects of breathing techniques. These are called hand **mudras** (see Figure 13.5). For example, gently pressing palms together at the level of one's heart can add to a sense of calm, and spreading fingers wide while inhaling deeply can add to a feeling of being more energetic. There are no high-quality research studies of hand mudras. However, in my clinical experience, many clients report greater calmness in body, thoughts, and emotions with their use. Regardless of the biological mechanism, this is advantageous for the person in pain.

Asana

In yoga, the physical postures have many purposes. Flexibility, strength, and balance are obvious

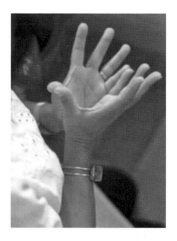

Figure 13.5
Mudras: Hand movements and positions can be used to enhance the effectiveness of breathing techniques, thanks to their large representation on the brain.
(Reprinted with permission, Life Is Now Pain Care Inc.)

effects. Yet these same postures can assist with regaining a sense of confidence, combating feelings of fragility, overcoming fear, improving body awareness, and learning how to create a sense of peacefulness (Mohri et al. 2005; Turnakar et al. 2005; Turnakar et al. 2013) in the face of persisting pain (see Figure 13.6). Yoga postures can also be used to progressively increase physical activity and desensitize to movement.

Yoga postures can be modified, allowing variations to accommodate physical ability. Individuals can perform postures from a chair or from a reclined position. Those with multiple sclerosis who cannot sit unsupported, and those with paraplegia or amputations who cannot stand, report many of the same positive effects from practicing modified yoga postures. Brain imaging and motor performance research clearly show similar benefits from visualization of a movement versus physically performing of that movement (Malouin, Jackson, and Richards 2013). When the client informs me that movement

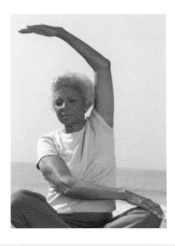

Figure 13.6
Asana—kind challenge: Yoga postures require just the right amount of challenge, and just the right amount of ease. Kind challenge provides greater benefits than forcing oneself to endure more pain.
(Reprinted with permission, Life Is Now Pain Care Inc.)

is not possible, I guide them in imagery. Once it is possible to keep body tension, breath, pain, and the mind calm, clients can progress from the mind to actual movements.

When individuals with persistent pain begin asana, it is important to provide instructions on how much pain should be present during recovery movements. Butler and Moseley (2003), in their excellent book, *Explain Pain*, point out that pain is not an accurate indication of tissue health. As such, by itself, pain is not able to accurately tell us when to stop a movement.

Stated another way, because pain does not accurately let us know when to stop and when to push further, our breath, body tension, and mind can be useful alarm systems. If any of these alarms increases in intensity during an asana, I would guide the client to scan through each to see if there is a way to stay with the posture or movement while at the same time calming the alarms. This is the process

by which I find that most clients make the greatest improvements towards their recovery goals.

I have developed the following guidelines as a four-point interoceptive guide to keep sensitized nervous systems calm while regaining ease of movement.

First, I guide the client to move mindfully into the yoga posture, to the point at which there is a slight increase in pain intensity, just above baseline pain intensity. Once there, I ask the client to ask two questions intended to calm the mind: "Is this safe for my physical body?" and "Will I regret moving this much, later?"

When the client finds a position that feels safe, and won't likely flare the pain, I ask that attention is divided between the remaining three points: keeping the breath calm, keeping muscle tension low, and monitoring the pain. Thus, the four-point guide includes awareness and regulation of mind, breath, body tension, and the pain. Nudging into the edge of the pain like this can be very challenging at the outset. Also, it can feel as if such small movements will never make any changes to the body. Patience, practice and persistence are necessary to be successful.

There may be other barriers to recovery; many of us learn how to ignore pain. It is important to guide clients to awareness of whether they have become masterful at distracting from pain and their body, and have learned how to breathe calmly in the face of pain. These techniques may help with the immediacy of a pain flare-up; however, they are not

Sidebar 13.7 Patient Interviews
When asked, "Do you feel different about yourself or your pain?", a 62-year-old woman with multiple pain conditions replied: "I feel that there is some control that I have and I am not a victim to my pain. I also know that I am merely human and that good days and bad days happen. I am definitely not as anxious about having pain as I was, which of course, lessens my pain."

effective for decreasing chronic pain and improving function over time. I focus the yoga therapy sessions on moving in the face of pain as an approach to recovering function, based on current understanding of pain physiology.

Savasana

The final posture of yoga practice is **savasana**. One rests, supine on the floor, letting the body, breath, and mind rest for 10 or more minutes. The purpose of this posture is deep relaxation, letting body and mind rest. Of all the postures and processes of asana practice, savasana differentiates yoga practice considerably from other exercise regimens. Clients can expect to receive as much benefit from what they let go in savasana at the end of the yoga therapy session as they gain in the other physical postures of yoga.

Hands-on adjustments and physical treatments

Yoga therapists provide hands-on guidance to assist clients with numerous aspects of pain management during asana practice (Mancini et al. 2014; McGlone, Wessberg, and Olausson 2014). When a client holds too much tension in their body, is positioned suboptimally, or when breathing has become shallow or tense, hands-on contact can provide the biofeedback needed to alleviate pain, and find greater ease of movement. Hands-on techniques can also be provided by yoga therapists to assist with stretching, muscle relaxation, and range of motion, within their scope of practice.

Pratyahara

This aspect of yoga translates as drawing one's attention inward. Persistent pain is associated with reports of being less able to feel the physical body in the area of pain. Growing evidence suggests that many people with persistent pain experience distortions of body awareness (Moseley 2008), body image, and the space around the physical body (Moseley, Gallance, and Spence 2012). Feeling anything other than pain in the painful area can seem difficult or impossible, or the body may feel larger, smaller, swollen, fragile, or more like an inanimate structure than dynamic human tissue.

Pratyahara, like sensory discrimination techniques, provides the brain with repeated and non-nociceptive interoceptive and exteroceptive inputs. This may be one key mechanism through which greater awareness is associated with decreased pain.

I prescribe pratyahara techniques such as body scans and progressive muscle contract–relax techniques to all my clients. Body scans involve noticing sensations that arise from the body. While breathing calmly, attention is drawn to the feet, and then slowly through all areas of the body. Both pleasurable and painful sensations are noticed; then attention is drawn back to the area, exploring with the mind for other sensations. Traditional body scans can last 35 minutes or more, and encourage awareness of thoughts, emotions, colors, or images. I modify the practice of body scans for people in pain: initially the focus is on physical sensations, less than 10 minutes long.

Progressive contract–relax practices involve gently contracting muscles in an area of the body, and then intentionally letting the muscle tension release. This can be a very effective body awareness technique. When individuals learn how to let muscle tension release, they may experience a reduction of pain related to both improved body awareness and decreased muscle guarding.

Finally, it is important to consider how body awareness and body image can affect the brain's ability to plan physical movement. If the brain's conclusion is that the body is broken, or disrupted, this may perpetuate painful movement as a protective measure. Accurate sensory input and sensory processing are required to plan, initiate, and sustain appropriate body movements. As such, pratyahara practices may also decrease pain by providing the brain with more accurate interoceptive sensory inputs.

Dharana

This aspect of yoga translates as focus or concentration. It is a step toward learning meditation. When pain demands so much attention, practice is required to relearn attention control. Yoga techniques provide the opportunity to practice concentration. Initially, it is necessary to find engaging or multiple sensations to focus on, especially when pain is demanding attention. Endless options are available for practicing dharana during breathing techniques—focusing on the sound of our breath, length, pace, and smoothness—during asana—attending to such things as one's feet on the floor, relaxation of shoulders, jaw and tongue, or gentle engagement of lower abdominals.

Dhyana

This aspect of yoga translates as meditation. There are many meditation techniques within yoga, each with different intentions. Meditation techniques can be used as a guide toward exploration of aspects of pain related to mind and spirit. Here, I may ask the client to notice thoughts or emotions that arise when focusing attention to the pain. Exploring more deeply, I guide the client to breathe calmly and focus outward. Then, I suggest the client focuses internally, considering body, mind, and spirit, to see what has changed and what has not. Or the meditation might address the yamas or niyamas, such as finding contentment and acceptance, while also holding the fiery determination to recover a sense of peace and purpose in life.

Specific modalities

Specific yoga therapy processes have been developed to guide clients in exploration and processing of thoughts, emotions, and spirit. Yoga nidra, is one example. This provides a vivid guided meditation, often allowing a sense of deep inner peacefulness, previously unattainable by those in pain. Phoenix Rising Yoga Therapy is another example, incorporating yoga postures supported by the therapist, while also guiding the client to deeper awareness. The techniques support the client in awareness, regulation, and processing of important aspects of the lived experience of pain. Although beneficial for anyone in a yoga therapy process, they are especially helpful for difficult-to-change cognitive, emotional, and spiritual aspects of pain.

Outcome Measures

The most important measurement of therapeutic success is defined by the goals of the individual. In the area of pain management, improved function in life is a critical outcome. We can use changes in the client's initial questionnaire scores as measures of therapy success; however, their value to the client, or ability to effectively guide ongoing therapy, must be considered.

Specific to yoga therapy and pain, awareness and self-regulation of breathing, body tension, thoughts, and emotions are important outcomes. Equally important are the client's report of being able to move with more ease, increasing and maintaining function without pain-flares, and finding purpose again in life despite the extent to which the pain changes.

In yoga, ascertaining the root cause of the client's suffering can be an important outcome. Individuals explore whether there is a deeper meaning to their persistent pain during meditative aspects of yoga. Some clients report that the pain has guided them to changes they believe are essential to make in their life, including exercise, diet, lifestyle, or occupation. From a yoga philosophy perspective, such realization guides us more towards self-realization, and can prevent further suffering.

Case Study

Kay is a 48-year-old woman who was hit by a car 2 years ago while crossing a road on foot. She healed well from the abrasions, contusions, and concussion, but experienced unresolved neck pain that spread to her left, dominant shoulder and upper back. She was working as a general manager at a landscaping business. The constant pain made it difficult for her to focus and stay calm. Specialist consultations concluded she had medically unexplained pain. She received weekly physical therapy treatments, and performed daily home exercises, but was not gaining ease of movement or lasting pain relief. She persisted because she did not want to lose any progress.

Her goals in yoga therapy were to strengthen her neck and shoulders, and return to swimming. She expressed grief from the loss of socializing with her swimming friends, and from losing the sense of strength and confidence gained from "strong swimmer's shoulders." Interestingly, pain control was not one of her goals. Like many clients, she believed she must "learn to live with it."

My Initial assessment findings included:

- Kay suffered from increased muscle tension and decreased body awareness in her left shoulder girdle and neck.

- She had a shallow, rapid, and apical breathing pattern, engaging upper trapezius and scalene muscles during inhale, and breath holding with left shoulder movements.

- Small shoulder movements created large increases in her pain. Light touch, superior to the spine of her left scapula, was painful (allodynia).

- Low pain self-efficacy.

- Difficulty concentrating.

- Social isolation.

During the initial treatment, I instructed Kay in two breathing techniques and a body awareness technique. She practiced breathing "longer, smoother, and softer." The goal was to use this technique as she recommended moving her shoulder. Alternate nostril breath was added to create a sense of calmness and peacefulness. This allowed her to feel how

pain is both changeable and an experience over which she has some influence. In the body scan, I initially guided her to focus on the sensations felt in her body. She was asked to pay attention to both the pain and the non-painful sensations in the left neck and shoulder. Kay's homework was to perform these techniques three times each day, in preparation for commencing the physical practice of yoga.

One week later, Kay expressed surprise at how different her left shoulder felt compared to the right during the body scan. She was already feeling improvement in her ability to concentrate, and reported the breathing techniques were more effective when she practiced longer than 5 minutes.

I then instructed Kay in yoga asana. Postures were chosen based on her physical assessment and her belief that they were both safe and unlikely to exacerbate her pain. The asana practice progressively applied more movement and more stress to the tissues of her shoulder and neck. She was guided to focus on keeping her breath, her body tension, and her mind calm during the asana. Her homework was to perform this sequence twice each day for 20 minutes, along with breathing and body scan techniques. Over the next few appointments, Kay was able to move her shoulder and neck with more ease, while breathing calmly. The allodynia was decreasing.

During the third appointment, I guided Kay in a breathing and meditation technique, allowing her the opportunity to explore interactions between the pain, her thoughts, emotions, and current life. Kay realized she was still the same competent person she was before the injury. This awareness gave her confidence in her own capacity to recover. She also reported that it was time to get back to the swimming pool and be around her friends, even if she couldn't swim like she used to.

I suggested Kay join a gentle yoga class three times each week to provide a chance to practice all she had learned in the one-to-one appointments.

Chapter 13

Kay realized the importance of spending time each day, not just moving her body, but doing so in a way that allows her more awareness of body and breath, and how these interact with her thoughts, emotions, and all the things that are really important in her life. My assessment of the important changes were Kay's ability to show that she could move without flaring the pain, without muscles becoming tight and guarding, and while keeping her breath pattern calm.

Conclusion

Modern science tells us that yoga can be effective for people with chronic pain, including difficult-to-change conditions. As a therapeutic intervention, yoga allows individuals to address important aspects of persistent pain in a manner aligned with active self-management components of current pain management programs. As such, yoga therapy is both an **evidence-informed** practice and a key component of current and effective pain care strategies.

The most compelling reason to include yoga in **integrative medicine** relates to an understanding that *pain changes everything*. Yoga offers opportunities to practice techniques not only aimed at changing pain and suffering, but also regaining influence over these individual, multifaceted and interacting pain-related changes.

The descriptions of yoga techniques and the case study here have provided explanations for the benefits of yoga for people with pain and pain-related disabilities. Yet, considerable research will be required to complete our understanding of how yoga truly works biologically. Perhaps the breathing techniques, or body awareness, or optimistic message, or the therapist–client interaction are its most powerful factors. Anecdotally, yoga's positive effects are most likely created through a complex interplay of body-mind-spirit practices and its biopsychosocial perspective.

References

American Yoga Association. 2006. www.americanyogaassociation.org (accessed December 14, 2014).

Buhrman, S. 1997. www.ayurvedicsolutions.com (accessed December 14, 2014).

Busch, V., W. Magerl, U. Kern, J. Haas, G. Hajak, and P. Eichhammer. 2012. The effect of deep and slow breathing on pain perception, autonomic activity, and mood processing—an experimental study. *Pain Medicine* 13(2):215–28.

Bussing, A., T. Osterman, R. Ludtke, and A. Michalsen. 2012. Effects of yoga interventions on pain and pain-associated disability: a meta-analysis. *The Journal of Pain* 13(1):1–9.

Butler, D., and L. Moseley. 2003. *Explain Pain.* Adelaide: NoiGroup Publishing.

Campbell, C., and R. Edwards. 2009. Mind-body interactions in pain: the neurophysiology of anxious and catastrophic pain-related thoughts. *Transl Res* 153(3):97–101.

Chou, K. 2007. Reciprocal relationship between pain and depression in older adults: evidence from the English Longitudinal Study of Ageing. *J Affect Disord* 102(1):115–23.

Chou, R., A. Qaseem, V. Snow, D. Casey, J. Cross Jr., P. Shekelle, and D. Owens. 2007. Diagnosis and treatment of low back pain: a joint clinical practice guideline from the American College of Physicians and the American Pain Society. *Ann Intern Med* 147(7):478–91.

Cramer, H., R. Lauche, H. Haller, and G. Dobos. 2013. Systematic review and meta-analysis of yoga for low back pain. *Clinical Journal of Pain* 29(5):450–60.

Crombez, G., C. Eccleston, S. Van Damme, J. Vlaeyen, and P. Karoly. 2012. Fear-avoidance model of chronic pain: the next generation. *The Clinical Journal of Pain* 28(6):475–83.

Holtzman, S., and R. Beggs. 2013. Yoga for chronic low back pain: A meta-analysis of randomized controlled trials. *Pain Res Management* 18(5):267–72.

International Association for the Study of Pain (IASP). 1986. Classification of chronic pain: Descriptions of chronic pain syndromes and definitions of pain terms. *Pain Suppl.* 3:1–222.

International Association for the Study of Pain (IASP). 2014. www.iasp-pain.org/Education/Content.aspx?Item-Number=1698&navItemNumber=576 (accessed July 13, 2015).

International Association of Yoga Therapists. 2014. www.iayt.org (accessed December 14, 2014).

Jackson, M. 2002. *Pain: the fifth vital sign: the science and culture of why we hurt.* New York: Crown Publishers.

Kolár, P., J. Êulc, M. Kyncl, J. Êanda, O. Cakrt, R. Andel, K. Kumagai, and A. Kobesová. 2012. Postural function of the diaphragm in persons with and without chronic low back pain. *J Orthop Sports Phys Ther* 42(4):352–62.

Lotze, M., and L. Moseley. 2007. Role of distorted body image in pain. *Current Rheumatology Reports* 9(6):488–96.

Malouin, F., P. Jackson, and C. Richards. 2013. Towards the integration of mental practice in rehabilitation programs. A critical review. *Front Hum Neurosci* 19(7):576–81.

Mancini, F., T. Nash, G. Lanneetti, and P. Haggard. 2014. Pain relief by touch: a quantitative approach. *Pain* 155(3):635–42.

Marchand, W. 2014. Neural mechanisms of mindfulness and meditation: Evidence from neuroimaging studies. *World J Radiol* 6(7):471–9.

McGlone, F., J. Wessberg, and H. Olausson. 2014. Discriminative and affective touch: sensing and feeling. *Neuron* 82(4):737–55.

Melzack, R. 1999. From the gate to the neuromatrix. *Pain* Suppl. 6:S121–6.

Mohri, Y. I., M. Fumoto, I. Sato-Suzuki, M. Ummino, and H. Arita. 2005. Prolonged rhythmic gum chewing suppresses nociceptive response via serotonergic descending inhibitory pathway in humans. *Pain* 118(2):35–42.

Moseley, L. 2008. I can't find it! Distorted body image and tactile dysfunction in patients with chronic back pain. *Pain* 140(1):239–43.

Moseley, L., A. Gallance, and C. Spence. 2012. Bodily illusions in health and disease: Physiological and clinical perspectives and the concept of a cortical "body matrix". *Neuroscience and Biobehavioral Reviews* 36(1):34–46.

Mostoufi, S., N. Afari, S. Ahumada, V. Reis, and J. Wetherell. 2012. Health and distress predictors of heart rate variability in fibromyalgia and other forms of chronic pain. *Journal of Psychosomatic Research* 72(1):39–42.

National Institutes of Health (NIH). 2015. National Center for Complementary and Integrative Health. https://nccih.nih.gov/health/yoga/introduction.htm#hed5 (accessed July 2, 2015).

Perl, E. R. 2007. Ideas about pain, a historical view. *Neuroscience* 8(Jan):71–80.

Plach, S., S. Heidrich, and R. Waite. 2003. Relationship of social role quality to psychological well-being in women with rheumatoid arthritis. *Res Nurs Health* 26(3):190–202.

Roland, M. 1986. A critical review of the evidence for pain-spasm-pain cycle in spinal disorders. *Clin Biomech* 1(2):102–9.

Schleicher, H., C. Alonso, E. Shirtcloff, D. Muller, B. Loevinger, and C. Coe. 2005. In the face of pain: The relationship between psychological well-being and disability in women with fibromyalgia. *Psychother Psychosom* 74(4):231–9.

Seminowicz, D., T. Wideman, L. Naso, Z. Hatami-Khoroushahi, S. Fallatah, M. Ware, P. Jarzem, M. Bushnell, Y. Shir, J. Ouellet, and L. Stone. 2011. Effective treatment of chronic low back pain in humans reverses abnormal brain anatomy and function. *J Neurosci* 31(20):7540–50.

Sherman, K. J., D. C. Cherkin, J. Erro, D. L. Miglioretti, and R. A. Deyo. 2005. Comparing yoga, exercise, and a self-care book for chronic low back pain: a randomized, controlled trial. *Ann Intern Med* 143(12):849–56. doi:10.7326/0003-4819-143-12-200512200-00003.

Siddall, P. J. 2013. Neuroplasticity and pain. What does it all mean? *The Medical Journal of Australia* 198(4):177–8.

Silverman, M., and P. Deuster. 2014. Biological mechanisms underlying the role of physical fitness in health and resilience. *Interface Focus* 4(5):201–4.

Smith, J., and M. Osborn. 2007. Pain as an assault on the self: An interpretative phenomenological analysis of the psychological impact of chronic benign low back pain. *Psychol Health* 22(5):517–34.

Smith, A., P. O'Sullivan, and L. Straker. 2008. Classification of sagittal thoraco-lumbo-pelvic alignment of the adolescent spine in standing and its relationship to low back pain. *Spine* 33(19):2101–7.

Smith, M., A. Russell, and P. Hodges. 2014. The relationship between incontinence, breathing disorders, gastrointestinal symptoms, and back pain in women: a longitudinal cohort study. *Clin J Pain* 30(2):162–7.

Snelling, J. 1994. The effect of chronic pain on the family unit. *J Adv Nurs* 19(3):543–51.

Sturgeon, J. A., and A. J. Zautra. 2010. Resilience: a new paradigm for adaptation to chronic pain. *Currrent Pain and Headache Reports* 14(2):105–12.

Terekhin, P., and C. Forster. 2006. Hypocapnia related changes in pain-induced brain activation as measured by functional MRI. *Neuroscience Letters* 400(29):110–14.

Turankar, A., S. Jain, S. Patel, S. Sinha, A. Joshi, B. Vallish, P. Mane, and S. Turankar. 2013. Effects of slow breathing exercise on cardiovascular functions, pulmonary functions and galvanic skin resistance in healthy human volunteers–a pilot study. *Indian J Med Res* 137(5):916–21.

Wallwork, T. L., W. R. Stanton, M. Freke, and J. A. Hides. 2009. The effect of chronic low back pain on size and contraction of the lumbar multifidus muscle. *Manual Therapy* 14(5):496–500.

Wand, B., L. Parkitny, N. O'Connell, H. Luomajoki, J. McAuley, M. Thacker, and L. Moseley. 2011. Cortical changes in chronic low back pain: Current state of the art and implications for clinical practice. *Manual Therapy* 16:15–20.

Ward, L., S. Stebbings, D. Cherkin, and G. D. Baxter. 2013. Yoga for functional ability, pain and psychosocial outcomes in musculoskeletal conditions: a systematic review and meta-analysis. *Musculoskeletal Care* 11(4):203–17.

Wideman, T., G. Asmundson, R. Smeets, A. Zautra, M. Simmonds, M. Sullivan, J. Haythornwaite, and R. Edwards. 2013. Re-thinking the fear avoidance model: toward amulti-dimensional framework of pain-related disability. *Pain* 54(11):2262–5.

Chenchen WANG   Ramel RONES

Chapter 14

Tai Chi/Qi Gong

Introduction

Chronic pain consists of a complex interplay between biological and psychological aspects, resulting in therapeutically challenging conditions. Clinical trials and observational studies provide encouraging evidence suggesting that Tai Chi/Qi Gong, a multi-component traditional Chinese mind–body exercise, has clinical benefits for patients with a variety of chronic disorders, particularly those involving chronic pain. Tai Chi, with its physical and mental components, uniquely promotes the integration of mind and body, and may improve function, self-efficacy, psychological well-being, and life satisfaction. In addition, Tai Chi may slow the progression of the disease and the disabilities associated with chronic pain (Wang, Collett, and Lau 2004; Wang et al. 2005, 2009b, 2010a, 2010b; Wang 2008, 2011, 2012).

Tai Chi is a mind–body exercise that originated in China as a martial art and is thought to have been created by Sanfeng Zhang in the twelfth century. The martial art is now one of the most popular mind–body exercises in the world (Birdee et al. 2009; Wang et al. 2014; Clarke et al. 2015). Tai Chi was developed in Daoist monasteries and its ultimate goal was enlightenment. Those who practice Tai Chi must regularly follow the fundamental principles of Qi Gong practice, which uses breathing techniques, gentle movement, and meditation to cleanse, strengthen, and circulate Qi (pronounced "chi"), the life energy. Qi Gong includes not only healing exercises and meditations but also any practices that contribute to physical, mental, emotional, and spiritual balance to promote health.

Tai Chi/Qi Gong is considered a complex multi-component intervention integrating physical, psychosocial, emotional, spiritual, and behavioral elements (China Sports 1983; Wayne and Kaptchuk 2008). These include a number of essential components from both external and internal exercises such as mind–body interaction, breathing regulation, hand–eye coordination, visualization, and relaxation that may lead to better health and vitality and a tranquil state of mind. The most important aspect of Tai Chi/Qi Gong is the calming and relaxing effect it can have on the mind and body that may help participants sense the Qi circulating within. Those who practice this type of meditative movement believe that sensing the internal energy may help them achieve pain relief and peace of mind. In addition, as a form of physical exercise, Tai Chi/Qi Gong may enhance cardiovascular fitness, muscular strength, balance, and physical function. Tai Chi/Qi Gong can be practiced safely and may be recommended to patients with chronic pain conditions as a complementary and alternative medical approach to affect patient overall well-being (Wang 2008, 2011, 2012; Wang et al. 2009b, 2010a, 2010b).

The overall field of Tai Chi/Qi Gong contains many components that may be beneficial in treating chronic pain. In this chapter, we offer a description of particular elements of our rationale and expertise, as well as information common to the overall field. This section highlights the current body of knowledge about the role of this ancient Chinese mind–body medicine as an effective treatment of chronic pain conditions that can lead to better informed clinical decision-making for treating chronic pain.

History and Overview of Tai Chi/Qi Gong

Originating as a Chinese martial art, Tai Chi/Qi Gong has been practiced in China for many centuries.

It has been valued as one of the most effective ways of self-healing in Chinese culture. However, it was not until the beginning of the twentieth century that Tai Chi became available to the the general public in China. While accounts of Tai Chi's history often differ, the most consistently documented history points to Sanfeng Zhang, a Daoist monk in the twelfth century, as the founder. Zhang developed an initial set of exercises that imitated the movements of animals. It is said that he observed five animals—tiger, dragon, leopard, snake, and crane—and concluded that the snake (see Figure 14.1) and the crane (snake with its evasive movements and crane with its deflective strategies) were the ones most capable of overcoming strong, unyielding opponents. In developing Tai Chi, Zhang brought flexibility and suppleness to the martial arts, in addition to some key philosophical concepts. The health-related benefits of Qi Gong have been widely accepted in China for thousands of years.

The term "Tai Chi" has been translated in various ways, such as "internal martial art," "supreme ultimate boxing," "boundless fist," and "balance of the opposing forces of nature." The techniques include bending, expanding, condensing, and extending movements of the body, and conscious regulation of breathing. They also include various forms of meditation; moving slowly, a unique characteristic of the Tai Chi form and practice; sitting; and standing (China Sports 1983; Wang et al. 2004; Rones, 2007, 2011).

A person practicing Tai Chi moves the body in a slow, relaxed, and graceful series of movements. These movements comprise what are called forms (or routines). Some movements are named for the animal the movement is based on, as in "White Crane Spreads Its Wings" (see Figure 14.2). The simplest style of Tai Chi uses thirteen movements; more complex styles offer dozens.

There has always been some controversy concerning which style represents the "truest" form of Tai Chi. There are many different styles of Tai Chi, including Chen (also known as Wu or Hao), Sun, and Yang styles. Although they are all based on the

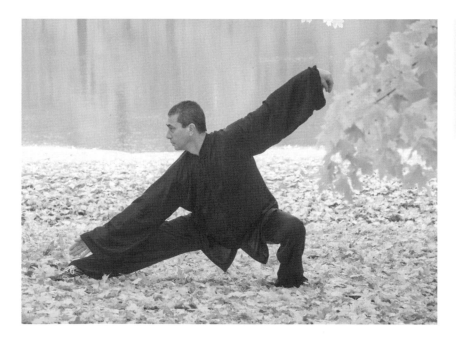

Figure 14.1
The Tai Chi move: Snake creeps down.
(From Yang Style Tai Chi Chuan, photograph by Clifford J. Snider.)

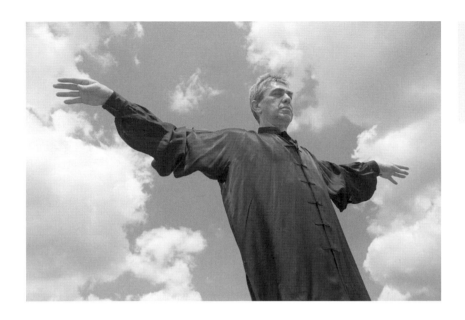

Figure 14.2
Tai Chi move: White crane spreads its wings.
(Photograph by Clifford J. Snider.)

same principles and theory of traditional Chinese medicine, each differs in the structure of its forms. Among those styles, Chen style is the oldest, while Yang style is the most popular. The Yang style consists of a classical long form of 108 postures or a simplified short form of 24 postures. The simplified short form is claimed to be the best style for beginners because it is easier to learn and practice (Wang et al. 2004; China Sports 1983; Rones 2007; Wang et al. 2004).

Various forms and styles of Tai Chi have been formulated and modified for different reasons such as general health promotion and easier learning, but the general principle and theory remain the same. Tai Chi can be practiced in almost any setting because it requires no equipment and minimal space (see Figure 14.3). The following concepts are universally important to both Tai Chi instructors and participants.

The Mind–body Prescriptions
Tai Chi is different from most ordinary martial arts, or ordinary sports for that matter. Tai Chi mind–body exercise is systematically based on

> **Sidebar 14.1 Patient Interviews**
> In response to the question, "Do you feel different about yourself or your pain since receiving this care?" a 35-year-old woman with fibromyalgia replied: "I see my pain as a sensation trying to communicate something to me. It causes me to stop what I'm doing and pay attention to my body. I see the sensation as an asset to my overall health instead of a constant nuisance. The pain is an indicator that I need to pay attention to something going on inside of me. Once I pay attention, I can make a choice in how to respond to the pain."

the mind, energy, and intention, not speed or brute force. It is based on qualities that promote a more spiritual tone relaxation, calmness, and stillness rather than tension, violence, or aggression. Therefore, these qualities promote a more spiritual tone than many other varieties of martial arts do.

The Meaning of Tai Chi
To implement and integrate Tai Chi principles into routine practice, we must focus on how to

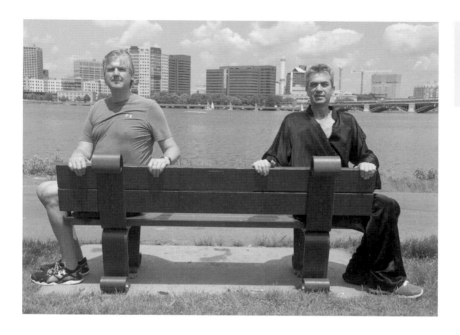

Figure 14.3
The bench/chair twist.
(Photograph by Clifford
J. Snider.)

optimize the important yin-yang relationships within ourselves. By practicing Tai Chi, one may:

- make the body conscious

- separate any specific yin-yang relationship into its constituent parts

- comprehend how internal energy/Qi and the physical tissue of the body work with or against each other

- navigate the relationships between intent and the manifestation Qi or physical movement.

The Meaning of Qi
Qi is a strong life force that makes a human being alive, alert, and present. Tai Chi mind–body exercises may help develop the Qi energy. The "life force" is found in most of the ancient cultures of the world. Some believe that a weak life force results in sluggishness and devolves into chronic pain and this energy can be increased in a human being. Consequently, the development of Qi may make an ill or weak person vibrant and robust, improving

both physical and mental capacity (Rones 2007; Yang 2010).

The Mind and Body are Composed of Qi
Many people consider the body, thoughts, and emotions as being separate entities. Many believe that the body is "real" because it is physical matter, while thoughts and emotions are not and are mere creations of the mind that can be modified. However, according to Chinese medicine, both the body and mind are composed of Qi and are controlled by the state of that Qi. Through the medium of Qi, the mind can affect the physical body positively or negatively. Balance and smooth flow of Qi in one creates balance and wellness. Imbalance, agitation, and uneven flow create discomfort and illness. Thus, according to Chinese medicine, mental and emotional stress may create physical illness.

The Yin and Yang
Philosophically, Tai Chi involves the opposite forces of yin and yang, as well as the balance and integration of both. From many Western perspectives,

night–day, up–down, strong–weak, or right–wrong connote parts that oppose each other. From an Eastern perspective, however, these opposites are thought to naturally complement each other, rather than oppose or conflict, and have a common source that is beyond dualistic opposites. This source is called Tai Chi. Tai Chi has many methods that are extremely effective in helping maintain the balance of yin and yang, which, from the position of traditional Chinese medicine, determines the state of one's health (China Sports 1983; Wayne and Kaptchuk 2008).

Imbued over thousands of years of Chinese culture and philosophy, Tai Chi now is considered a complex, multicomponent intervention. It integrates physical, psychosocial, emotional, spiritual, and behavioral elements that promote a mind–body interaction for health (China Sports 1983; Wang et al. 2004).

Theory and Philosophy in Treating Pain

Tai Chi has become widely accepted as the most popular martial Qi Gong exercise. In Tai Chi, each movement flows naturally, smoothly, and effortlessly into the next. The entire body is always in motion, with the movements performed gently at a uniform speed. It is considered important to keep the body upright. Many Tai Chi instructors use the image of pearls on a string ascending from the soles of the feet to the top of the head (see Figure 14.4); the mind extends from the center of the earth and up into the heavens. In addition to movement, two

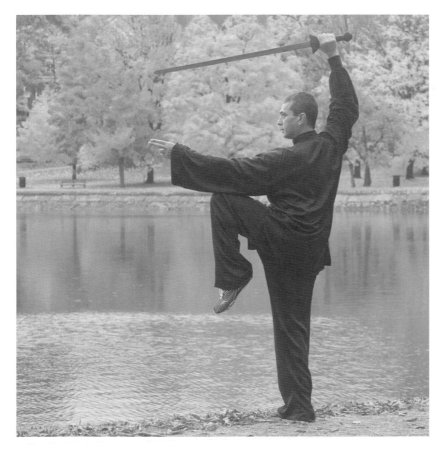

Figure 14.4
Yang-style the Tai Chi sword move "big chief star." (Photograph by Clifford J. Snyder.)

other essential elements in Tai Chi are breathing and meditation. A conscious mental process using certain techniques such as focusing attention or maintaining a steady posture helps suspend the consciousness of thoughts, and relax the body and mind. In Tai Chi practice, it is necessary to concentrate, to cancel distracting thoughts, and to breathe wholesomely in a deep, relaxed, and laserly focused manner. Tai Chi instructors as well as the Tai Chi philosophy, believe that this kind of breathing, coordinating the movements of the lungs with the movements of the abdominal and back muscles with deep meditation, contains a multitude of benefits which include increasing calmness and awareness (China Sports 1983; Rones 2007).

To understand the philosophy of Tai Chi, one needs to observe that the practice adheres closely to the theory of yin and yang, the foundational concepts of Chinese philosophy. The yin-yang theory represents all phenomena in the universe; individually, yin and yang are monitors of opposing concepts. **Yin** is believed to have the qualities of water, such as coolness, darkness, stillness, inward/downward directions, and tends to be feminine in character. **Yang** is believed to possess the qualities of fire such as heat, light, action, upward/outward movement, and tends to be masculine. The Chinese have long believed that the universe and humankind are formed from opposing forces that should counterbalance each other. In this belief system, each person's yin and yang need to be in perfect balance in order to be healthy.

Consequently, from the traditional Chinese medicine perspective, disease or pain is understood as a loss of balance between the yin and yang. This destructive imbalance leads to the blocking of the flow of "Qi," also known as vital energy, along pathways (channels) known as meridians. Specifically, certain concepts from Chinese philosophy, which are the key beliefs in Tai Chi/Qi Gong, act within that construct by normalizing the free flow of "Qi" throughout the body for pain reduction. Tai Chi masters believed that the careful, controlled breathing of Tai Chi might result in a rested body, a peaceful mind, and progressive relaxation that might break the "pain cycle." Pain, stress, melancholy, and depression all might interfere with typical functional capabilities (Wang et al. 2010b).

Tai Chi is a Qi Gong training that leads to a calm and peaceful mind as well as a relaxed, healthy body. These elements are most critical to health, both mental and physical. Tai Chi was developed following the natural cultivation and training procedures of Qi Gong, also known as the five regulations listed below:

- *Regulating the Body*: A deep level of physical and mental relaxation is emphasized in the first step of learning Tai Chi. It is believed that once one relaxes deeply, the blood and Qi circulation can begin to flow smoothly.

- *Regulating the Breathing*: Breathing plays a very important role in Tai Chi/Qi Gong practice. The Tai Chi philosophy has many breathing techniques performed in various postures while shaping the Tai Chi form. Breathing should be deep, relaxed, and regular. Over time, with practice, the breathing can be longer, deeper, quieter, and more peaceful. Holding different positions while sustaining deep breathing over time will fortify the lungs and improve their capacity. The breath is a pathway linking the external and the internal universes, and serves many purposes in Tai Chi. This pathway makes it possible for the Qi to circulate smoothly, and helps the mind to focus and lead the Qi, whenever desired, to reduce both physical and mental stress (Rones 2007; Wang et al. 2010a).

- *Regulating the Mind*: Regulating the mind is a key element for achieving optimum health in the practice of Tai Chi. Recognizing the emotional mind, learning to have a calm mind, as well as reducing stress, greatly improves health outcomes.

- *Regulating the Qi*: A relaxed body, a peaceful mind, and correct breathing can direct the Qi to any place in the body.

- *Regulating the Spirit*: The final stage of Tai Chi practice is regulating and evoking the spirit while strengthening the spiritual center.

From the Western Medicine perspective, evidence suggests that Tai Chi/Qi Gong mind–body exercise might influence the immunological functions. For example, it has been hypothesized that Tai Chi reduces the circulating levels of interleukin-6, a marker of inflammation in older adults (Irwin et al. 2012). By reducing inflammatory signaling molecules such as interleukin-6, Tai Chi may reduce the risk of aberrant inflammation, thereby decreasing the risk of diseases such as cardiovascular disease. In addition, it has been shown that Tai Chi improves pain and physical function in rheumatoid arthritis, suggesting its potential as a therapeutic option for improving functionality in chronic pain (Wang, 2008).

Indeed, both the physical and mental components of the mind–body interaction play major roles in diminishing the sensation of pain (Wang, 2011, 2012). Tai Chi and Qi Gong are a form of physical exercise, which might enhance cardiovascular health, muscular strength, balance, coordination, and physical function. Strong evidence from other studies suggests that mechanisms might exist by which the brain and central nervous system influence immune, endocrine, and autonomic functioning, which is known to impact health outcomes (Irwin et al. 2003; Irwin, Wang et al. 2010a; Irwin and Cole 2011; Wang and An 2011; Irwin and Olmstead 2012; Wang 2012). From the psychological and psychosocial perspectives, improving self-efficacy, social function, and depression can help patients build confidence, reach out for support, and overcome the fear of pain, which by itself causes physical malfunction and debility (Wang et al. 2010b).

Thus, Tai Chi/Qi Gong, beyond its universally accepted multicomponent mind–body theory based on historical multidimensional principles, has also become an accepted and welcome therapeutic for addressing stress management, relaxation, and coping skills. It might be the appropriate adjunctive treatment for pain-related disorders and a variety of chronic pain conditions. It has been shown to be safe and to promote aerobic cardiovascular fitness, muscle strength, emotional functioning, and quality of life in patients with chronic conditions (Wang et al. 2003, 2004, 2005, 2009a, 2009b, 2010b; Yeh et al. 2008, 2009). In fact, Tai Chi is practiced preferentially in the United Status among individuals with musculoskeletal pain and mental health conditions (Barnes and Nahin 2007; Birdee et al. 2009; Wang et al. 2010a, 2010b).

Over the past decades, Tai Chi has been proven to be a useful treatment with potential therapeutic benefits in chronic rheumatic pain conditions, such as rheumatoid arthritis, osteoarthritis, and fibromyalgia (Wang 2008, 2011, 2012; Wang et al. 2005, 2009b, 2010b). Because of its powerful mind–body attributes and the positive results gained from clinical trials, the use of Tai Chi is justified for the treatment of chronic pain. The masters utilize the

Sidebar 14.2 Research
In a recent chronic pain hypothesis proposed by Mosely and Vlaeyen (2015), the authors summarize the literature: "people in chronic pain have lower proprioceptive acuity, disruptions in perceived size and alignment of body parts, and show poor ability to mentally maneuver the painful body part" (Mosely and Vlaeyen 2015, 37).

relevant Tai Chi/ Qi Gong principles and techniques to alleviate pain and improve physical and mental health.

Methodology

In this section, we offer a description of particular elements of our rationale and expertise, as well as information common to the overall field. Specifically, we present information on how our patients improve through our teaching experience, and how our actual practice better informs clinical decision-making. The Tai Chi program highlights the role of the mind and spirit as healing tools; many Tai Chi masters attempt to address both mind and body, emphasizing the individual approach and the individual's journey.

A mind–body-Tai Chi approach could easily be integrated into conventional treatment approaches for chronic pain in clinics and especially households. Most importantly, a mind–body-Tai Chi approach empowers individuals to play an active role in their own personal journey to better health, an action which is beneficial to all involved (e.g. patients, families, nurses, and doctors). Additionally, we present information on assisting healthcare practitioners with referring patients with pain to Tai Chi.

- *Patient Safety*: Patient safety is a primary concern when implementing a specialized practice such as Tai Chi into a treatment plan for people suffering from pain. The risks for Tai Chi mind–body exercise are minimal; however, there is some potential for injury from the exercise, including muscle soreness (mild muscle pain or discomfort occurring after exercise), muscle tears, strain, sprains, and joint pain. In case of injury during exercise, patients will be asked to immediately notify the Tai Chi masters if their pain symptoms do not remit promptly with rest and conservative measures. Warm-up and stretching before exercise are integral to the training program, as these maneuvers may prevent such injuries. Thus, they are incorporated into the exercise routine; instructors will inquire about the occurrence of potential side effects at each class and take necessary measures. The instructors will specifically ask patients about adverse events that might be associated with Tai Chi exercises (i.e. falling down, joint swelling, muscle ache).

- *Patient Education*: Patient education helps ensure safe participation in a Tai Chi program. In the first session of the group intervention, the Tai Chi instructors explain the mind/body exercise theory and procedures of Tai Chi. They briefly discuss the historical background of Tai Chi during the introductory class as well as at least one essential principle, explaining why it is important. We provide printed materials about the Tai Chi mind–body program for patients with chronic pain and other disease conditions, such as osteoarthritis, rheumatoid arthritis, and fibromyalgia.

- *Belief and Outcome Expectation*: Before the group session begins, we interview patients to learn their disease conditions, diagnoses, previous treatments, symptoms, and treatment goals. We also provide questionnaires to assess patients' beliefs and outcome expectations to estimate if their ideas will affect their treatment outcomes.

Treatment Goals and Strategy

We prepare, organize, and review our teaching curriculum, homework, and any other materials relevant to the Tai Chi treatment. We use our findings to generate treatment goals and strategies for one or more sessions. At the beginning of class, approximately ten patients will be briefed on the lesson for the day, including how many movements will be taught. For the remaining sessions, each patient practices Tai Chi/Qi Gong under the instruction of the Tai Chi instructor in a group setting. Every session will include the following components:

- warm up, self-massage, and a review of Tai Chi principles (10 minutes)

- Tai Chi movements (30 minutes)

- breathing technique (10 minutes)

- relaxation (10 minutes).

Each component of the program derives from the classical Yang style of Tai Chi which contains 108 postures.

Treatment Methods

Tai Chi is designed to affect a person on any level one chooses or allows. It physically strengthens the body while encouraging flexibility and ease of movement. It is designed to increase internal energy of "Qi" flow within the body, thereby increasing vitality. It will clean, relax, and focus the mind, promoting creativity, sensitivity, and optimism. It provides emotional balance and spiritual guidance. A convenient aspect of Tai Chi is that most people are able to do it.

Important principles of Tai Chi

To fully derive the benefits of Tai Chi, it is essential to incorporate certain philosophical and ethical principles into the Tai Chi form. The practice of Tai Chi teaches the patient to realize relaxed, smooth, and graceful movements. The feeling of the Qi circulation, balance, body connectedness, body

Sidebar 14.4 Research

Tai Chi Research Intervention: Selection of ten forms from 108 postures of Classical Yang style Tai Chi Chuan. To reduce stress on the leg joints, and due to the time constraints, we condensed the 108 forms to ten forms that could be learned by patients with chronic pain within 12 weeks, during which time total contact and training was restricted to 1 hour sessions, twice a week based on literature. The ten forms were selected because: (1) they are easily comprehensible, (2) they clearly represent progressive degrees of difficulty concerning postural stability, with weight-bearing moving from bilateral to unilateral supports, and (3) they seem to emphasize increasing magnitude of trunk and arm rotation with diminishing base of support and, as such, potentially improve physical function without excessively stressing the joints.

awareness, and structural alignment increases as one integrates each principle. The Tai Chi masters will teach patients to absorb just one principle per week and allow that particular principle to become a habit so that it no longer requires conscious effort. All Tai Chi forms tend to operate on the following three principles:

- The extended and relaxed body: Awareness of trunk alignment and deep breathing are necessary prerequisites to achieving a proper posture before forms can be practiced and learned.

- The alert but calm mind: One becomes more aware of the presence and movement of the body within its own space.

- The well-coordinated body movements require sequencing of segments:

  - Keep the knees aligned with the feet: This is important in order to reduce stress applied to your knees (see Figure 14.5).

- The tip of the tongue touches the roof of the mouth: This action connects the main Qi pathway that is called the "Small Heavenly Circle."

- Lightly close the anal sphincter: This completes the "Small Heavenly Circle" pathway. If the anal sphincter is open the Qi will not accumulate nearly as quickly.

- Push the lower back out and keep the buttocks tucked in: Over time, dropping the tailbone down versus tucking it in; relaxed versus coerced. Feel the weight of the body in the heels. This structurally connects the upper and lower body. It stabilizes one's balance and allows the leverage and power of the movement to come from the legs. It also allows the chi to circulate upwards from the feet to the head and back down to the feet.

- Tuck the chin in and push up the crown point of the head: This motion stabilizes the head and permits the Qi to flow up the back of the neck.

- Let the shoulders and elbows drop and sink: This motion structurally connects the arms to the torso and allows the chi to flow to the hands (Rones 2007).

Home practice and self-care

Ending on an affirmative note, we review what was taught during the class period, and discuss homework and what will happen at the next lesson. We encourage participants to form "buddy" groups to practice together during the week (see Figures 14.6 a and b) and to check on each other if they miss class—social interaction is an excellent way to help patients follow through with their exercises when not in class. We inspire and motivate participants to stay on and to practice after class. This gives

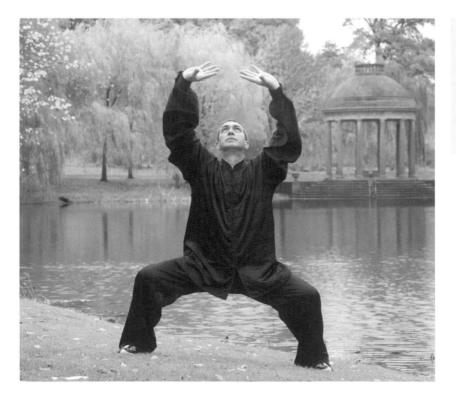

Figure 14.5
The Chi Kung posture: Holding the heavens. From Martial Chi Kung/ Yang Style Tai Chi Chuan. (Photograph by Clifford J. Snider.)

participants something to look forward to in their next lesson. Note: this is not a general exercise program for the public, but with some modifications, it can easily be used as one.

Practical Aspects of Accessing Tai Chi/ Qi Gong Treatments

From the results of our previous work as well as the work of many others, Tai Chi appears to provide both physical and mental benefits for a variety of chronic pain conditions (Wang et al. 2004, 2010b). The physical component provides exercise that is consistent with recommendations for elderly subjects (muscle conditioning and aerobic cardiovascular exercise), while the mental component has the potential to improve psychological well-being, life satisfaction, and perceptions of health (Wang et al. 2004, 2005, 2009b, 2010a, 2010b; Li et al. 2005, 2008, 2012; Wayne and Kaptchuk 2008; Wang 2011, 2012).

Participants and providers alike are increasingly interested in integrative therapies because of the potential as effective remedies for reducing pain while simultaneously improving physical and psychological health and well-being. The principal barriers preventing patients from accessing these treatments in the United States include uncertainties about the methods and costs, and where to find these services. Thus, it is important that the evidence behind these treatments be discussed openly with patients so that they can make an informed decision. Many health insurance plans are beginning to include some discounts, rebates, or even benefit coverage for these services, as the evidence for efficacy grows.

Finding an experienced provider of Tai Chi/ Qi Gong therapies might be difficult. A growing number of physicians are receiving dual training in both Western and Eastern medicine, which benefits patients who are uncertain how to integrate the two philosophies. When selecting a Tai Chi instructor, the two most important characteristics for patients and referring providers to consider are general experience as well as experience in treating chronic pain disorders. Tai Chi should not be a replacement for conventional Western care or be

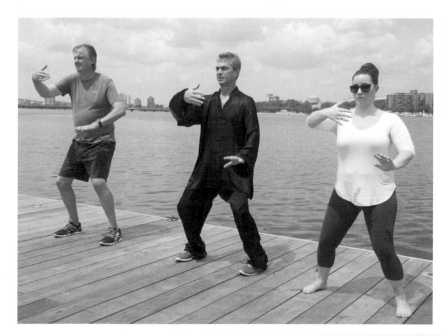

Figure 14.6a
The Tai Chi move: Cloud hands.
(Photograph by Clifford J. Snider.)

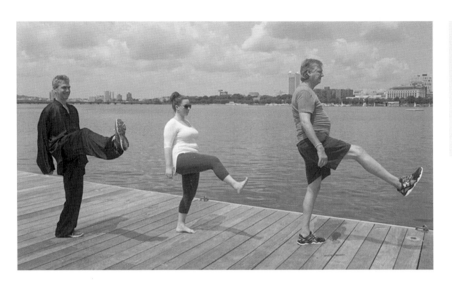

Figure 14.6 b
Tai Chi Walking from the Tai Chi philosophy. From Martial Chi Kung/Yang Style Tai Chi Chuan.
(Photograph by Clifford J. Snider.)

Sidebar 14.5 Patient Interviews

When asked, "Is there anything I haven't asked about your experience that you feel is important to share with referring healthcare providers?", a 28-year-old man receiving care for pain replied: "Pain can be all-consuming. It can be the first thing that you think about when you wake up, the last thing you think about when you go to sleep and something that prevents you from getting a good night sleep. It can become a full-time job trying to manage your pain and I can understand why people with chronic pain become dependent on narcotics, are disabled to the point where they can't work and are labeled by the healthcare system as 'drug seekers' and by society as 'deadbeats.' These words might be strong but as a healthcare provider, I hear them every day as they are muttered by colleagues, nurses, and ancillary medical staff. I am fortunate because I have the financial resources and work flexibility to manage my pain in a more positive and therapeutic fashion but I am also aware that I am in the minority. Expanding medical benefits costs money that we don't have. Information can be free. I didn't know that these resources were available to me until I asked and looked. Perhaps more outreach to primary care providers and to the general public would help."

used to postpone seeing a Western doctor about a medical condition.

Standards for training Tai Chi instructors do not currently exist, so providing patients with access to experienced Tai Chi instructors is essential. Ideally, instructors should have at least 5 to 10 years of experience working with the specific patient populations. Additionally, patients should inquire as to ways in which the therapy might be modified to accommodate their conditions. For example, some Tai Chi forms require deep knee bending, which could be painful or harmful to patients with knee arthritis. We expect that experienced Tai Chi instructors will be able to embrace this issue and find ways to adapt their principles in a safe manner while preserving the therapeutic value and philosophy of the therapy.

As the demand and evidence for integrative medical therapies grow, educating healthcare providers and patients about the known evidence and clinical implications for these remedies is vital. Healthcare providers should be able to discuss the evidence behind these treatments with patients to enable them to make informed decisions. Furthermore, by providing practical information about methods, costs, and experience, providers can effectively encourage their patients to explore the options for integrating Western and Eastern medicines.

Case Study

Mary's story was published in the *New York Times* 2010. A 59-year-old, retired phone company employee from Massachusetts, Mary was one of sixty-six participants in a research study conducted by Tufts University in 2008. We measured the fibromyalgia impact questionnaire (FIQ) score between baseline and the end of the 12-week intervention. The FIQ is a well-validated multidimensional measure for participant-rated overall severity of fibromyalgia. It includes intensity of pain, physical functioning, fatigue, morning tiredness, stiffness, depression, anxiety, job difficulty, and overall well-being (Burckhardt, Clark, and Bennett 1991). The total score ranges between 0 and 100, with higher scores indicating more severe symptoms. After 12 weeks of Tai Chi intervention (condensed the 108 movement Yang style long form to ten forms), patients with fibromyalgia, a chronic pain condition, did significantly better in measurements of pain, fatigue, physical functioning, sleeplessness, and depression than a comparable group given stretching exercises and wellness education. Tai Chi patients were also more likely to sustain improvement 3 months later.

The therapy impressed Mary, who said that before participating in the 2008 study, "I couldn't walk half a mile," and it "hurt me so much just to put my hands over my head." Sleeping was difficult, and she was overweight. "There was no joy to life," she said. "I was an entire mess from head to foot." She had tried and rejected medication, physical therapy, swimming, and other approaches. "I was used to being treated in a condescending manner because they couldn't diagnose me: 'She's menopausal, she's crazy.' Before the study, I didn't know Tai Chi from a sneeze," said Ms. Petersen, who had diabetes and other conditions. "I was like, 'Well, OK, I'll get to meet some people, it will

get me out of the house.' I didn't believe any of it. I thought this is so minimal, it's stupid." After a few weeks, she said she began to feel better, and after 12 weeks "the pain had diminished 90 percent." She has continued Tai Chi, lost 50 pounds and can walk 3 to 7 miles a day. "You could not have convinced me that I would ever have done this or continued with this," she said. "I wouldn't say it's a cure. I will say it's an effective method of controlling pain."

At the 6-months follow-up, Mary continues to practice Tai Chi (five classes/wk, practice at home). Her pain relief from fibromyalgia is significant and she is experiencing improvements in related areas: more flexibility, range of motion, strength, improved energy, and no headaches in the last 2 months. Anxiety is no longer a problem and her sleep has improved and is more restful (6–7 hours). She has a more positive attitude, and her pain medications are significantly reduced. Her primary care physician for 7 years is so impressed with her improved condition, on all levels, that she asked Mary to share her story and offer hope to other patients with fibromyalgia.

Conclusion

Overall, based on the current body of knowledge on the therapeutic benefits of Tai Chi/Qi Gong for pain and symptom relief, Tai Chi/Qi Gong training might provide an ideal form of exercise for individuals suffering from chronic pain. Our chapter not only offers a brief history and a theoretical conceptual overview of Tai Chi/Qi Gong, but also elucidates the methodology for implementing complementary and integrative approaches into clinical practice. Therefore, integrative approaches combine the best of conventional medicine and the wisdom of traditional Chinese medicine. These modalities might lead to the development of better disease-modifying strategies that could improve symptoms and decrease the progression of chronic pain.

Chapter 14

References

Barnes, P. M., E. Powerll-Griner, R. L. McFann. Complementary and alternative medicine use among adults: United States, 2002. *Seminars in Integrative Medicine*. Vol. 2. No. 2. WB Saunders, 2004.

Birdee, G. S., P. M. Wayne, R. B. Davis, R. S. Phillips, and G. Y. Yeh. 2009. T'ai chi and qigong for health: patterns of use in the United States. *J Altern Complement Med* 15(9):969–973.

Burckhardt, C. S., S. R. Clark, and R. M. Bennett. 1991. The fibromyalgia impact questionnaire: development and validation. *J Rheumatol* 18(5):728–733.

China Sports. 1983. Simplified "Taijiquan", 2nd edn. Beijing, China: China Publications Center.

Christian, G., 2011. Sunset Tai Chi: Simplified Tai Chi for Relaxation and Longevity.

Clarke, T. C., L. I. Black, B. J. Stussman, P. M. Barnes, and R. L. Nahin, 2015. Trends in the use of complementary health approaches among adults: United States, 2002–2012. *National Health Statistics Reports*, (79), p.1.

Hochberg, M. C., R. D. Altman, K. T. April, M. Benkhalti, G. Guyatt, J. McGowan, T. Towheed, V. Welch, G. Wells, and P. Tugwell. 2012. American College of Rheumatology 2012 recommendations for the use of nonpharmacologic and pharmacologic therapies in osteoarthritis of the hand, hip, and knee. *Arthritis Care & Research*, 64(4): 465–474.

Irwin, M. R. and S. W. Cole. 2011. Reciprocal regulation of the neural and innate immune systems. *Nature Reviews Immunology*, 11(9): 625–632.

Irwin, M. R. and R. Olmstead. 2012. Mitigating cellular inflammation in older adults: a randomized controlled trial of Tai Chi Chih. *The American Journal of Geriatric Psychiatry*, 20(9): 764–772.

Irwin, M. R., R. Olmstead, and M. N. Oxman. 2007. Augmenting immune responses to varicella zoster virus in older adults: a randomized, controlled trial of Tai Chi. *Journal of the American Geriatrics Society*, 55(4): 511–517.

Irwin, M. R., J. L. Pike, J. C. Cole, and M. N. Oxman. 2003. Effects of a behavioral intervention, Tai Chi Chih, on varicella-zoster virus specific immunity and health functioning in older adults. *Psychosomatic Medicine*, 65(5): 824–830.

Li, F., P. Harmer, K. J. Fisher, E. McAuley, N. Chaumeton, E. Eckstrom, and N. L. Wilson. 2005. Tai Chi and fall reductions in older adults: a randomized controlled trial. *The Journals of Gerontology Series A: Biological Sciences and Medical Sciences*, 60(2):187–194.

Li, F., P. Harmer, K. Fitzgerald, E. Eckstrom, R. Stock, J. Galver, G. Maddalozzo, and S. S. Batya. 2012. Tai chi and postural stability in patients with Parkinson's disease. *New England Journal of Medicine*, 366(6): 511–519.

Li, F., P. Harmer, R. Glasgow, K. A. Mack, D. Sleet, K. J. Fisher, M. A. Kohn, L. M. Millet, J. Mead, J. Xu, and M. L. Lin. 2008. Translation of an effective Tai Chi intervention into a community-based falls-prevention program. *American Journal of Public Health*, 98(7):1195–1198.

Morgan, N., M. R. Irwin, M. Chung, and C. Wang. 2014. The effects of mind-body therapies on the immune system: meta-analysis. *PloS one*, 9(7):e100903.

Moseley, G. L. and J. W. Vlaeyen. 2015. Beyond nociception: the imprecision hypothesis of chronic pain. *Pain*, 156(1):35–38.

National Institutes of Health (NIH), National Center for Complementary and Integrative Health: https://nccih.nih.gov/health/arthritis/osteoarthritis#science (accessed July 4, 2015).

Rones, R., 2006. *Sunrise Tai Chi: simplified Tai Chi for health and longevity*. YMAA Publication Center, Inc..

Wang, C., 2008. Tai Chi improves pain and functional status in adults with rheumatoid arthritis: results of a pilot single-blinded randomized controlled trial.

Wang, C., 2011. Tai Chi and rheumatic diseases. *Rheumatic Disease Clinics of North America*, 37(1):19–32.

Wang, C., 2012. Role of Tai Chi in the treatment of rheumatologic diseases. *Current Rheumatology Reports*, 14(6):598–603.

Wang, C., R. Bannuru, J. Ramel, B. Kupelnick, T. Scott, and C. H. Schmid. 2010a. Tai Chi on psychological well-being: systematic review and meta-analysis. *BMC Complementary and Alternative Medicine*, 10(1):1.

Wang, C., J. P. Collet, and J. Lau. 2004. The effect of Tai Chi on health outcomes in patients with chronic conditions: a systematic review. *Archives of Internal Medicine*, 164(5):493–501.

Wang, C., M. D. Iversen, T. McAlindon, W. F. Harvey, J. B. Wong, R. A. Fielding, J. B. Driban, L. L. Price, R. Rones, T. Gamache, and C. H. Schmid. 2014. Assessing the comparative effectiveness of Tai Chi versus physical therapy for knee osteoarthritis: design and rationale for a randomized trial. *BMC Complementary and Alternative Medicine*, 14(1):1.

Wang, C., R. Roubenoff, J. Lau, R. Kalish, C. H. Schmid, H. Tighiouart, R. Rones, and P. L. Hibberd. 2005. Effect of Tai Chi in adults with rheumatoid arthritis. *Rheumatology*, 44(5): 685–687.

Wang, C., C. H. Schmid, P. L. Hibberd, R. Kalish, R. Roubenoff, R., Rones, and T. McAlindon. 2009 a. Tai Chi is effective in treating knee osteoarthritis: a randomized controlled trial. *Arthritis Care & Research*, 61(11):1545–1553.

Wang, C., C. H. Schmid, R. Kalish, J. Yinh, D. L. Goldenberg, R. Rones, and T. McAlindon. 2009b. Tai Chi is effective in treating fibromyalgia: a randomized controlled trial. *Arthritis Rheum*, 60:S526.

Wang, C., C. H. Schmid, R. Rones, R., Kalish, J. Yinh, D. L. Goldenberg, Y. Lee, and T. McAlindon. 2010b. A randomized trial of tai chi for fibromyalgia. *New England Journal of Medicine*, 363(8):743–754.

Wang, M. Y. and L. G. An. 2011. Effects of 12 weeks Tai Chi Chuan practice on the immune function of female college students who lack physical exercise. *Biology of Sport*, 28(1): 45.

Wayne, P. M. and T. J. Kaptchuk. 2008. Challenges inherent to T'ai Chi research: part I-T'ai Chi as a complex multicomponent intervention. *The Journal of Alternative and Complementary Medicine*, 14(1): 95–102.

Yang, J. -M. 2010. Tai Chi Chuan: Clasical Yang Style, 2nd edn. Wolfeboro, NH: YMAA

Yeh, G. Y., C. Wang, P. M. Wayne, and R. Phillips. 2009. Tai chi exercise for patients with cardiovascular conditions and risk factors: a systematic review. *Journal of Cardiopulmonary Rehabilitation and Prevention*, 29(3):152.

Yeh, G. Y., C. Wang, P. M. Wayne, and R. S. Phillips. 2008. The effect of Tai Chi exercise on blood pressure: a systematic review. *Preventive cardiology*, 11(2):82–89.

Introduction

Mindful awareness has been defined as "the awareness that emerges through paying attention on purpose, in the present moment and nonjudgmentally to the unfolding experience, moment by moment" (Kabat-Zinn 2013, xxxv.) Two components of mindful awareness have been suggested: sustained attention to present moment experience, and the deliberate adoption of specific attitudes (Bishop et al. 2004). The first component, a sustained attention to present-moment experience, includes the observation of thoughts, emotions, and sensations as they arise moment by moment with a stable and unwavering quality of attention. Often, the mind is not in the present moment, but rather reflecting on the past, planning for the future, or lost in a narrative *about* life. In truth, the past exists only as a memory, and the future, only a fantasy. Life happens in the present moment. To experience life fully, the mind must be in the here and now.

People can have a misperception of the present moment as inadequate and in need of constant improvement. They believe life and themselves to be insufficient, and constantly push themselves to improve and accomplish more and more. An underlying tension and anxiety drives their efforts while inner peace remains elusive. When mindful, the "to do" list is not abandoned, but is not an obstacle to a direct experience of ease or peace available in the present moment with things just as they are. To touch life fully and deeply, it is necessary to stop running, stop doing, and touch life just as it is.

In addition, persistent pain can make the present moment uncomfortable, unpleasant, and unwanted. People can react to the disagreeable quality of their experience with struggle, hostility, and/or distraction. These reactions take energy, cloud the mind, and undermine possibilities for insights, choices, and peace that are available in the present moment, even in the presence of persistent pain. Mindfulness offers a practical strategy to cultivate mental stability while simultaneously experiencing pain.

The second component of mindful awareness is the deliberate adoption of specific attitudes (Kabat-Zinn 2013, 21–30; Bishop et al. 2004). Our attitude toward an experience will directly influence our perception and response to the experience. Mindful attitudes include acceptance, friendliness, curiosity, nonjudging, and nonstriving. All perceptions, whether pleasant, unpleasant, or neutral, are consistently met with this orientation. These attitudes do not exist separate from each other, but rather are interdependent, overlap, and influence each other.

Mindful awareness is cultivated through training in sitting meditation, mindful body scan, walking meditation, and mindful movement. Two styles of **mindful meditation** training, focused attention and open monitoring, can be applied to these practices (Lutz et al. 2014). Focused-attention meditation is the practice of maintaining attention on a specific object, such as on the sensation of the breath. When attention moves away from the object to a distracting sensory, cognitive, or emotional event, that event is acknowledged. The practitioner disengages his or her attention from the distracting event and returns to focus on the object of meditation.

Open monitoring meditation involves the nonreactive, nondirective observation of the present-moment content of the mind. The practitioner observes sensory, emotional, and cognitive events as they arise without bias or cognitive elaboration.

Although rooted in the Buddhist spiritual tradition, training the mind to abide in the present moment with acceptance, nonjudgment, and curiosity does not require a religious affiliation and has been introduced as a secular practice to the general public and medical populations. In 1979, Jon Kabat-Zinn, PhD, pioneered **Mindfulness-Based Stress Reduction (MBSR)**, a patient-centered educational program designed to instruct people with chronic medical conditions, including chronic pain, in mindful awareness. This program is described in detail in Kabat-Zinn's book, *Full Catastrophe Living* (Kabat-Zinn 2013). Interest in MBSR has continued to grow and the program is now offered throughout the United States and internationally.

Mindfulness-based interventions are intended to complement a patient's medical treatment and are not an alternative to allopathic medical care. Participants are encouraged to inform their medical team of their participation in the program and may simultaneously receive physical therapy, occupational therapy, psychotherapy, massage, acupuncture, or other medical treatments while enrolled.

Over the past three decades, a growing body of research has identified multiple health benefits resulting from formal training in mindful awareness (Keng, Smoski, and Robins 2011; Cramer et al. 2012a; Lakhan and Schofield 2013; Witkiewitz, Lustyk, and Bowen 2013). This chapter offers the reader an introduction to the history of mindful awareness, a discussion of pertinent research, a theoretical model for its applications to the treatment of persistent pain conditions, and a case study.

History of Mindfulness

Mindful awareness takes its origins 2500 years ago in the insights of an Indian prince, Siddhartha Guatama (Nhat Hanh 1991). Leaving the comfort and shelter of his royal home, Siddhartha ventured into the surrounding community where he witnessed human illness, aging, and death. Confronted with the depths of human suffering, he abandoned his privileged living conditions and embraced a spiritual journey that led him to liberating insights into the roots and ultimate relief of human suffering.

His insights became the foundation of Buddhism, a religion that flourished throughout Asia. Mindful awareness and its role in relieving suffering are among his insights.

Buddhism came to the West in the 1800s when North Americans and Europeans returned from visits to Asia with Buddhist texts (Duerr 2010). In addition, Chinese immigrants brought Buddhism to the United States in the 1940s when they settled in western parts of the country (Duerr 2010). Interest in the religion gradually grew and, by the 1960s, Buddhist teachers had emigrated from Asia to establish Buddhist centers and offer instruction in Buddhism in the United States and Europe.

In 1979, Jon Kabat-Zinn, PhD, successfully translated the basic principles of mindful awareness found in Buddhism into secular language and concepts accessible to clinical populations at the University of Massachusetts Medical Center in an eight-session course, MBSR. He provided instruction in sitting meditation, mindful body scan, walking meditation, and mindful movement to patients with a wide range of medical conditions, including chronic pain. This initial program grew and developed to become the University of Massachusetts Medical School Center for Mindfulness in Medicine, Health Care, and Society. Presently, the center provides MBSR programs, MBSR professional training and certification for professionals, and supports basic science and clinical research related to MBSR. The success of the program has led to the establishment of MBSR programs throughout the United States and around the world.

The evidence-based benefits of MBSR led to the development of additional group interventions that offer training in mindful awareness as a central program component. These include Mindfulness-Based Cognitive Behavioral Therapy (Segal, Williams, and Teasdale 2012), Mindfulness-Based Relapse Prevention (Bowen et al. 2014), Mindfulness-Based Childbirth and Parenting (Duncan and Bardacke 2010), Mindfulness-Based Functional Therapy

(Schutze et al. 2104), and Mindfulness-Based Living Well with Pain and Illness (Doran 2014). In addition to programs for clinical populations, the growing popularity of mindfulness training led to programs tailored for healthcare professionals (Fortney et al. 2013; Zeller and Levin 2013). Mindfulness training is also available for students on many college and university campuses.

Loving kindness meditation (LKM) and **compassion meditation (CM)** also originated in the Buddhist tradition and are closely associated with mindful meditation (Hofmann, Grossman, and Hinton 2011; Holzel et al. 2011). Building on the success of MBSR, secular training in LKM and CM was developed. LKM is practiced with the intent to develop and experience a fundamental goodwill and kindness toward oneself and other people. CM invites the practitioner to open the heart toward oneself and other people in distress. Preliminary research suggests that both LKM and CM broaden attention, enhance positive emotions, and reduce negative emotions (Carson et al. 2005; Hofmann et al. 2011; Kearney et al., 2014) and may reduce pain in patients with chronic back pain (Carson et al. 2005). Given that higher levels of positive

affect in women with chronic pain conditions have been shown to predict lower levels of pain in subsequent weeks (Zautra, Johnson, and Davis 2005), the deliberate cultivation of positive emotional states through LKM and CM offers potential strategies for the self-management of chronic pain.

Theoretical Approaches to Pain Management

The experience of persistent pain results from a complex interaction of sensory, cognitive, and affective elements. Mindful awareness, with its emphasis on the nonjudging observation of sensations, thoughts, and emotions, offers a unique mechanism to bring these elements into conscious awareness and modulate nociceptive processing. This awareness provides a first step to the self-regulation of reflexive habit patterns that escalate pain, suffering, and contribute to disability (Doran 2014).

Clinical Populations

Literature reviews suggest that mindfulness-based therapies may be effective in reducing pain intensity in individuals with chronic pain (Lakhan and Schofield 2013; Reiner, Tibi, and Lipsitz 2103) and in reducing symptom severity, depression, and anxiety and improving quality of life in individuals suffering from somatization disorders, such as fibromyalgia, chronic fatigue, and irritable bowel syndrome (Lakhan and Schofield 2013). Slightly earlier reviews suggest there is not yet sufficient evidence to determine the magnitude of the effects of mindfulness-based therapies on chronic pain conditions (Chiesa and Serretti 2011; Cramer et al. 2012b). Although the current research is positive and promising, further research trials with a larger sample size, active control groups, and longer follow-up are needed to clarify the advantages of mindfulness-based interventions for the pain patient population (Chiesa and Serrette 2011; Cramer et al. 2012b; Lakhan and Schofield 2013; Reiner et al. 2103).

Sidebar 15.1 Patient Interviews

In response to the question, "Have your condition or symptoms or ability to function changed since receiving care?" a 53-year-old woman receiving care for neck pain and depression resulting from a traumatic brain injury replied: "My ability to function has increased. Several things occurred in close proximity that helped me. My pain was reduced by medication. I learned to meditate and think about pain differently. I learned how to handle pain signals. I learned the 'loving kindness' meditation which is my favorite. Meditation allows me to go into an altered state as it were. I focus on different things—or perhaps I don't focus on the pain. The workshop was a focused effort to take care of myself and learning tools to do so. I am so thankful I took the course."

Sidebar 15.2 Research
A small trial reported significant decreases in pain with multiple sclerosis patients and those with peripheral neuropathy (Tavee et al. 2011). This trial, along with two other studies summarized by Simpson and colleagues in a systematic review, reported benefits in quality of life, depression, and anxiety in study populations. The interventions were described as mindfulness meditation classes spanning 6 to 8 weeks (Simpson et al. 2014).

In a randomized controlled trial investigating the effects of MBSR on patients with nonspecific chronic pain, 109 patients, with a mean pain duration of 19.21 months, were randomized to either MBSR or to a wait list control group (la Cour and Petersen 2014). Significant medium to large size effects were found for vitality, general anxiety, depression, feeling in control of pain, and higher pain acceptance.

A promising pilot study for individuals with chronic low back pain combined mindfulness training with pain neurophysiology education, functional movement training, graduated cardiovascular exercise, and group support (Schutze et al. 2014). Significant improvements in physical function, role limitations, and catastrophizing were noted at 6 months. This multifaceted therapeutic protocol that combines mindfulness training with other evidence-based approaches might best address the multiple, complex factors that give rise to the chronic pain experience.

Qualitative research reveals positive cognitive and behavioral changes in patients with chronic low back pain who are trained in mindfulness (Doran 2014). Participants in this study reported they:

- became familiar with the pattern of pain and habitual reactions to pain

- recognized the difference between being tense and being relaxed in relation to pain

- identified early warning signs that preceded a flare-up

- stopped the cycle of projecting past experience of pain onto a fear of future pain

- changed maladaptive attitudes and approaches to pain

- reduced identification with diagnostic labeling or story about the pain

- increased flexibility in attitude toward pain

- reduced self-blame and inner conflict

- felt less "fragmented," greater integration of mind and body, and experience of wellness within illness.

In addition, mindfulness-based therapies might have a role in addressing the abuse and long-term use of **opioids** in the treatment of chronic pain conditions. From 1999 to 2010, the USA experienced a fourfold increase in prescriptions for opioids and an alarming rise in deaths and emergency department

Sidebar 15.3 Patient Interviews
When asked, "What have you learned about this treatment approach or self-care that you would like healthcare providers to know about?", a 35-year-old woman with fibromyalgia replied: "Mindfulness empowers the patient and gives them tools they can use to be proactive with their physical and mental health. I was very skeptical about this approach when my counselor recommended it because it's not part of mainstream medicine. I realized mindfulness exercises could have prevented my medical conditions before they started, but I'm thankful I was able to learn them early on into my diagnosis. Now I have seen the results of this treatment, I feel equipped to take control of my health and I feel like I have more control over managing my pain without medication. I think every patient dealing with pain has a right to know mindfulness is an effective treatment option."

visits due to opioid abuse (Cobaugh et al. 2014). While some individuals are able to take opioid medications as prescribed, others demonstrate addictive tendencies (Fishbain et al. 2008). Also, the extended use of opioids can contribute to nociceptive sensitization and loss of opioid efficacy (Lee et al. 2011). In response to these concerns, researchers developed a randomized controlled trial to pilot a mindfulness-based intervention targeting the underlying mechanisms of chronic pain and opioid misuse (Garland et al. 2014). At 3 months, when compared with a support group intervention, the mindfulness group reported significantly greater reductions in pain severity and interference. These results were mediated by increased nonreactivity and reinterpretation of pain sensations.

Possible Mechanisms
Leading researchers suggest training in mindful meditation results in beneficial health consequences through four mechanisms: improved attention regulation, increased body awareness, enhanced emotional regulation, and changes in perspective on self (Holzel et al. 2011).

Attention regulation
The consistent practice of mindfulness meditation improves a person's ability to rest the mind in the present moment in an uninterrupted manner for increasing periods of time (Jha, Krompinger, and Baime 2007; van den Hurk et al. 2010). This improved cognitive control has been suggested to generate less negative appraisal of pain by cultivating acceptance and reducing anticipation or expectation (Brown and Jones 2010).

Body awareness
Body awareness is hypothesized to be the outcome of a dynamic process that reflects afferent and efferent neural processes, includes cognitive appraisal and unconscious modulation, and is shaped by a person's attitudes, beliefs, and experience in a social and cultural context (Mehling et. al. 2009). Participants in an MBSR course demonstrated

significant increases in body awareness self-report measures (Carmdy and Baer 2008).

When practicing mindful breathing, body scan, walking, and movement, patients pay attention to physical sensations with acceptance, friendliness, and curiosity. They learn to experience physical sensations as separate from thinking about, or emotional reactions to, the sensations. They become aware of pain-free body areas. This enhanced body awareness is a necessary step in controlling muscle tension levels in reaction to pain. In addition, body awareness enables patients to better pace activities and appropriately adjust posture and body position as a means to prevent pain and tension escalation (Doran 2014). Body awareness is also necessary for the awareness and regulation of emotions (Pollatos, Gramann, and Schandry 2007; Holzel et al. 2011).

Emotional regulation
Mindfulness training has been shown to enhance emotional regulation, improve mood, and reduce anxiety and depression in patients with chronic pain (Brown and Jones 2013; Doran 2014; Song et al. 2014). Researchers postulate that this improved emotional regulation occurs through two possible mechanisms: reappraisal and extinction (Holzel et al. 2011).

Reappraisal is an active, adaptive coping strategy by which stressful events are reinterpreted to be beneficial, meaningful, or benign. Mindfulness is associated with positive reappraisal (Garland, Gaylord, and Park 2009). For example, patients learn to label pain as "sensation" rather than use the term "pain." "Sensation" is a benign term that does not carry the threat value associated with the word "pain."

Extinction learning allows an individual to eliminate a fear response to a stimulus when fear is not an adaptive response to that stimulus (Quirk and Mueller 2008). Fear extinction requires a continual exposure to the stimulus. This repeated exposure is hypothesized to create a new memory or reconfigure the old memory with new contextual associations. In the case of chronic pain, fear is a maladaptive response to the unpleasant sensation. When mindful, patients expose themselves to the sensation and emotional reaction again and again, moment by moment. The emotion is continually witnessed within a larger field of an accepting, kind, curious attention. Patients are trained to turn toward rather than away from emotions, even the most difficult ones. This repeated exposure might have the effect of reducing fear of the emotion and sensation through extinction learning.

In addition, extinction mechanisms are thought to be enhanced by the experience of relaxation while the individual encounters the feared stimulus. Mindfulness meditation is associated with increased parasympathetic activity and decreased sympathetic activity, and might contribute to fear extinction through evoking greater relaxation in response to pain and fear (Holzel et al. 2011).

Changes in perspective on the self

Mindfulness meditation trains the practitioner to observe, without judgment or reactivity, sensory, cognitive, and emotional experiences as they appear and disappear in the mind. Practitioners are aware of these events as they arise and pass but do not identify with them. What was previously perceived as "subject" now becomes an observable "object." Self is experienced as disengaged from transitory sensations, cognitions, and emotions. This ability to mindfully observe experience but not identify with it has been termed "reperceiving" (Shapiro et al. 2006). Although difficult to quantify through quantitative research, qualitative investigations suggest that mindfulness training contributes to the development of this nonreacting, observing self (Kerr, Josyula, and Littenberg 2011; Doran 2014).

Consistent with this reperceiving model, patients with chronic pain who completed a mindfulness training intervention describe shifting perceptions of pain from "unchanging," "solid," or "everlasting" to pain as a process and something in a constant state of flux (Doran 2014). Participants in this qualitative study also report becoming less identified with their pain condition or diagnostic label.

Methodology

I teach **mindful awareness** to patients with chronic pain in a group format and through individual training. Both forms of mindful awareness instruction require the active involvement of the patient. This treatment approach is not suitable for a patient with a passive, unengaged attitude. For success, patients must be motivated to learn and experiment with new approaches to pain and to life. They must be willing to participate in a home program that requires commitment, time, and effort. Patients identify escalating and de-escalating responses to pain and stress for themselves. They take responsibility for the choices they make and learn skills that will serve them for life.

> **Sidebar 15.4 Patient Interviews**
> When asked, "Do you feel different about yourself or your pain since receiving care?", a 53-year-old woman with a traumatic brain injury replied: "I know that it is my duty to take care of myself first and foremost. I alter my behavior to be conducive to identifying pain before it ramps up too much. It is necessary for me to have down time—for both my mental functioning and my pain management. Certain things are challenging such as travel. I have to maintain a consistent schedule. This is a cognitive compensatory method as well as pain management. I lie down as much as I can. The biggest thing I learned is that I can affect my pain by meditating."

Important Principles Conveyed in Both Formats

Whether delivered in a group or individual format, I teach patients to identify the immediate sensory experience of pain and automatic physical, cognitive, and emotional reactions to pain. This calm observation enables patients to directly witness their experience but not identify with it. The accepting, curious, observing mind is unperturbed by the unpleasant sensation. Patients experience the pain as a constantly changing sensation rather than something fixed and solid. This ability to distinguish between the sensation and reactions to the sensation is a necessary step in the self-regulation of these reactions. I invite patients to more closely examine reflexive reactions and their influence on pain intensity and overall well-being. This investigation includes the following elements.

Physical

Patients can observe the sensation of pain and their physical reaction to the pain. What is happening with their breathing? Are muscles tense or relaxed? What posture are they adopting? Out of this stable observation, patients recognize new conscious choices that can impact the experience. For example, if a patient notices she is shallow breathing, she could deliberately take a deep breath. If she is clenching her teeth, she could relax her jaw. If she is drawing her shoulders up and curling her spine forward, she could adopt an upright posture.

Cognitive

Patients can observe the sensation and the story they tell themselves *about* the sensation. They observe the story without attaching to or identifying with the story. For example, a patient can observe an unrealistic catastrophic statement about pain as just a thought. He does not identify with the thought or believe it as an infallible reflection of the truth. The thought is observed as a cloud is observed in the sky. This ability to detach from the narrative about the pain illuminates the distinction between the sensation and language about the sensation that escalates the pain experience. In addition, patients can be taught to substitute the word "sensation" for the word "pain." I also encourage patients to develop kind and compassionate self-talk by talking to themselves as they would to a good friend.

Emotional

Patients can observe the sensation of pain and their emotional reaction to the pain. As with cognitions, the emotion can be observed without identifying with or being swept away by the emotion. All emotions are allowed without judgment or censorship. There is no deliberate effort made to change or reduce an emotion. The emotion is accepted with friendliness and curiosity. Patients can discover for themselves how some emotions escalate their pain while others de-escalate their pain.

I teach additional strategies for emotional regulation such as:

- Repeat to yourself:

  - "Breathing in, I am aware I feel angry. Breathing out, I meet myself with compassion."

  - "Right now there are other people just like me, in pain and feeling fear. I send compassion to myself and to everyone else in pain who feels fear."

- Explore the emotion more closely as a scientist might explore a new object. Ask yourself, "What is anger anyway? Where do I feel it in my body? What is the energy like moment to moment? How does the emotion influence the pain sensation? How do my thoughts impact my emotions?"

The ability to recognize and accept emotions takes practice and patience. Training to mindfully observe and investigate emotions contributes to emotional intelligence and improved emotional regulation (Holzel et al. 2011). Patients can more readily discern which emotions they need to just observe and which are an invitation to action. The mindful observation of an emotion enables a patient to take a more thoughtful response to a situation rather than act in an automatic, reflexive manner. Sometimes, a new insight into a situation or the root of the emotion is recognized. Other times, the emotion is observed but not amplified and pro-longed by additional thoughts and mental images.

In the course of mindfulness training, patients frequently identify body parts that are pain free. This is a revelation for many and can support a more realistic and balanced view of the body.

In addition, I discuss the application of mindfulness to stressful situations. I introduce the equation: Stress = Situation + Your Reaction to the Situation. Just as patients learn to observe the sensation of pain and their physical, cognitive, and emotional reactions to pain, so too they learn to observe stressful situations and their automatic reactions to those stressful situations. By bringing awareness to these reactions, patients can make conscious choices that de-escalate stress.

Sidebar 15.5 Research
The American College of Chest Physicians include Mindfulness-Based Stress Reduction (MBSR) and meditation in their 2013 clinical guidelines to reduce pain, anxiety, depression, stress, and enhance mood and self-esteem in people suffering from lung cancer. Additionally, the 2014 clinical practice guidelines from the Society for Integrative Oncology recommend meditation to address stress, anxiety, and depression and to improve overall quality of life in breast cancer patients (Get the Facts 2014).

The Group Model
A popular and widely offered model for mindful awareness instruction, and the one I teach, is MBSR. For a complete and comprehensive description of this program, the reader is referred to the book *Full Catastrophe Living* by Kabat-Zinn (2013). Participants meet once a week for 2.5 hours for eight consecutive weeks. A day of mindfulness is offered between classes 6 and 7. Participants enrolling have a wide range of physical and mental health conditions including chronic pain, cancer, cardiovascular

disease, anxiety, and depression. The program offers instruction in sitting meditation, mindful body scan, walking meditation, and mindful movement or yoga. A structured home program is provided that includes a workbook, guided audio recordings for daily practice, and instructions to incorporate mindfulness into neutral, pleasant, and unpleasant daily experiences.

To enroll in MBSR, programs offer an orientation session or have an individual pre-program screening. I provide a pre-program screening interview by phone. Both formats offer the prospective participant an opportunity to learn about the program and connect with the program instructor. The interested individual and instructor together can determine if the program is a fit.

Although the MBSR program is described in detail in Kabat-Zinn's book, *Full Catastrophe Living*, and the course curriculum is included in MBSR professional training, no two programs are the same. The present moment is always new, fresh, and unique. No two moments are precisely the same. No two teachers or groups are identical. Mindfulness instruction is not offered in a cookie-cutter, one-size-fits-all fashion but is shared in a dynamic, living manner that emerges from the experience of the instructor and the contributions of the group, moment by moment. To teach mindfulness, I not only offer skill instruction, but aspire to embody mindfulness and respond to the unique needs of the group in each moment.

My average class size is eighteen participants. Other programs can have classes as large as thirty participants. A significant benefit of the program comes from the group discussion in a supportive community. Participants learn from each other's experiences and insights. While sharing in the large group is encouraged, I acknowledge the discomfort some people experience when speaking in a large group, and suggest that talking to the whole group is optional and participants can always choose not to share.

Class Content

In the first class, participants have an opportunity to introduce themselves and talk about their motivation for participating. I introduce mindfulness and lead an exercise in mindful eating. I provide instruction and lead guided practices in sitting meditation and body scan. Participants discuss their experiences and ask questions. They receive a workbook with educational materials, home program guidelines, and instructions to access online audio recordings of guided meditation practices. I emphasize the importance of actively following the home program recommendations.

Classes 2 through 7 begin with a meditation practice and a question and answer period about the practice. The group breaks into pairs and participants talk with one another about their week's experiences. We then gather as a large group and participants share their experiences in the larger group. Following this discussion, I introduce additional information related to mindfulness and health. The themes I introduce in each class are as follows:

- Class 2: Stress and our reaction to stress
- Class 3: Movement and gentle yoga
- Class 4: Mindfulness of thoughts
- Class 5; Mindfulness of emotions
- Class 6: Mindful communication
- Class 7: Kindness meditation.

Following the introduction of new material, I lead anther meditation practice and discussion. I then review the upcoming week's home program. Over the 8 weeks, participants practice 40–60 minutes of sitting meditation, body scan, walking meditation, gentle yoga, and kindness meditation in class. They are given handouts each week that include material related to the week's theme, and instructions for the home practice.

The weekly home program will include instructions to practice 30–45 minutes of a formal mindfulness practice daily and to apply mindfulness to routine activities, such as when washing hands or brushing teeth. In addition, the home practice will include specific topics, guidelines, and worksheets to more fully integrate mindfulness into daily life. These topics include bringing mindful attention to:

- one pleasant event each day, as it is happening
- one unpleasant event each day, as it is happening
- thoughts throughout the day
- moods and emotions throughout the day
- listening and self-expression.

Between weeks 6 and 7, I offer a day of mindfulness on a Saturday. This is a day spent in silence from 10 a.m. to 4 p.m. during which I guide participants in sitting meditation, walking meditation, gentle yoga, and kindness meditation. Lunch is spent in silence, practicing mindful eating. Previous program participants are invited to attend the day of mindfulness on a donation basis. At 3:30 the silence is broken and we go around the circle, giving each participant the opportunity to share something of their experience.

The eighth class begins with a sitting meditation and opportunity to discuss the practice, the day of mindfulness, and the week in the large group. Participants then break into dyads and share their experience of the program with one other person. They explore what they learned, how they changed, and what are areas for continued growth and learning. We gather as a large group and go around the circle, giving each participant the opportunity to share something from their experience of the program. I then introduce additional resources that support their continued practice. These include my future days of mindfulness, local meditation groups, yoga and Tai Chi instructors, books and audio recordings. We do a short closing practice that includes the dedication of our efforts to the benefit of all beings.

Chapter 15

The Individual Model

Healthcare professionals, with advanced training and experience in mindfulness, can include instruction in mindful awareness as a component of their individual patient care. In my own case, mindfulness training is a core skill I teach in my physical therapy chronic pain treatment program. I also use surface electromyography (EMG) biofeedback to evaluate resting muscle tension and assist patients to build body awareness and relaxation skills.

Individual mindfulness training enables me to tailor my instruction to a patient's specific goals and needs. I usually see people for three to six 1-hour training sessions. In the first visit, I take the patient's history and identify the patient's present activity level and goals. The patient identifies functional goals. Examples of common functional goals include return to work, socialize with friends, and accomplish household chores. I evaluate the patient's resting muscle tension using surface EMG biofeedback, breathing pattern, and posture. I provide patient education on the topics of pain neurophysiology, central sensitization, the modulation of pain by cognitions and emotions, and the basic science of stress-induced hyperalgesia. I teach principles of mindful awareness and mindful breathing. I guide the patient to rest the mind in the present moment, observing sensations of breathing in and breathing out. I help the patient identify the difference between diaphragmatic breathing and shallow breathing. I introduce the patient to the difference between the sensation of pain and his or her reaction to the sensation and offer the equation:

Pain = Sensation + Your Reaction.

The patient brings previously unconscious, automatic physical, cognitive, and emotional reactions to pain into awareness. These unconscious, automatic reactions are discussed, and alternatives are explored.

The majority of my patients breathe in a shallow manner, have poor body awareness and carry abnormal, elevated resting tension levels in major muscle groups. I use surface EMG biofeedback to assist patients in building body awareness, releasing excessive muscle tension, and in learning diaphragmatic breathing and muscle relaxation.

I guide a brief, 5- or 10-minute, progressive muscle relaxation exercise integrating mindful principles. I emphasize that being tense is not bad or wrong. It just is. I suggest that the patient can meet both areas of tension and relaxation with the same nonjudging, open, accepting, curious mind.

I develop a home program with the patient, based on his or her goals. This will often include:

- mindful breathing throughout the day

- labeling pain "sensation" and incorporating imagery, for example, thinking of it like a cloud in the sky

- talking to yourself as you would a good friend who was in your shoes

- integrating mindful awareness into routine activities such as when washing your hands

- planning a pleasant activity and being mindful of the experience

- bringing mindful awareness to your experience of pain

- practicing 10–30 minutes of a mindful meditation or relaxation daily; for the latter, I suggest trying the 10-minute guided relaxation and meditation practices at my website and other online resources, and I also recommend a mindfulness app if a patient is interested: https://itunes.apple.com/us/app/the-mindfulness-app/id417071430?mt=8

In the second visit, I review the patient's goals and invite the patient to talk about his or her experience of the home program. We explore, in a collaborative manner, what went well and what was challenging. I respond to a patient's questions and clarify areas of confusion. I review main themes of pain neuroscience (Louw et al. 2011; Woolf 2011; Jennings et al. 2014). These include:

- Stress can amplify pain.

- Pain can arise in the absence of tissue damage.

- A sensitive nervous system can generate pain in response to normal movement.

- The nervous system is always changing and nerve sensitivity is reversible.

- For optimal healing, you need to calm your nervous system.

I explain that mindfulness can help reduce the stress reaction, change pain-related brain activation, and reduce nerve sensitivity.

We explore the role of mindfulness in illuminating new ways to physically, cognitively, and emotionally respond to pain. I explain the role of these reactions in changing brain activation and escalating or de-escalating the stress response and nerve sensitivity. We develop a home program for the week suitable to the patient's unique goals and needs.

During the second and successive visits, I respond to the individual needs of the patient and find ways for the patient to successfully practice and integrate mindfulness in response to pain, stress, and daily life. For example, if a patient has not followed the home program, I guide a discussion exploring the patient's motivation to change and strategies to practice home program recommendations in the future. If a patient describes being tense and worried about pain when working, we examine practical strategies to integrate mindful awareness and mindful breathing in the workplace. These subsequent visits involve a combination of patient education, neuromuscular re-education, diaphragmatic breathing instruction and practice, posture guidelines, guided relaxation and mindfulness meditation, pacing and pleasant activity instruction, and applying mindful awareness to movement and exercise.

Some patients are highly motivated, quick learners, and require only two or three visits to achieve their goals and become independent on a home mindfulness program. Other patients are slower to grasp the concept of mindfulness, develop a consistent mindfulness practice, and successfully integrate mindfulness into pain management, movement and exercise, and activities of daily living. These patients may require four to six individual visits.

Case Study

David was a 38-year-old man with a 4-year history of chronic neck, upper back, and arm pain. The initial onset was gradual and had become more severe in the past 2 years. He described the pain as a constant, dull, throbbing ache with intermittent, shock-like bursts of pain. His pain intensity ranged 4–9/10 and averaged 5/10. His pain was aggravated by working at a computer for greater than 30 minutes and carrying anything. His pain was eased with rest, ice, and heat. On a pain interference scale where 1 indicates no interference and 10 indicates maximum interference, David rated the following: general activity 7, relationships 4, mood 9, normal work 6, and enjoyment of life 9. His MRI was normal.

David's treatment included a 2-hour pain neurophysiology education class, three individual physical therapy treatments, followed by his participation in an eight-session MBSR program. David's individual physical therapy included instruction in pain neurophysiology education, progressive muscle relaxation, and the application of mindful awareness, diaphragmatic breathing, and relaxation to pain and activities of daily living.

Within 3 months, David was pain free. He had no pain when working on a computer or with other upper extremity activity, including lifting. On the pain interference scale, he identified 1, no interference, with general activity, relationships, mood, normal work, and enjoyment of life.

In his own words:

"Everything I did was fast. I was supercharged and constantly pressured. I took on as much as I could and then more. It slowly started catching up with me.

"The pain came on slowly. A tingling in the wrists and then up to my elbows. After a few years my neck and upper back were in trouble. It didn't stop me. I kept going. When the pain got scary, I took breaks to feel better and then would get right back to it.

"I went to several doctors and had four different courses of physical therapy that included stretching, ultrasound, manual therapy, traction, and wrist splints. Nothing helped, and as the years progressed I got worse and worse. I was aging exponentially and losing weight. I was in total despair.

"Then I was referred for mindfulness instruction. As a workaholic, I was resistant. I was scared that if I slowed down I would lose things I loved and not get as much done. Wow, was I wrong. Now, I don't work as much but I get more done. My life is more full and I enjoy so much more of everything. I don't even stress about things that would have driven me crazy before. I am more compassionate, patient, and deliberate.

"Through learning more about pain and receiving mindfulness instruction, I was taught a different way of looking at pain. My pain was due to sensitive nerves caused by stress and compounded by my reaction to pain and stressful situations. After a few weeks of practicing mindfulness, I found amazing results. By the time I finished the course I was pain free.

"The pain I experienced was something I had to go through to grow and change my life for the better. Now I feel I have a long happy and healthy life ahead."

Conclusion

The experience of pain is the outcome of the complex interaction of sensory, cognitive, and emotional variables. Mindful awareness, with its emphasis on the nonjudgmental, curious observation of sensations, thoughts, and emotions, offers a practical approach to the self-management and relief of chronic pain. Mindfulness-based therapies teach patients with chronic pain to observe maladaptive physical, cognitive, and emotional habit patterns that escalate pain, suffering, and disability with acceptance, friendliness, and curiosity. This alone is a valuable skill. In addition, patients learn to make new physical, cognitive, and emotional choices that reduce pain and improve mood and physical function. A growing body of research provides evidence for the effectiveness of mindfulness-based therapies in the treatment of chronic pain.

References

Bishop, S. R., M. Lau, S. Shapiro, L. Carlson, N. D. Anderson, J. Carmody, Z. V. Segal, S. Abbey, M. Speca, D. Velting, et al. 2004. Mindfulness: A proposed operational definition. *Clinical Psychology: Science and Practice* 11(3):230–41.

Bowen, S., K. Witkiewitz, S. L. Clifasefi, J. Grow, N. Chawla, S. H. Hsu, H. A. Carroll, E. Harrop, S. E. Collins, M. K. Lustyk, et al. 2014. Relative efficacy of mindfulness-based relapse prevention, standard relapse prevention, and treatment as usual for substance use disorders: a randomized clinical trial. *JAMA Psychiatry* 71(5):547–56.

Brown, C. A., and A. K. Jones. 2010. Meditation experience predicts less negative appraisal of pain: electrophysiological evidence for the involvement of anticipatory neural responses. *Pain* 150(3):428–38.

Brown, C. A., and A. K. Jones, 2013. Psychobiological correlates of improved mental health in patients with musculoskeletal pain after a mindfulness based pain management program. 2013. *Clin J Pain*, 29(3):233–44.

Carmdy, J., and R. A. Baer. 2008. Relationships between mindfulness practice and levels of mindfulness, medical and psychological symptoms and well-being in mindfulness-based stress reduction. *J Behav Med* 31(1):23–33.

Carson, J. W., F. J. Keefe, T. R. Lynch, K. M. Carsoon, V. Goli, A. M. Fras, and S. R. Thorp. 2005. Loving kindness meditation for chronic low back pain: Results from a pilot trial. *J Holistic Nurs* 23(3):287–304.

Chiesa, A., and A. Serretti. 2011. Mindfulness-based interventions for chronic pain: A systematic review of the evidence. *J Altern Complement Med* 17(1):83–93.

Cobaugh, D. J., C. Gainor, C. L. Gaston, T. C. Kwong, B. Magnani, M. L. McPherson, J. T. Painter, and E. P. Krenzelok. 2014. The opioid abuse and misuse epidemic: implications for pharmacists in hospitals and health systems. *Am J Health Syst Pharm* 71(18):1539–54.

Cramer, H., R. Lauche, A. Paul, and G. Dubos. 2012a. Mindfulness based stress reduction for breast cancer: A systematic review and meta-analysis. *Curr Oncol* 19(5):343–52.

Cramer, H., H. Heidemarie, R. Lauche, and G. Dobos. 2012b. Mindfulness-based stress reduction for low back pain. A systematic review. *BMC Complement Altern Med* (12):162.

Doran, N. J. 2014. Experiencing wellness within illness: Exploring a mindfulness-based approach to chronic back pain. *Qual Health Res* 24(6):749–60.

Duerr, M. 2010. How Buddhism came to the west. http://www.pbs.org/thebuddha/blog/2010/mar/17/how-buddhism-came-west-maia-duerr/.

Duncan, L. G. and N. Bardacke. 2010. Mindfulness-based childbirth and parenting education: Promoting family mindfulness during the perinatal period. *J Child Fam Stud* 19(2):190–202.

Fishbain, D. A., B. Cole, J. E. Lewis, H. L. Rosomoff, and R. S. Rosomoff. 2008. What percentage of chronic nonmalignant pain patients exposed to chronic opioid analgesic therapy develop abuse/addiction and/or aberrant drug-related behaviors? A structured evidence-based review. *Pain Med* 9(2):149–60.

Fortney, L. C. Luchterhand, L. Zakletskaia, A. Zierska, and D. Rakel. 2013. Abbreviated mindfulness intervention for job satisfaction, quality of life, and compassion in primary care clinicians: a pilot study. *Ann Fam Med* 11(5):412–20.

Garland, E., S. Gaylord, and L. Park. 2009. The role of mindfulness in positive reappraisal. *Explore (NY)* 5(1):37–44.

Garland, E. L., E. G. Manusov, B. Froeliger, A. Kelly, J. M. Williams, and M. O. Howard. 2014. Mindfulness-oriented recovery enhancement for chronic pain and prescription opioid use: results from an early-stage randomized controlled trial. *J Consult Clin Psychol* 82(3):448–59.

Get The Facts. 2014. US Department of Health and Human Services. National Institutes of Health. National Center for Complementary and Integrative Health. https://nccih.nih.gov/sites/nccam.nih.gov/files/Get_The_Facts_Meditation_12-18-2014.pdf (accessed July 10, 2015).

Hofmann, S. G., P. Grossman, and D. E. Hinton. 2011. Loving kindness and compassion meditation: Potential for psychological interventions. *Clin Psychol Rev* 31(7):1126–32.

Holzel, B. K., S. W. Lazar, T. Guard, Z. Schuman, D. R. Vago, and U. Ott. 2011. How does mindfulness meditation work? Proposing mechanisms of action from a conceptual and neural perspective. *Perspect Psychol Science* 6:537–59.

Jennings, E. M., B. N. Okine, M. Roche, and D. P. Finn. 2014. Stress-induced hyperalgesia. *Prog Neurobiol* 121:1–18.

Jha, A. P., J. Krompinger, and M. J. Baime. 2007. Mindfulness training modifies subsystems of attention. *Cogn Affect Behav Neurosci* 7(2):109–19.

Kabat-Zinn, J. 2013. *Full Catastrophe Living: Using the Wisdom of Your Body and Mind to Face Stress, Pain and Illness*, 2nd edn. New York: Bantam.

Kearney, D. J., C. A. McManus, C. A. Malte, M. E. Martinez, B. Felleman, and T. L. Simpson. 2014. Loving-kindness meditation and broaden-and-build theory of positive emotions among veterans with posttraumatic stress disorder. *Med Care I* 52(12)S5:S32–8.

Keng, S. L., M. J. Smoski, and C. J. Robins. 2011. Effects of mindfulness on psychological health: a review of empirical studies. *Clin Psychol Rev* 31(6):1041–56.

Kerr, C. E., K. Josyula, and R. Littenberg. 2011. Developing an observing attitude: an analysis of meditation diaries in an MBRS clinical trial. *Clin Psychol Psychother* 18(1):80–93.

la Cour, P., and M. Petersen. 2014. Effects of mindfulness meditation on chronic pain: A randomized controlled trial. *Pain Med* Nov 7. doi: 10.1111/pme.12605.

Lakhan, S. E., and K. L. Schofield, K. 2013. Mindfulness-based therapies in the treatment of somatization disorders: a systematic review and meta-analysis. *PLoS One* 8(8):e71834.

Lee, M., S. M. Silverman, H. Hansen, V. B. Patel, and L. Manchikanti. 2011. A comprehensive review of opioid-induced hyperalgesia. *Pain Physician* 2011 Mar–Apr;14(2):145–61. Review.

Louw A., I. Diener, D. Butler, and E. J. Puentedura. 2011. The effect of neuroscience education on pain, disability, anxiety and stress in chronic musculoskeletal pain. *Arch Phys Med Rehabil* 92(12):2041–56.

Lutz, J., U. Herwig, S. Opialla, A. Hittmeyer, L. Jancke, M. Rufer, M. Grosse Holtforth, and A. Bruhl. 2014. Mindfulness and emotion regulation – an fMRI study. *Soc Cogn Affect Neurosci* 9(6):776–85

Mehling, W. E., V. Gopisetty, J. Daubenmier, C. J. Price, F. M. Hecht, and A. Stewart. 2009. Body awareness: construct and self-report measures. *PLoS One* 4(5):5614.

Nhat Hanh, T. 1991. *Old Path White Clouds: Walking in the Footsteps of the Buddha.* Berkeley: Parallax Press.

Pollatos, O., K. Gramann, and R. Schandry. 2007. Neural systems connecting interoceptive awareness and feelings. *Hum Brain Mapp* 28(1):9–18.

Quirk, G. J., and D. Mueller. 2008. Neural mechanisms of extinction learning and retrieval. *Neuropsychopharmacology* 33(1):56–72.

Reiner, K., L. Tibi, and J. D. Lipsitz. 2013. Do mindfulness-based interventions reduce pain intensity? A critical review of the literature. *Pain Med* 14(2):230–42.

Schutze, R., H. Slater, P. O'Sullivan, J. Thornton, A. Finlay-Jones, and C. S. Rees. 2014. Mindfulness-based functional therapy: A preliminary open trial of an integrated model of care for people with persistent low back pain. *Front Psychol* 4(5):839.

Segal, Z. J., M. G. Williams, and J. D. Teasdale. 2012. *Mindfulness based Cognitive Therapy*, 2nd edn. New York: Guilford Press.

Shapiro, S. L., L. E. Carlson, J. A. Astin, and B. Freedman. 2006. Mechanisms of mindfulness. *J Clin Psych* 62(3):373–86.

Simpson, R., J. Booth, M. Lawrence, S. Byrne, F. Mair, and S. Mercer. 2014. Mindfulness based interventions in multiple sclerosis — a systematic review. *BMC. Neurology* **14**:15. doi:10.1186/1471-2377-14-15.

Song, Y., H. Lu, H. Chen, G. Geng, and J. Wang. 2014. Mindfulness intervention in the management of chronic pain and psychological comorbidity: A meta-analysis. *Int J Nurs Sci* 1(2):215–23.

van den Hurk, P. A., F. Giommi, S. C. Gielen, A. E. Speckens, and H. P. Barendregt. 2010. Greater efficiency in attentional processing related to mindfulness meditation. *Q J Exp Psychol* 63(6): 168–80.

Tavee, J., M. Rensel, S. Pope Planchon, and L. Stone. 2011. Effects of meditation on pain and quality of life in multiple sclerosis and polyneuropathy: a controlled study. *Int J MS Care* 13(S2):163–8.

Witkiewitz, K., M. K. Lustyk, and S. Bowen. 2013. Retraining the addicted brain: a review of hypothesized neurobiological mechanisms of mindfulness-based relapse prevention. *Psychol Addict Behav* 27(2):37–44.

Woolf, C. J. 2011. Central senitization: implications for the diagnosis and treatment of pain. *Pain* 152(3 Suppl):S2–15.

Zautra, A. J., L. M. Johnson, and M. C. Davis. 2005. Positive affect as a source of resilience for women in chronic pain. *J Consult Clin Psychol* 73(2); 2012–20.

Zeller, J. M. and P. F. Levin. 2013. Mindfulness interventions to reduce stress among nursing personnel: an occupational health perspective. *Workplace Health Saf* 61(2):85–9.

Additional Resources

https://itunes.apple.com/us/app/the-mindfulness-app/id417071430?mt=8

Books on Mindfulness

Chodron, P. 2013. *How to meditate.* Sounds True.

Kabat-Zinn, J. 2013. *Full catastrophe living: using the wisdom of your body and mind to face stress, pain and illness,* updated edition. New York: Bantam.

Salzberg, S. 2010. *Real happiness: the power of meditation: A 28-Day Program.* Workman Publishing Company.

Review of Mindfulness Apps

Mani, M., D. J. Kavanagh, L. Hides, and S. R. Stoyanov. 2015. Review and evaluation of mindfulness-based iphone apps. *JMIR Mhealth Uhealth* 19(3): e82.

Introduction

Body awareness is a complex construct at the interface of mind and body. Depending where it is discussed, whether in primary care medicine, behavioral science, health psychology, cognitive neuroscience, anthropology, massage therapy, physical therapy, body-oriented psychotherapy, martial arts, or in various mind–body approaches, we hear quite divergent views about it. Historically, it has commonly been associated with hypervigilance and hypochondriasis and thereby been viewed as a proxy for anxiety (Cioffi 1991; Porges 1993); however, conversely, it can be associated with mindfulness and discriminative attunement to subtle bodily cues and then it becomes a powerful tool in self-regulation. As one view describes it as maladaptive and the other as beneficial, there may still remain substantial confusion despite recent attempts at a more differentiated understanding of the body awareness construct (Mehling et al. 2009). We define body awareness as sensory awareness that originates from the body's physiological state, involving interactive processes (including pain and emotion), actions (including movement), and appraisal (as well as complex bottom-up and top-down neural activities) shaped by the person's attitudes, beliefs, and experience in their social and cultural context (Mehling et al. 2009).These top-down activities determine whether body awareness is maladaptive or beneficial.

Neurophysiology of Pain as it Relates to Body Awareness

From a neurophysiological viewpoint, body awareness includes both proprioception and interoception. **Proprioception** is the perception of joint angles and muscle tensions, of movement, posture, and balance. **Interoception** is the perception of all sensations from inside the body and includes the perception of physical sensations related to internal organ function such as heart beat, respiration, satiety, and the autonomic nervous system symptoms related to emotions (Vaitl 1996; Cameron 2001; Craig 2002; Barrett et al. 2004). Many of these perceptions remain unconscious; what becomes conscious enters proprioceptive and interoceptive *awareness*, which involves higher mental processes such as emotions, memories, attitudes, beliefs, and behavior (Cameron 2001). Neuroscience has revealed how and in which areas of the brain interoception is processed and how it relates to emotion and pain (Bechara and Naqvi 2004; Critchley et al. 2004; Wiens 2005; Naqvi , Shiv, and Bechara 2006). In this chapter, however, we will emphasize the first-person phenomenology of massage and body therapy experiences, an area that is of yet not within the purview of current brain science.

Pain, particularly chronic pain, is a highly complex subjective experience with sensory discriminative, affective, and behavioral aspects, and distinguishable neural pathways for each. The last decades have provided important new insight into pain and the ways it is neurologically processed. Both pain in its *affective* component and interoception use identical neural pathways (Craig 2003a, 2003b) and converge in a cortex region of the brain that processes the physical and sensory aspects of emotions and their autonomic nervous system correlates (Craig 2003a). Pain as a bodily sensation is part of interoception and has intriguing parallels to emotions. As both pain and emotions have sensory, affective, and motivational-behavioral aspects and common neurological pathways, some neuroscientists now view pain as a "homeostatic emotion:" pain is a signal from the body that motivates behavior to maintain or restore the system's energetic balance and integrity, e.g. protect a wound or avoid potentially damaging situations. Pain—often quite dramatically—demands our attention, enters consciousness and, thereby, emerges as an experience we access through interoceptive body awareness.

Chapter 16

In response to the question, "Have your condition or symptoms or ability to function changed since receiving care?" replies included:

- "I am far more knowledgeable about my health issues since I am afforded more time, expertise, guidance, and overall sensitivity as compared to most available practitioners within traditional UCMC medical environment. I also am alerted to less invasive and effective approaches outside of the realm of healthcare offerings. [Regarding how I feel about myself or my pain since receiving care:] I feel I am more in control of my health condition since I am more aware of my health issues. I am more proactive, have greater options as a result."

- "I am in less pain and can resume many of my normal activities. In past years I have dealt with the pain as it was just part of what I had to do. I needed additional help and not shots for pain and spine. [Regarding how I feel about myself or my pain since receiving care:] I can function in day-to-day life without as much pain. I have slowly started to add activities back in my life—spin, hiking within moderation. I feel like I am getting my life back."

Developmental Phenomenology of Body Awareness

How pain and body awareness interact and unfold for our patients has been beautifully described by Sally Gadow as a dialectic of self and body (Gadow 1980). In a first level or stage of that dialectic labeled by her "the lived body," the body is taken for granted: we are unaware of it. The philosopher Drew Leder described the body in that first stage simply as "absent" (Leder 1990). We and our patients might live in this state before pain occurs and demands our attention. In a second level labeled "the objective body" by Sally Gadow, the body is experienced as opposed to the self. We are forced to pay attention to the pain in our body. Body and self are in tension with each other or in a state of disunity, the body as the new object of our attention is "symptomatic" and patients experience functional constraints from pain. This state is the situation that brings patients into therapy, either with the medical system or with practitioners who use the approaches described in this book. None of us likes to pay attention to our pain; we experience it as an aversive stimulus that preferably is dealt with through distraction. When we seek to give pain our attention, often by asking another person, a loved one, or a professional to do so, the helping person or a practitioner is tasked to look at our body where it hurts, as we have a hard time focusing our attention on it ourselves. In a third developmental stage, if reached, labeled as "cultivated immediacy" (Gadow 1980), we then may experience a new relationship to the body characterized by acceptance and immediacy. We now accept that the body may have had its good "reasons" to start hurting, for example, when we had ignored our physical limits, believing we can do whatever we want. In a fourth state labeled "the subjective body," the body may be experienced without objectification as a source of learning and meaning. In focus groups we have conducted with practitioners, they described the body experienced in that stage as endowed with "intelligence" and having an "innate tendency towards embodiment" (Mehling et al. 2011). The body then is no longer (a) just the means by which the self carries out its projects, or (b) the source of pain, constraints, and limits to the self's goals, but rather an integral and equal part of the self and the locus of consciousness and subjectivity with its own perspective (Hudak, McKeever, and Wright 2007).

Relevance of Body Awareness for Body Therapy Approaches to Pain Management

Because everyday body awareness—in the way we understand it and defined it above—includes the filters and modifications from our deep beliefs, biases, expectations, and attitudes, it might play an important role in our perception of pain (Cioffi and Holloway 1993; Zeidan et al. 2011). Pain is intimately entwined with emotions (Wade et al. 1990; Cauda et al. 2012), and pain management has much in common with emotion regulation. Attention, how we direct and focus it, plays a key role in both emotion and pain regulation.

A pain patient can focus attention, e.g. on low back pain, in quite different ways: (a) ignore the pain (distraction, endurance; first stage in the developmental model above) (Hasenbring and Verbunt 2010), (b) focus on it with worry and anxiety-driven hypervigilance (fear-avoidance; the second stage) (Vlaeyen and Linton 2012), or (c) focus on it with mindful attention (the third or fourth stage) (McCracken and Keogh 2009). These different styles of attention versus distraction have a major impact on the perceived intensity of chronic pain (see Sidebar 16.2) (Eccleston et al. 1997; Hasenbring 2000; Eccleston and Crombez 2005; Flink et al. 2009; Hasenbring, Hallner, and Rusu 2009; Gard et al. 2011; Johnston, Atlas, and Wager 2012).

Most of the therapeutic approaches discussed in this book have developed outside of medical and behavioral science. When the efficacy or effectiveness of these methods is investigated in research, the mechanisms of action are generally unknown. However, when taking a broader perspective, we argue that the development of body awareness, moving along the stages described above, might be a common denominator of these therapies' mechanism of action for their various benefits (Shusterman 2008; Fogel 2009; Mehling et al. 2011). Indeed, body-based approaches can provide patients with a unique opportunity to learn interoceptive awareness as a tool for pain management.

History of Body Awareness: Applications in Related Modalities

While the majority of body-based approaches claim to enhance body awareness, the explicit focus on body awareness varies greatly (Smith et al. 1999;

Sidebar 16.2 Research

Psychologists studying the effect of mindfulness—mostly in the form of mindfulness-based stress reduction (MBSR)—on emotions and pain found that "one problem in chronic pain is not only the pain itself, but the 'turning away' from, the averting of attention from, the regions that give rise to painful sensations, either through deliberate distraction, or by thinking about the pain (conceptually) rather than experiencing the sensations directly" (Williams 2010). Intriguingly, this psychologist describes two ways of distraction from pain: first, the common mechanisms of the deliberative diversion of attention, for example, by watching a movie or cracking jokes with friends; but second, an often unrealized mechanism of distraction, that of thinking about the pain rather than directly feeling it, a distinction that we will see is of major importance. Recent research findings suggest that focusing on sensory/discriminative aspects of acute experimental pain may be useful pain-regulation strategies when severe pain is expected (Johnston et al. 2012). It implies that directing attention in specific ways towards sensations of pain may be a promising way of coping with chronic pain. Thus, attention regulation appears to be a critical element of interoception for pain management and may determine whether body awareness is beneficial or maladaptive in a given situation. This has been known by healers and clinicians over the ages, including many practitioners of the approaches presented in this book, expressed in Nietzsche's remarks that great pain may be the ultimate teacher (Nietzsche 1882), but medical and behavioral science may still have to catch up.

Mehling 2001; Ernst and Canter 2003; Ives 2003; Daubenmier 2005; Lazar et al. 2005; Mehling, Diblasi, and Hecht 2005; Price 2005; Sherman et al. 2005; Kahn 2007; Holzel et al. 2011). In Feldenkrais and Alexander Technique and Mindful Awareness in Body-oriented Therapy, there is an explicit and active focus on teaching and developing interoceptive awareness as an integral aspect of each therapeutic approach. For practices such as yoga, Tai Chi, Qi Gong, and mindfulness meditation, body awareness is fundamental to the practice, and the degree to which this is explicitly taught and developed varies by teacher and practice style. Approaches in which the patient is more receptive (vs. active) such as in massage, structural work, energy work, and Asian modalities, body awareness is considered important yet is often implicit versus an integral educational focus.

It is important to touch on the role of culture. Many of the approaches in this book originated in the East (e.g. Tai Chi, yoga, acupressure, tui na, shiatsu, Qi Gong), where there was not the Cartesian split between mind and body. As these traditions came to the West, the need to address body awareness for health and healing was more clearly identified (Benson 1985), and was picked up in experiential psychology (Gendlin 2012), mind–body practices to treat medical conditions (Kabat-Zinn 1982), and lead to the development of new body therapy approaches, many of which are highlighted in this book.

As indicated above, the use of focused attention to the body to attend to sensory experience is critical to pain management. Touch, either from a practitioner or self-touch, can be used to increase attention to an area of the body and to increase interoceptive awareness of sensations. For patients in pain, it is much easier for them to focus on their pain when supported by a therapist who can meet them with touch right where it hurts. In massage, patients can gain this awareness if they attend to their bodily sensations in response to the activity of the massage practitioner. More direct guidance from the practitioner aids this process by bringing increased intention and conscious attention to bodily experience. This can require that the practitioner have/ use a psycho-educational approach, particularly if the patient is not able to easily attend to bodily

experience. Difficulty attending to bodily experience is common among patients who have habits of disconnection or dissociation from the body—due to chronic pain, trauma, or other mental health challenges. The dimensions of body awareness that we think are integral from a theoretical/educational perspective are outlined in the next section.

Body Awareness for the Treatment of Pain: Theory and Research
Theoretical Framework
Body awareness can be understood in theory as a construct of multiple dimensions (Mehling et al. 2009):

- *Noticing* body sensations includes bodily sensations that are viewed as negative, positive, and neutral (e.g. from breathing).

- *Emotional reaction and attentional response* to these sensations include: (a) suppressing, ignoring, or avoiding perceptions of sensations such as by distracting oneself; (b) worrying that something is wrong; and (c) present-moment awareness with nonjudgmental awareness of sensations, i.e. a mindful presence.

- *Capacity to regulate attention* pertains to various ways of controlling one's attention as an active regulatory process. These include the ability to (a) sustain awareness, (b) actively direct attention to various parts of the body, (c) narrow or widen the focus of attention, and (d) allow sensations without trying to change them.

- *Mind–body integration* is viewed as the goal of mind–body therapies and includes: (a) emotional awareness, the awareness that certain physical sensations are the sensory aspect of emotions; (b) self-regulation of emotions, sensations, and behavior; and (c) ability to feel a sense of an embodied self, representing a sense of the interconnectedness of mental, emotional, and physical processes as opposed to a disembodied sense of alienation and of being disconnected from one's body.

- *Trusting* body sensations reflects beliefs about the importance of sensations and the extent to which one views awareness of bodily sensations as helpful for decision making or health.

All of these dimensions of body awareness can be useful in pain management. We may better understand how by first starting with a brief overview of well-known key psychological factors for the trajectory of pain, including research on low back pain as an example and then, second, relating the elements of body awareness to the psychology of pain.

- *Depression*, although preferably viewed more as a consequence rather than an antecedent of chronic pain, distress (complaining of physical symptoms associated with depression and anxiety), depressive mood, and somatization are all implicated in the transition from acute to chronic low back pain. Longitudinal studies have yielded somewhat contradictory results, and some researchers postulate that this is because people with chronic pain can be divided into two groups that appear quite different. In one group, pain symptoms are associated with other somatic symptoms and symptoms of depression and anxiety, heightened stress reactivity, and a sense of overwhelm. In the second group, individuals tend to stoically ignore symptoms of discomfort and pain and make a "happy face" in response to stress or pain, thereby appearing quite the opposite of depressed. Persons with this latter endurance coping style have been found to be equally at risk of longer pain duration (Hasenbring 2000).

- *Pain catastrophizing* is conceptualized with three components: magnification or amplification of pain, ruminating thoughts

about pain, and perceived helplessness in the face of pain. It appears to be the strongest and most consistent psychosocial factor associated with persistence of pain and poor function in persons with chronic pain, even after controlling for depression. Catastrophizing is modifiable, and, if addressed in therapy, pain has been shown to improve when catastrophizing decreases.

- *Fear-avoidance* is the behavior of avoiding work, movement, or other activities due to fearful beliefs that they may damage the body or worsen pain. Fear-avoidance is associated with catastrophic misinterpretations of pain, increased escape and avoidance behaviors, and increased pain intensity and functional disability, and increases the risk for developing new-onset back pain, for its chronification, and for its persistence. The value of changing beliefs about pain early in its course has been shown in studies involving patient education in physician and physical therapy offices, and even over the public radio (Buchbinder, Jolly, and Wyatt 2001; Buchbinder 2008).

- *Distraction* is a coping style that generally is favored by many patients, which is most consistently advantageous with *acute* pain. Its opposite, a hypervigilant attention style towards pain, is related to anxiety and clearly maladaptive. In research studies of chronic pain, however, distraction appears to have no consistent proven benefits (Goubert et al. 2004), although music, providing distraction combined with positive affect and relaxation, appears to diminish pain. Whether an attention focus towards pain is beneficial or maladaptive may be mediated by the attention style. An anxiety-driven and hypervigilant attention style is likely maladaptive, while accepting and mindful attention may be beneficial (Mehling et al. 2013). Research on this question is underway.

- *Ignoring* pain is generally considered an adaptive coping style, particularly with the use of cognitive distraction, a focused approach to diverting attention from pain used by cognitive behavioral therapy (CBT). Yet, suppressing the perception of pain to avoid interruptions in daily activities, a more disorganized and nonfocused search for distraction that often fails and causes feelings of emotional distress, is a form of distressed endurance behavior and task persistence that has been shown to lead to chronic pain, possibly via physical overload (Hasenbring and Verbunt 2010). There are, however, studies indicating that the opposite of ignoring and suppression, an in-vivo exposure approach such as acceptance and mindfulness training, may be effective in pain patients (Linton et al. 2008; Flink et al. 2009; Johnston et al. 2012).

- *Recovery expectation* is one of the strongest predictors of chronic pain. Expectation itself is strongly influenced by concerns and worries about pain exacerbations, recurrent pain, financial security, support at work, and self-confidence.

- *Maladaptive body perception*: A 2012 review of current behavioral pain research and treatments showed, that "important contributors to chronic pain may be disturbed processing of the body image, impaired multisensory integration and faulty feedback from interoceptive processes," which has led to new treatment approaches, such as sensory discrimination training, that focus on a restoration of the body image and "the alteration of maladaptive changes in body perception" (Flor 2012).

We can now theorize how various therapeutic approaches discussed above and in previous chapters of this book may aid pain management by modifying these key psychological factors through improving various dimensions of body awareness. A mindful focus on pain with non-judgmental present-moment awareness would diminish ignoring, distraction, and catastrophizing. Differentiating variations in pain intensity and the felt experience helps the patient gain insight into how these variations correlate to activity and movement, and allows for fine-tuning of personal activities and modification of any fear-avoidance beliefs and behavior. If pain is acknowledged as real but impermanent and fluctuating, like every emotion, the pain patient learns that emotion and pain regulation skills can change the intensity or bothersomeness of pain and expectations about the pain duration. The sense of overwhelm and helplessness (catastrophizing) can then improve. If patients learn to listen to their body, if they ultimately learn to trust that the body can be a source of insight rather than merely a mean adversary, then negative emotions (anxiety-fear, depression) and catastrophizing can improve. If present-moment awareness and direct immediate felt experience can be learned, and if the patient can learn to choose between thinking about pain and sensing pain, a tendency for rumination (part of catastrophizing) can be positively influenced. These are some theoretical ways in which body awareness skills might benefit pain management.

Research

Our research group compared a group of primary care patients with current or past low back pain with a group of individuals with professional clinical experience in mind–body therapies on levels of self-reported body awareness using the Multidimensional Assessment of Interoceptive Awareness (MAIA) scales (see Figure 16.1) (Mehling et al. 2013). The therapies were the ones described in this book, e.g. meditation, yoga, and bodywork therapy. We found that "mind–body trained individuals scored significantly higher on all eight scales, suggesting they may be more often aware of body sensations, tend to ignore or distract themselves less often from pain or discomfort, tend to worry less often with sensations of pain and discomfort, are more often able to sustain and control attention to body sensation, are more often aware of the connection between body sensations and emotional states, listen more often to the body for insight, and experience their body more often as safe and trustworthy." The difference was particularly large for the scale assessing distraction habits, which is in line with Gadow's developmental stage model of body awareness and the difference between the second and third stages.

Neuroimaging studies have shown that mindfulness meditators might be able to downregulate painful stimuli by increased sensory processing of the pain sensation itself, rather than by distraction away from it, and by replacing attempts to exert more cognitive control over the pain with a distinct brain state of cognitive disengagement (Gard et al. 2011). This is consistent with the view that "turning away" from pain can be a problematic coping style, particularly with chronic pain, and that body awareness approaches might facilitate direct experience of pain, thereby introducing an advantageous coping style for pain and discomfort (see Sidebar 16.3.).

Clinical Trials

As researchers, we use the MAIA (Mehling et al. 2012) or the **Scale of Body Connection (SBC)** (Price and Thompson 2007) to assess body awareness. The SBC has two scales: body awareness and bodily dissociation. The SBC was developed prior to the MAIA and the majority of the SBC body awareness items have been incorporated into the MAIA. The body dissociation scale is relevant to pain because disconnection or dissociation from the body can

---

Sidebar 16.3 Research

Until now, few research studies have addressed the topic of a mindful attention focus on pain versus distraction as a coping mechanism for pain, and how these two modes of attention might modify the experience of pain. A group of Swedish pain behavior scientists used a technique intended to help people suffering from chronic back pain and low pain acceptance to alter the aversiveness or threat value of their persisting pain. A small pilot study compared a form of "interoceptive exposure" to a relaxation/distraction breathing-based technique, both over 3 weeks, in the presence of their chronic pain (Flink et al. 2009). Additionally, a larger study compared interoceptive exposure to waitlist control (Linton et al. 2008). Both studies showed benefits for function and fear in these chronic pain patients. A few studies have addressed this question with experimentally induced pain. Another group showed that attention to the body reduced pain, partially suppressing the effects of high-pain expectancy, which commonly increases pain and pain-related brain activity, and thereby creates a vicious cycle of psychologically maintained pain (Johnston et al. 2012). An increased body-focus had larger pain-reducing effects when pain expectancy was high, suggesting that a focus on external distractors can be counterproductive. Overall, the results of that study show that focusing on sensory/discriminative aspects of pain might be a useful pain-regulation strategy when severe pain is expected. A Belgian group investigated the effects of distraction from pain during and after a pain-inducing lifting task in patients with chronic low back pain (Goubert et al. 2004). Distraction was associated with more pain immediately after the lifting task. Catastrophizing about pain worsened pain through hypervigilance to pain. A 2012 review of current behavioral pain research and treatments showed that "important contributors to chronic pain may be disturbed processing of the body image, impaired multisensory integration and faulty feedback from interoceptive processes," which has led to new treatment approaches that focus, among other things, on a restoration of the body image and "the alteration of maladaptive changes in body perception" (Flor 2012).

Chapter 16

Scoring instructions Take the average of the terms on each scale

Note: reverse-score items 5, 6, and 7 on Non-distracting, and items 8 and 9 on Not-worrying

1 **Noticing** Awareness of uncomfortable, comfortable, and neutral body sensations
Q1 ☐ + Q2 ☐ + Q3 ☐ + Q4 ☐ / 4 = ☐

2 **Not-distracting** Tendency not to ignore or distract oneself from sensations of pain or discomfort
Q5 (reverse) ☐ + Q6 (reverse) ☐ + Q7 (reverse) ☐ / 3 = ☐

3 **Not-worrying** Tendency not to worry or experience emotional distress with sensations of pain or discomfort
Q8 (reverse) ☐ + Q9 (reverse) ☐ + Q10 ☐ / 3 = ☐

4 **Attention regulation** Ability to sustain and control attention to body sensations
Q11 ☐ + Q12 ☐ + Q13 ☐ + Q14 ☐ + Q15 ☐ + Q16 ☐ + Q17 ☐ / 7 = ☐

5 **Emotional awareness** Awareness of the connection between body sensations and emotional states
Q18 ☐ + Q19 ☐ + Q20 ☐ + Q21 ☐ + Q22 ☐ / 5 = ☐

6 **Self regulation** Ability to regulate distress by attention to body sensations
Q23 ☐ + Q24 ☐ + Q25 ☐ + Q26 ☐ / 4 = ☐

7 **Body listening** Active listening to the body for insight
Q27 ☐ + Q28 ☐ + Q29 ☐ / 3 = ☐

8 **Trusting** Experience of one's body as safe and trustworthy
Q30 ☐ + Q31 ☐ + Q32 ☐ / 3 = ☐

Below you will find a list of statements.
Please indicate how often each statement applies to you generally in daily life

Circle one number on each line

		Never					Always
1	When I am tense I notice where the tension is located in my body	0	1	2	3	4	5
2	I notice when I am uncomfortable in my body	0	1	2	3	4	5
3	I notice where in my body I am comfortable	0	1	2	3	4	5
4	I notice changes in my breathing, such as whether it slows down or speeds up	0	1	2	3	4	5
5	I do not notice (I ignore) physical tension or discomfort until they become more severe	0	1	2	3	4	5
6	I distract myself from sensations of discomfort	0	1	2	3	4	5
7	When I feel pain or discomfort, I try to power through it	0	1	2	3	4	5
8	When I feel physical pain, I become upset	0	1	2	3	4	5
9	I start to worry that something is wrong if I feel any discomfort	0	1	2	3	4	5

Figure 16.1 (Continued)

10	I can notice an unpleasant body sensation without worrying about it	0	1	2	3	4	5
11	I can pay attention to my breath without being distracted by things happening around me	0	1	2	3	4	5
12	I can maintain awareness of my inner bodily sensations even when there is a lot going on around me	0	1	2	3	4	5
13	When I am in conversation with someone, I can pay attention to my posture	0	1	2	3	4	5
14	I can return awareness to my body if I am distracted	0	1	2	3	4	5
15	I can refocus my attention from thinking to sensing my body	0	1	2	3	4	5
16	I can maintain awareness of my whole body even when a part of me is in pain or discomfort	0	1	2	3	4	5
17	I am able to consciously focus on my body as a whole	0	1	2	3	4	5
18	I notice how my body changes when I am angry	0	1	2	3	4	5
19	When something is wrong in my life, I can feel it in my body	0	1	2	3	4	5
20	I notice that my body feels different after a peaceful experience	0	1	2	3	4	5
21	I notice that my breathing becomes free and easy when I feel comfortable	0	1	2	3	4	5
22	I notice how my body changes when I feel happy/joyful	0	1	2	3	4	5
23	When I feel overwhelmed, I can find a calm place inside	0	1	2	3	4	5
24	When I bring awareness to my body, I feel a sense of calm	0	1	2	3	4	5
25	I can use my breath to reduce tension	0	1	2	3	4	5
26	When I am caught up in thoughts, I can calm my mind by focusing on my body/breathing	0	1	2	3	4	5
27	I listen for information from my body about my emotional state	0	1	2	3	4	5
28	When I am upset, I take time to explore how my body feels	0	1	2	3	4	5
29	I listen to my body to inform me about what to do	0	1	2	3	4	5
30	I am at home in my body	0	1	2	3	4	5
31	I feel my body is a safe place	0	1	2	3	4	5
32	I trust my body sensations	0	1	2	3	4	5

Chapter 16

be understood as avoidance/distraction strategies for coping with pain, involving a level of separation from bodily sense-of-self (Price and Thompson 2007). There has been a number of body therapy clinical trials that have used the SBC and have examined pain outcomes (see Sidebar 16.4).

Summary

Based on the research (see sidebars), we can argue: (1) undergoing and learning the methods presented in this book are associated with higher body awareness in those aspects that are captured by self-report with the MAIA, at least cross-sectionally (longitudinal studies of mind–body therapies that used the MAIA (Bornemann et al. 2015)) and with the SBC longitudinally; (2) increases in body awareness through experimental behavior modifications can reduce pain; and (3) mindfulness training appears to reduce pain in association with increased activity in brain areas related to interoceptive awareness and decreased activity in areas related to rumination.

Methodology

Our work is intimately involved in the assessment and treatment of pain using body awareness. As researchers, we use the MAIA or the SBC to assess patient self-reported change in body awareness. As clinicians, we teach body or interoceptive awareness to our patients to help them address their pain. Patients are guided into a relaxed state and learn to maintain attention on the subtle sensations in the body despite constant distracting sensory stimuli from the outside and their untamed, freely associating thoughts. With this mindful attention, an important goal is to learn to distinguish between (a) experiencing the sensations from within the body and (b) thoughts, beliefs, emotions, stories, and reactions about these sensations. A primary goal is to allow and be aware of body sensations as they come into awareness at any given moment without controlling or manipulating them. The advanced mode of awareness is to become non-dual: instead of a mental self as a subject attending to the body as an object, the goal is to learn to be present and "collected" within the body, fully experientially embodied, which is a transition from the stage of disunity between body and mind to become a conscious unity, the spiritual meaning of "yoga." Below is a brief outline of how we address body awareness in practice:

- *Intake Assessment*: At the first session, in addition to an interview to learn the patient's history (injuries, diagnoses, previous treatments, symptoms, and treatment goals), we also ask a series of questions to assess how easily the patient can engage in body awareness activities and self-care. At subsequent visits, we ask about their use of body awareness practices in daily life since the previous session.

- *Treatment Methods*: At the table, we engage the patient in body awareness activities.

- *Patient Education*: If a patient is new to this work or finds body awareness challenging, we educate about the purpose of body awareness and engage in educational strategies to facilitate the ability to access and incrementally increase body awareness.

- *Patient Self-care*: Integral to learning body awareness practices, we encourage the patient to use these practices in daily life for self-care. Building on what the patient learns and on changes that occur during the session, we encourage the practice of simple body awareness exercises during daily life.

- *Monitoring Patient Outcomes and Safety*: We constantly assess the patient's ability to engage in body awareness activities during the session through the patient's use of language, ability to bring mindful attention to the body, and presence in the body which we can monitor through touch. During our sessions we pay close attention to imagery, memories, and emotions our patient may

experience, and the arousal level that may be associated with these in order to gauge the patient's ability to process these without being overwhelmed.

To understand the process involved in body awareness during bodywork practice, several aspects of clinical practice are presented below in further detail:

- *Intake Assessment*: It is important early on to know how easily our patient can engage in body awareness activities and self-care. In the intake, questions related to body awareness are helpful. For example, we might ask the following questions to better understand the patient's awareness of his or her body:

  - How would you describe your pain or the discomfort you feel in your body?

  - Where are you aware of holding tension in your body?

  - What do you do in your daily life to relieve physical discomfort?

  - Are you aware of anything that makes your pain or discomfort increase?

  - Do you feel connected to your body—in other words, do you listen to your body for cues about how you are feeling?

- *Treatment (On the Table)*: To facilitate body awareness in pain patients, we ask the patient to attend to their bodily experience, particularly in areas in which they experience physical discomfort. As we both use touch in our clinical work, we typically place our hands on the patient's body to facilitate patient's ability to focus attention on his or her inner body experience in the symptomatic area. We might begin by asking the patient to describe what she/he feels in the area (or space) of pain. Finding words to describe sensation requires the ability to access the internal experience of discomfort, or the "felt-sense" (Gendlin 2012) of an area within the body. This can take practice and guidance, as it can be difficult to bring awareness inside and to know *how* an area feels. We listen for the use of present-moment descriptive words that identify sensation.

We then guide the patient to attend to inner experience using mindful presence—a nonjudgmental and compassionate attitude of present-moment awareness. We guide the patient in observation of his or her inner body experience—sometimes using breath, and sometimes asking about awareness of various aspects of sensory awareness. For example, in MABT, we ask the patient to attend to interoceptive awareness by: (a) bringing awareness to a specific area within the body, (b) sustaining mindful present-moment awareness in the body, and (c) noticing specific aspects of sensory awareness (sensation, image, emotion, and form). This attention to inner experience involves accessing multiple sensory modes of sensory awareness (visual, kinesthetic, auditory, and emotional). Again, this can take a lot of guidance and practice. However, with successful practice, the capacity to attend with mindful awareness to internal experience expands, and with this can come the ability to notice increasing specificity or depth (sometimes referred to as granularity) of awareness, a sense of the body as a trusted resource, and associations between physical sensation, emotion, memory, and behavior.

- *Patient Education*: It is not uncommon that patients need to understand the concepts behind therapeutic strategies, particularly when they are experienced as challenging and/or include a psycho-educational component. We spend time talking with the patient prior to and after sessions to provide a conceptual framework, to discuss the experiences on the table, and to answer questions the patient may have. In small case series study, this aspect of the work was identified as important for trust and motivation to engage (Price et al. 2011).

Similarly, patients often find this work challenging as they are being asked to be active participants in a therapeutic process and to engage with their pain in a way that is often unfamiliar. Moving toward pain in openness and self-compassion can be a scary endeavor for those who typically avoid sensations to cope with discomfort. We must then facilitate the patient's development of this capacity with tremendous sensitivity, creativity, and patience. Each patient is different, and there are multiple strategies to engage and deepen interoceptive awareness.

- *Patient Self-care*: Interoceptive or body awareness is like anything else: practice helps to develop capacity and integration into daily life. We ask our patients to spend time every day engaged in a body awareness practice. It works best if they choose a process that appeals to them the most—something that they can easily achieve. For example, one person may choose to attend to an area of discomfort by placing a hand on this area and breathing into the area while attending to what she notices internally just before going to bed each night. Another person might choose to stop all activities for a few minutes every hour or two throughout the day and massage or stretch the tissue in an area of discomfort—tuning into the sensation, adjusting posture and activities accordingly.

- *Monitoring Patient Outcomes*: We attend to our patient's ability to access and engage in interoceptive or body awareness to help facilitate this engagement, to guide the therapeutic process, and to monitor change over time. Our work involves a mindful approach in which presence is a key factor. Presence is what allows for awareness of inner body sensation. As practitioners, we can monitor presence in multiple ways including body language, voice quality, word choice/language, energy, and touch.

Practitioner skills are needed to teach and facilitate patient body awareness. With skilful assessment, the practitioner can learn to distinguish the patient's presence from a lack of presence. When a patient is in presence, the practitioner should notice a change of tonus in the bodily tissue. To the practitioner this may feel like increased vitality in the tissue, and is typically accompanied by a shift in the patient's overall demeanor toward a state of deep inner attention. The patient's ability to maintain presence activity is also something that can be "felt" through the practitioner's hands. When the patient "leaves"—(i.e. awareness absences the inner body), this can often be sensed immediately by the practitioner: there is a reduction in the élan vital in the tissue. In addition, the practitioner's ability to maintain presence during the session can enhance patient presence (Blackburn and Price 2007).

Case Study

A 45-year-old single woman named Carol has a 15-year history of chronic pain. She has not been employed for 10 years due to debilitating back pain and is prescribed opiates to manage the pain. She no longer finds the medication to be efficacious and has reduced her opioid use significantly over time. She now uses opioids occasionally and gets by with over-the-counter analgesics on most days. Carol is fairly inactive; she gets around her house to accomplish simple household tasks and will take an occasional walk around the block. When her pain is severe, she stays on the couch and watches TV or reads.

On her first appointment, Carol reports that she has had a couple of massages in her life but is seeking body-oriented therapy on the basis of a friend's referral. She doesn't know what to expect but she is willing to try something new, almost out of a sense of desperation. She is dreaming of having movement back in her life, to have the possibility of travel and more fun times. Carol can't remember an event that explains the onset of her symptoms; rather, increasing spasms in her back over the course of a year to the point that she was unable to continue normal daily activities. She receives disability benefits. Carol also reports a history of depression and has taken anti-depressants for 6 years.

In response to Intake questions, Carol indicates that she took a course on pain management many years ago and that she learned distraction techniques, which she finds useful and continues to practice. She said that she ignores her body when she can, and that she doesn't engage in many body self-care activities. She is, however, able to describe her back pain. She says that it is a constant ache and that she experiences sharp twinges that cause her to double over. She says she never feels relaxed in her body, except for an occasional moment when she first wakes up in the morning and before she moves. I administer the SBC, and her scores are moderate (score of 3 on a 5-point scale) for body awareness and high (score of 4) for bodily dissociation, indicating that, although she has some body awareness, she feels separated from or not very connected to her body.

On the table, I begin with massage to get a sense of where she holds tension, asking her about what she senses as we go along. She is able to describe sensation in some areas and not in others. She holds her body tight and every muscle group feels tense. She is so habitually tense that, at times, she has trouble noticing my touch. When working on her back, I simply hold my hands on the areas that cause her the most pain. After many minutes her breathing relaxes and I notice the smallest hint of give in her tissue. I ask her how she would describe this area and she says, "It is like having two boulders in there." I ask her to bring her attention to the space underneath my hands. Carol concentrates on bringing her attention into the space in her back. When she has connected in a bit, I ask how she would describe the space—would she still say that it feels like two boulders? She slowly replies, "No … actually it feels more dark and thick with spiky things nearby." Carol's response lets me know that she is both visual and kinesthetic in her sensory orientation. She is also able to access interoceptive awareness, even if for just a brief moment at a time.

Carol and I work together for many months; each session, she seems to relax a bit more and to feel/sense a bit more into her body. Her muscles become more pliable. She is increasingly able to follow along with her attention to various parts of her body, and to describe what she feels. In our work on her back she learns to bring her awareness deeply into the areas where she has pain. At first, she can only come to the edges of it; but with time, patience, and persistence, she is able to bring her awareness inside the areas where she experiences the most pain (or perhaps it is more accurate to say that these areas of her back open to her). She develops the capacity to sustain her mindful attention in these areas of her body and to notice sensation within. She practices at home on a regular basis, and more when the pain is severe. She notices that when she brings her attention inside to her back, that the sensations shift and the pain lessens. She begins to have thoughts and memories associated with her childhood come forth, sometimes during her body awareness practice and sometimes at any time during the day. They are uncomfortable memories of her angry father, of being punished, or feeling bad. She begins to paint, to use watercolors: abstract paintings that are dark and intense. She starts psychotherapy and begins to explore her memories, her art, her emotions.

Carol is now engaged in a journey that leads her to a new sense of self. Her back becomes a place in her body that she goes to; a place that helps her to unfold from. She has shifted from relating to her body as dangerous to a place of resource. Her back doesn't always hurt and, although it often aches, it no longer spasms. She can move and begins to explore stretching and dancing on her own. She can take long walks. She does not use opioids at all and only occasionally over-the-counter analgesics. She is thinking about working again. A year after our first session, her body awareness score on the 5-point SBC is increased (from 3 to 4.5) and her bodily dissociation score is reduced (from 4 to 2), indicating a meaningful change that confirms my observations and her reports. Carol has developed a daily body awareness practice that has become second-nature to her. She no longer needs my assistance although she still comes in for the occasional session.

Conclusion

In this chapter we have outlined the positive role of body/interoceptive awareness for pain management. With practitioner guidance, a patient can learn to shift from thinking to sensing, from attention that is directed outwards to attention directed inwards on to subtle body sensations (from **exteroception** to **interoception**). Body-based approaches can play a unique role in teaching body awareness and can facilitate our patient's engagement with dimensions of body awareness that are linked to regulation, self-care, and stages of acceptance and change in relationship to both the experience of pain and the experience of self.

References

Barrett, L. F., K. S. Quigley, E. Bliss-Moreau, and K. R. Aronson. 2004. Interoceptive sensitivity and self-reports of emotional experience. *J Pers Soc Psychol* 87:684–97.

Bechara, A., and N. Naqvi. 2004. Listening to your heart: interoceptive awareness as a gateway to feeling. *Nat Neurosci* 7, 102–3.

Benson, H. 1985. *Beyond the relaxation response*. New York: Berkeley Press.

Blackburn, J., and C. Price. 2007. Implications of presence in manual therapy . *J Bodywork Movement Therapies* 11(1):68–77.

Bornemann, B., B. Herbert, W. E. Mehling, and T. Singer. 2015. Interoceptive awareness and contemplative training. *Frontiers in Psychology* 5(15o4):1–13.

Buchbinder, R. 2008. Self-management education en masse: effectiveness of the back pain: Don't Take It Lying Down mass media campaign. *Med J Aus* 189:S29–32.

Buchbinder, R., D. Jolley, and M. Wyatt. 2001. 2001 Volvo Award Winner in Clinical Studies: Effects of a media campaign on back pain beliefs and its potential influence on management of low back pain in general practice. *Spine (Phila Pa 1976)* 26:2535–42.

Cameron, O. 2001. Interoception: The inside story – a model for psychosomatic processes. *Psychosom Med* 63:697–710.

Cauda, F., D. K. Torta, E. Sacco, F. Geda, F. D'agata, T. Costa, S. Duca, G. Geminiani, G., and M. Amanzio. 2012. Shared "core" areas between the pain and other task-related networks. *PLoS ONE* 7:e41929.

Cioffi, D. 1991. Beyond attentional strategies: cognitive-perceptual model of somatic interpretation. *Psychol Bull* 109:25–41.

Cioffi, D., and J. Holloway. 1993. Delayed costs of suppressed pain. *J Pers Soc Psychol* 64:274–82.

Craig, A. D. 2002. How do you feel? Interoception: the sense of the physiological condition of the body. *Nat Rev Neurosci* 3:655–66.

Craig, A. D. 2003a. A new view of pain as a homeostatic emotion. *Trends Neurosc* 26:303–7.

Craig, A. D. 2003b. Pain mechanisms: labeled lines versus convergence in central processing. *Annu Rev Neurosci* 26:1–30.

Critchley, H. D., S. Wiens, P. Rotshtein, A. Ohman, and R. J. Dolan. 2004. Neural systems supporting interoceptive awareness. *Nat Neurosci* 7:189–95.

Daubenmier, J. 2005. The relationship of yoga, body awareness, and body responsiveness to self-objectification and disordered eating. *Psychology of Women Quarterly* 29:207–19.

Eccleston, C., and G. Crombez. 2005. Attention and pain: merging behavioural and neuroscience investigations. *Pain* 113:7–8.

Eccleston, C., G. Crombez, S. Aldrich, and C. Stannard. 1997. Attention and somatic awareness in chronic pain. *Pain* 72: 209–15.

Ernst, E., and P. H. Canter. 2003. The Alexander technique: a systematic review of controlled clinical trials. *Forsch Komplementarmed Klass Naturheilkd* 10:325–9.

Flink, I. K., M. K. Nicholas, K. Boersma, and S. J. Linton. 2009. Reducing the threat value of chronic pain: A preliminary replicated single-case study of interoceptive exposure versus distraction in six individuals with chronic back pain. *Behav Res Ther* 47:721–8.

Flor, H. 2012. New developments in the understanding and management of persistent pain. *Curr Opin Psychiatry*. 25(2):109–13.

Fogel, A. 2009. *The Psychophysiology of Self-awareness: rediscovering the lost art of body sense.* New York: W. W. Norton.

Gadow, S. 1980. Body and self: a dialectic. *J Med Philos* 5:172–85.

Gard, T., B. K. Holzel, A. T. Sack, H. Hempel, S. W. Lazar, D. Vaitl, and U. Ott. 2011. Pain attenuation through mindfulness is associated with decreased cognitive control and increased sensory processing in the brain. *Cereb Cortex* 22(11):2692–702.

Gendlin, E. T. 2012. *Focusing.* New York: Bantam book. First published 1978.

Goubert, L., G. Crombez, C. Eccleston, and J. Devulder. 2004. Distraction from chronic pain during a pain-inducing activity is associated with greater post-activity pain. *Pain* 110:220–7.

Hasenbring, M. 2000. Attentional control of pain and the process of chronification. *Prog Brain Res* 129, 525–34.

Hasenbring, M. I., and J. A. Verbunt. 2010. Fear-avoidance and endurance-related responses to pain: new models of behavior and their consequences for clinical practice. *Clin J Pain* 26:747–53.

Hasenbring, M. I., D. Hallner, and A. C. Rusu. 2009. Fear-avoidance- and endurance-related responses to pain: development and validation of the Avoidance-Endurance Questionnaire (AEQ). *Eur J Pain* 13:620–8.

Holzel, B. K., S. W. Lazar, T. Gard, Z. Schuman-Oliver, D. R. Yago, and U. Ott. 2011. How does mindfulness meditation work? Proposing mechanisms of action from a conceptual and neural perspective. *Perspectives on Psychological Science* 6:537–59.

Hudak, P. L., P. McKeever, and J. G. Wright. 2007. Unstable embodiments: a phenomenological interpretation of patient satisfaction with treatment outcome. *J Med Humanit* 28:31–44.

Ives, J. C. 2003. Comments on "the Feldenkrais Method: a dynamic approach to changing motor behavior". *Res Q Exerc Sport* 74:116–23; discussion 124–6.

Johnston, N. E., L. Y. Atlas, and T. D. Wager. 2012. Opposing effects of expectancy and somatic focus on pain. *PLoS ONE* 7:e38854.

Kabat-Zinn, J. 1982. An outpatient program in behavioral medicine for chronic pain patients based on the practice of mindfulness meditation: theoretical considerations and preliminary results. *Gen Hosp Psychiatry* 4:33–47.

Kahn, J. 2007. Massage Clients' Perceptions of the Effects of Massage. Publication in preparation: *MTI Foundation and Massage Therapy Research Consortium.*

Lazar, S. W., C. E. Kerr, R. H. Wasserman, J. R. Gray, D. N. Greve, M. T. Treadway, M. McGarvey, B. T. Quinn, J. A. Dusek, H. Benson, S. L. Rauch, C. I. Moore, and B. Fischl.

2005. Meditation experience is associated with increased cortical thickness. *Neuroreport* 16:1893–7.

Leder, D. 1990. *The Absent Body*, 3. Chicago, London: The University of Chicago Press.

Linton, S. J., K. Boersma, M. Jansson, T. Overmeer, K. Lindblom, and J. W. Vlaeyen. 2008. A randomized controlled trial of exposure in vivo for patients with spinal pain reporting fear of work-related activities. *Eur J Pain* 12:722–30.

McCracken, L. M., and E. Keogh. 2009. Acceptance, mindfulness, and values-based action may counteract fear and avoidance of emotions in chronic pain: an analysis of anxiety sensitivity. *J Pain* 10:408–15.

Mehling, W. E. 2001. The experience of breath as a therapeutic intervention – psychosomatic forms of breath therapy. A descriptive study about the actual situation of breath therapy in Germany, its relation to medicine, and its application in patients with back pain. *Forsch Komplementarmed Klass Naturheilkd* 8:359–67.

Mehling, W. E., Z. Diblasi, and F. Hecht. 2005. Bias control in trials of bodywork: a review of methodological issues. *J Altern Complement Med* 11: 333–42.

Mehling, W. E., V. Gopisetty, J. Daubenmier, C. J. Price, F. M. Hecht, and A. Stewart. 2009. Body awareness: construct and self-report measures. *PLoS ONE* 4:e5614.

Mehling, W. E., J. Wrubel, J. J. Daubenmier, C. J. Price, C. E. Kerr, T. Silow, V. Gopisetty, and A. L. Stewart. 2011. Body Awareness: a phenomenological inquiry into the common ground of mind-body therapies. *Philos Ethics Humanit Med* 6:6.

Mehling, W. E., C. Price, J. J. Daubenmier, M. Acree, E. Bartmess, and A. Stewart. 2012. The Multidimensional Assessment of Interoceptive Awareness (MAIA). *PLoS ONE* 7:e48230.

Mehling, W. E., J. Daubenmier, C. J. Price, M. Acree, E. Bartmess, and A. L. Stewart. 2013. Self-reported interoceptive awareness in primary care patients with past or current low back pain. *J Pain Res* 6:403–18.

Naqvi, N., B. Shiv, and A. Bechara. 2006. The role of emotion in decision making. *Current Directions in Psychological Science* 15:260–4.

Nietzsche, F. 1882. The gay science [*die froehliche Wissenschaft*].

Porges, S. W. 1993. *Body Perception Questionnaire*. http:\\www.wam.umd.edu/~sporges/body/body.txt (accessed May, 2007).

Price, C. J. 2005. Body-oriented therapy in recovery from child sexual abuse: an efficacy study. *Altern Ther Health Med* 11:46–57.

Price, C. J. 2007. Dissociation reduction in body therapy during sexual abuse recovery. *Complement Ther Clin Pract* 13:116–28.

Price, C. J., and E. A. Thompson. 2007. Measuring dimensions of body connection: body awareness and bodily dissociation. *J Altern Complement Med* 13:945–53.

Price, C. J., B. Mcbride, L. Hyerle, and D. R. Kivlahan. 2007. Mindful awareness in body-oriented therapy for female veterans with post-traumatic stress disorder taking prescription analgesics for chronic pain: a feasibility study. *Altern Ther Health Med* 13:32–40.

Price, C., K. Krycka, T. Breitenbucher, and N. Brown. 2011. Perceived helpfulness and unfolding processes in body-oriented therapy practice. *Indo-Pacific J Phenomenology* 11:1–15.

Price, C., E. Wells, D. Donovan, and T. Rue. 2012. Mindful awareness in body-oriented therapy as an adjunct to women's substance use disorder treatment: a pilot feasibility study. *J Substance Abuse Treatment* 43:94–107.

Sherman, K. J., D. C. Cherkin, J. Erro, D. L. Miglioretti, and R. A. Deyo. 2005. Comparing yoga, exercise, and a self-care book for chronic low back pain: a randomized, controlled trial. *Ann Intern Med* 143:849–56.

Shusterman, R. 2008. *Body consciousness; a philosophy of mindfulness and somaesthetics*. New York: Cambridge University Press.

Smith, M. C., M. A. Stallings, S. Mariner, and M. Burrall. 1999. Benefits of massage therapy for hospitalized patients: a descriptive and qualitative evaluation. *Altern Ther Health Med* 5:64–71.

Vaitl, D. 1996. Interoception. *Biol Psychol* 42:1–27.

Vlaeyen, J. W., and S. J. Linton. 2012. Fear-avoidance model of chronic musculoskeletal pain: 12 years on. *Pain* 153(6):1144–7.

Wade, J. B., D. D. Price, R. M. Hamer, S. M. Schwartz, and R. P. Hart. 1990. An emotional component analysis of chronic pain. *Pain* 40:303–10.

Wiens, S. 2005. Interoception in emotional experience. *Curr Opin Neurol* 18:442–7.

Williams, J. M. 2010. Mindfulness and psychological process. *Emotion* 10:1–7.

Zeidan, F., K. T. Martucci, R. A. Kraft, N. S. Gordon, J. G. McHaffie, and R. C. Coghill. 2011. Brain mechanisms supporting the modulation of pain by mindfulness meditation. *J Neurosci* 31:5540–8.

Additional Resources

To obtain the complete Multidimensional Assessment of Interoceptive Awareness (MAIA) scale and for permission and copyright, please go to PLoS-ONE 2012, and www.osher.ucsf,edu/maia/

Pathways to integrative clinical care

Introduction

In this culminating chapter of *Integrative Pain Management*, we seek to provide primary **biomedical providers** a framework and guidelines with which to create pathways for patients in pain to access massage, movement, and mindfulness care. In addition, we offer complementary providers ways in which they can support, facilitate, and participate in these care pathways.

The Problem

Pain is an enormous global health problem. Estimates are that 1 in 5 adults suffer from pain and that another 1 in 10 adults are diagnosed with chronic pain each year (Goldberg and McGee 2011). The Institute of Medicine (IOM) reports that people in the USA whose income was below poverty level were more likely to report pain (IOM 2011). The World Health Organization (WHO) has recognized this plight by co-sponsoring the first Global Day Against Pain. "Chronic pain is one of the most underestimated healthcare problems in the world today, causing major consequences for the quality of life of the sufferer and a major burden on the healthcare system in the Western world" (WHO 2004).

Patients in pain

Despite significant developments in pharmacologic, behavioral, and rehabilitative pain treatment (Dubois, 2009), patients with chronic pain are often disappointed with biomedicine (Berman 2003). There is a growing body of evidence that prolonged use of pain medications can worsen pain symptoms and pose substantial risk (Menard et al. 2014; Fulton-Kehoe et al. 2015). Medication as a "sole" treatment "may be inadequate to effectively address persistent pain as a disease process ... comes with significant societal expense and treatment failure, and fails to treat the patient as a whole human being" (Dubois et al. 2009, 987).

Patients, using a method of trial and error, often combine biomedical and complementary treatment without counseling or advice from their primary providers (Launso and Haahr 2007). Accessing **integrative health care** can be complicated, with or without the support of a primary care provider. Complementary approaches to pain are often costly, particularly for lower-income populations with limited or no health insurance coverage, along with geographic challenges in finding qualified providers.

Functional interdisciplinary care teams

Interdisciplinary care is defined in a variety of ways, and implementation is often less than ideal. Interdisciplinary teams may comprise a primary care provider referring out to another primary care provider or to a different discipline within biomedicine. This chapter discusses the problem with this shortsighted, definition-in-practice and offers the reader a more holistic definition of an **interdisciplinary care team** within the context of integrative health care. The current problems include a limited or biased understanding of the complementary care approach, lack of communication between providers, challenges with referring to complementary providers, and an absence of systems for tracking outcomes, gauging success, and without evolving clinical expertise to inform future pain patients.

Communication as a Primary Solution

In this chapter, we propose solutions to the challenges of implementing functional interdisciplinary care: patient-centered communication strategies between biomedical and complementary providers.

While integration is challenging, it is important to maintain perspective: integration is necessary for the welfare of the patient. The move toward integrative health care is patient driven and supported by data. The number of people who are seeking approaches to complement their biomedical care is in the millions (Clarke et al. 2015). Evidence of positive outcomes regarding pain, function, and quality of life is cited in every chapter of this book. It makes good sense to support our patients and advance integration.

Effective communication takes time and energy. Biomedical providers must gain a working understanding of the approaches available in complementary care, and develop functional, interactive relationships with complementary colleagues.

Integrative clinical care pathways

Integrative clinical care pathways are a solution to ineffective pain care. The core of our definition comes from Vanhaecht: "The aim of a care pathway is to enhance the quality of care across the continuum by improving risk-adjusted patient outcomes, promoting patient safety, increasing patient satisfaction, and optimizing the use of resources" (Vanhaecht, De Witte, and Sermeus 2007). We added the terms "integrative" and "clinical" to represent the type of care (complementary) and how it is delivered (human interaction and relationship-oriented, rather than a form of technology or pharmacology).

Integrative pain management: massage, movement, and mindfulness-based approaches

Studies have shown the key to successful integration is provider education (Estrin Dashe 2012). This book aims to educate providers on various approaches to pain care, offering practical information based in clinical experience and available and emerging evidence. Issues with scope of practice are paramount to referring providers—each chapter describes the discipline's approach to pain management, its theoretical underpinnings, and outcome measures. Authors describe the clinical encounter from the initial intake to the application of techniques and self-care homework, and provide case studies to illustrate the patient experience. These components provide the information that

we believe is not only helpful, but instrumental in choosing a complementary approach and supporting the patient through the continuum of care.

The Role of Interdisciplinary Care in Integrative Pain Management

Within the context of integrative pain management, this section defines functional interdisciplinary care, describes current issues—from the team composition to the role of patient-centered care—and begins the conversation of how these might be addressed.

Functional Interdisciplinary Care

According to the National Institutes of Health, pain is the most common reason that people seek integrative health approaches and the most common reason for medical care (Pain Page 2015). This presents an opportunity to reconfigure care pathways and assemble functional interdisciplinary care teams to create successful patient outcomes. We posit that true interdisciplinary care is team-oriented, patient-centered (Drinka and Clark 2000), and has a biopsychosocial framework that includes biomedical, behavioral health, and complementary care (Kamper et al. 2014).

Current practice

Some interpret interdisciplinary care teams to be contained within biomedical care models: integrating allopathic primary care with specialty care. This might include a primary care provider (PCP) referring his pain patient to a surgeon to address the back pain she is experiencing. Other models include behavioral health with biomedical care. An example of this model is a PCP referring a patient to a psychologist to address emotional complications of pain. In the USA, the Affordable Care Act (ACA) provides direction, funding, and implementation support, bringing together biomedicine and behavioral health systems. These integration efforts provide the framework for medical homes, accountable care organizations, and accountable communities of health. This is a landmark, national effort of integrating behavioral health into primary allopathic care. Fortunately, in other sections, the ACA defines and directs complementary care inclusion. For example, section 2706 of the ACA includes nondiscrimination language for the purpose of healthcare coverage. This section states that health insurance companies cannot exclude a healthcare provider that is licensed, certified, or regulated and working within their scope of practice (IHPC 2015). The ACA was implemented January 1, 2014.

A dovetailing of integrative healthcare practices can also be seen today (Giannelli et al. 2007). Biomedical providers sometimes look internally to offer complementary care to their pain patients: nurses can massage, physical therapists prescribe movement, physicians provide meditation guidance, all within their scope of practice. Although this may provide an avenue of access to complementary care, we contend that the best interdisciplinary care practices include providers specifically trained in the complementary approaches they provide. For example, a medical doctor that took a weekend workshop on mindfulness-based stress reduction (MBSR) or a nurse who has 4 to 6 hours of hands-on training in massage may not provide the most effective care. This is especially true for the more complex cases of patients in pain. The better care option would be an MBSR teacher/certified provider and a licensed/certified massage therapy professional, respectively.

Sometimes biomedical providers just don't know enough to make an informed referral. Among physicians in an Italian survey, approximately one-third reported lack of knowledge as a reason for not recommending integrative health practices (Giannelli et al. 2007). When they did recommend these approaches, the most common reason was for pain (Giannelli et al. 2007). Another complication is deficient communication between providers. This is evidenced in a lack of a shared electronic medical record—or one that complementary providers have access to—and if clinical grand rounds or

meetings are called for a patient case review, the complementary providers are often not invited, or are not paid to attend.

Navigating treatment options

Biomedical providers can influence the treatment pathway a patient will take to address their pain and related health concerns. Some complementary providers may also influence care pathways and refer patients to biomedical providers or others within complementary care. This latter scenario is common when patients seek complementary care without the participation of their primary care provider. A massage therapist, for example, may not be getting the results expected, and refer the pain patient to a neurologist or complementary provider with diagnostic scope, such as a naturopath or chiropractor. Complementary professions with diagnostic scope may include naturopathic doctors, chiropractors, osteopaths, and acupuncturists. Biomedical and complementary providers have a responsibility and opportunity to play an active role in navigating treatment approaches for pain management (See Figure 17.1).

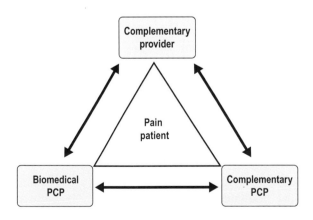

Figure 17.1

Communication and referrals between team members: Communication between all members of the care team should include and support the patient's preferences and needs.

Challenges in referring to complementary care include:

- professional turf:
  - fear of referring out and losing patient
  - scope of practice overlap
- understanding: lack of knowledge about various complementary approaches
- trust: lack of understanding plus no relationships with complementary providers
- time: managing an **interdisciplinary team** may not be financially supported or scheduled
- monitoring progress: responsibility, lack of communication and shared health records.

A fully functional interdisciplinary care team should include both biomedical and complementary providers who both refer within their discipline and out to their interdisciplinary team colleagues.

Individualized Care Team Approach

The specific members of the team should vary depending on the needs of the individual patient. A holistic team includes biomedical, behavioral health, and complementary providers, and also includes social supports such as family or loved ones. For example, an interdisciplinary team supporting a young woman with her first episode of back pain—the only medical issue she faces—may include her PCP, massage therapy provider, yoga teacher, and sister who goes to yoga with her each week. On the other hand, the team supporting a 65-year-old, type II diabetic, severely overweight man with osteoarthritis in one knee might include his PCP, rheumatologist, nutritionist, physical therapist, psychologist to address his depression, massage therapy provider, Tai Chi instructor, and wife for transportation to appointments and supporting his self-care plan.

While few functional interdisciplinary teams—as we define them—currently exist, promising efforts are taking place. The US Veterans Administration (Pain Management Task Force Report 2010) has recently published guidelines for integration, declaring that: "Pain medicine should be managed by integrated care teams which employ a biopsychosocial model of care. The standard of care should have objectives to decrease overreliance on medication driven solutions and create an interdisciplinary approach that encourages collaboration among providers from differing specialties" (Pain Management Task Force Report 2010). Our approach to team care is inclusive, employs a biopsychosocial framework, and should, at the very center, include the patient (see Figure 17.1).

Patient-centered Care

Previous chapters in this book describe approaches to patient-centered care. Explicit in these are a shared, passionate respect for patients as unique human beings. Therapeutic relationships are paramount, and cultivated in massage, movement, and mindfulness disciplines. With sessions averaging 60 minutes, a deep understanding of the individual patient is possible. **Patient-centered care** is a philosophical and moral approach to care (Epstein and Street 2011) and includes: respecting patients' preferences and facilitating positive outcomes; the patient feels understood, heard, involved, and uses the knowledge gained and is empowered and motivated to create and commit to the care plan, including actively engaging in self-care activities. Care is taken to get to know the patients, their thoughts, feelings, needs, wants, and desires and to work within those parameters to facilitate success toward the treatment goals and desired outcomes.

The provider focuses care on optimal health—encompassing the physical, emotional, mental, social, and spiritual aspects of a person—not on illness. Complementary providers often do not assume responsibility for healing, but empower the patient to recognize when their actions affect the outcomes, treatment, and life goals. Awareness is a large part of educating the patient, noticing when something they do increases or ameliorates their pain or dysfunction.

We are in the midst of a paradigm shift in health care; by employing a patient-centered approach in interdisciplinary care, and incorporating shared decision-making (Plastaras et al. 2013), the patient's values, knowledge, culture, and socioeconomic position necessitate consideration.

Integrative Practice Models

Providers trained in one discipline, massage therapy for example, often have solo practices and have established professional careers independent of biomedical environments (Smith, Sullivan, and Baxter 2011; AMTA 2014; Young 2015). Autonomy has its benefits, but does not naturally facilitate participation on a team where the practice model is hierarchical—decisions are, not surprisingly, made by a physician, given the inherent responsibility. Collaboration can be difficult for both complementary providers who work independently in their clinics and biomedical providers in hospital or group practice settings where care is solo rather than interdisciplinary.

Co-located practices are typically integrative health centers, either stand-alone centers or, more often, attached to a biomedical facility or academic medical university. These centers will have both biomedical and complementary care available to pain patients. This shared geography is sometimes considered integrative care (Soklaridis et al. 2009), but can fall short of fully functional care teams. Interestingly, only two of the eighteen *Integrative Pain Management* chapter authors who are still practicing are co-located with biomedical providers. Co-location is not always feasible, isn't always the patient's preference (Smithson et al. 2010) and doesn't inherently enhance communication.

Parallel care exists when biomedical providers refer out to complementary providers. Currently, this is the more common practice model for integrative care. These providers are geographically isolated, and don't typically have operationalized mechanisms for communication, making the team approach difficult. Off-site, parallel practice models are further removed from interprofessional relationships, hallway conversations, or meetings with collegial patient reviews. Further, complementary providers in solo practices may not have access to the full patient medical record or be able to chart complementary treatments in health records alongside primary care providers' notes, making this aspect of communication challenging.

Communication issues are similar regardless of the practice environment. Meetings are difficult on-site or off because of busy schedules. Often, complementary providers are not invited to or paid to attend meetings about patients. All integrative team members should be familiar with the variety of practice models and language subsets and create opportunities for communication, if true integration is to succeed.

Sidebar 17.1 Clinical Experience

I have been a licensed massage therapist in Washington State since 1984. In 1986, I moved my practice above a chiropractic clinic, and began treating patients referred not only from the chiropractors downstairs, but also from psychiatrists, surgeons, physical therapists, and nurses. I sublet space to mental health providers and a provider practicing Asian modalities. Over time, the clinic grew to include seventeen massage therapists, and the clinic's referring provider list expanded. Massage therapists were able to bill patients' insurance directly for on-the-job injuries and motor vehicle collisions since 1988, and because of the Every Category of Provider law (WA State Leg, accessed July 8, 2015), this extended to primary healthcare plans in 1997. It was not until 2011 that I was invited to my first patient consult meeting with a naturopath and an acupuncturist to discuss a complicated patient case, and it was the patient who initiated the meeting.

Access to Integrative Health Care

Accessing health care in general is a challenge for many (Davis and Ballreich 2014) and this issue becomes magnified with integrative health care services. Adequate access to integrative health care can be measured by what is offered and available to the patient and should include utilization, treatment completion, and pain outcomes. This section focuses on the providers' contribution to integrative healthcare access, and mentions the more complicated aspects of access that are beyond the scope of this book.

Components of Access

Access to integrative healthcare services is a complex problem and not merely about services offered. Accessing care requires economic, geographic, and time-of-day access, and cultural and socially acceptable considerations (see Figure 17.2). Although services are available, they may not be accessible to a pain patient who can't afford to pay out-of-pocket for a series of Feldenkrais sessions, for example.

Economic access to care includes insurance coverage (health, workers compensation, labor and industries coverage), the level of coverage, including deductibles, co-pays and co-insurance, and the pain patients' income. These are the primary financial considerations that a provider can integrate into care recommendations and referrals. Secondary economic considerations are the length of treatment or number of sessions, and the costs these create for the patient, along with the cost of work time or wages lost and travel to appointments. Some complementary care disciplines offer group sessions as a less costly option to private provider–patient sessions that are suitable for people in pain, such as yoga, Tai Chi, and Feldenkrais. Another option is to find a provider who has dual training and can bill health insurance for the treatments. A number of our authors and other professionals hold both biomedical and complementary licensure and certifications, and have access to well-established biomedical reimbursement procedures.

Geographic access can pose unique challenges for integrative health practices. Even when integrative care centers or sole providers offer care within a "reasonable" distance to the patient, some may be challenged by public transportation and travel time. Driving to an appointment that is 10 miles away may take 20 minutes in an urban environment. Taking the bus to that same location may take over an hour and require changing buses and walking—making the location inaccessible for the previously mentioned 65-year-old man with osteoarthritis.

Cultural and social considerations are an important component of patient-centered care and to successful access and utilization of health services. These considerations include the gender of the provider and patient, acceptability of the approach by the patient, family and loved ones, along with any potentially conflicting morals or values. For example, a provider refers a Hispanic woman to a male provider for massage therapy. This may be a perfectly acceptable referral. On the other hand, the woman may not feel it is appropriate to be alone with a male provider who is not her relative. The referring provider can be instrumental in successful access and utilization. By incorporating patient-centered care practices and including the patient in a shared decision-making process about her care, the provider can choose a female massage therapy provider to refer the pain patient to. "The availability of services, and barriers to access, have to be considered in the context of the differing perspectives, health needs and material and cultural settings of diverse groups in society" (Gulliford et al. 2002, 186).

Limitations to Accessing Integrative Health Care

There are aspects of access that we cannot cover. They require changes to systems that would provide more widespread health insurance coverage—both private (individual and employer offered) and public—for integrative health services, social supports to facilitate utilization of healthcare service, and culturally acceptable integrative healthcare approaches beneficial to pain patients. Complementary providers are scarce (in comparison to biomedical providers) in some geographic areas. This is a complex challenge that includes professionalization, employability, local cultural climate, government and insurance reimbursement opportunities, and public interest. These are all important aspects that contribute to accessing care, but are, however, beyond the scope and focus of this book.

Provider Role in Access to Care

There are many ways to address barriers to care. Some require patients to share personal information in a trusting relationship with her or his provider, such as divulging financial challenges and cultural considerations. Other solutions require the provider to find, build, and draw from networks of complementary providers that meet the needs of the individual patient. By operationalizing a patient-centered approach to shared decision-making regarding recommendations and referrals

to care, providers can help the pain patient effectively navigate a complex and often barrier-ridden healthcare system.

Communication as a Primary Solution

Solutions for the myriad of problems identified above are not simple, nor can they all be addressed through communication guidelines. However, by improving communication between providers, we begin to deepen provider understanding of massage, movement, and mindfulness-based approaches to pain, strengthen relationships, and contribute to improving the patients' experience with pain care.

Integrative Clinical Care Pathways

Characteristics of care pathways presented by Vanhaecht et al. (2007) include:

- "An explicit statement of the goals and key elements [treatment approaches] of care based on evidence, best practice, and patients' expectations and their characteristics;

- The facilitation of the communication among the team members and with patients and families;

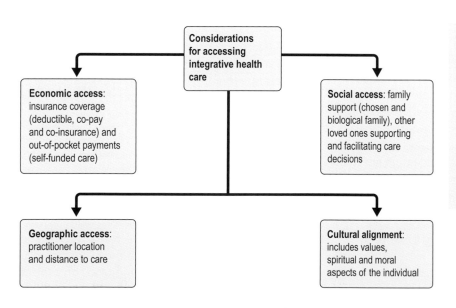

Considerations for accessing integrative health care

Economic access: insurance coverage (deductible, co-pay and co-insurance) and out-of-pocket payments (self-funded care)

Social access: family support (chosen and biological family), other loved ones supporting and facilitating care decisions

Geographic access: practitioner location and distance to care

Cultural alignment: includes values, spiritual and moral aspects of the individual

Figure 17.2
Components of access to integrative health care: Access is not merely about services offered. These four components of access can pose barriers to integrative healthcare utilization and good health outcomes.

- The coordination of the care process by coordinating the roles and sequencing the activities of the multidisciplinary care team, the patients and their relatives;

- The documentation, monitoring, and evaluation of variances and outcomes; and

- The identification of the appropriate resources." (Vanhaecht et al. 2007, 137–8).

Care pathways offer distinct advantages in health care (Shrijvers, van Hoorn, and Huiskes 2012):

- The sooner the integrative care team members can be identified, the sooner treatment can begin. (For example, lymphatic drainage and scar massage are much more effective immediately post mastectomy than a year later, after lymphedema has set in and the scar tissue has matured. That said, we acknowledge that care pathways develop as the patient condition shifts over time.)

- Greater coherence of care and communication between providers increases continuity of care and the opportunity for patient empowerment.

- Clear communication reduces the risk of errors.

There are disadvantages to care pathways—for example, patient choice can be bypassed because providers are busy defining care pathways and managing the team—that, with awareness and vigilance, can be mitigated. Most importantly, patient participation must be protected, and individualized care must be the focus. Providers should not rely on an existing care pathway that worked for one patient in pain without considering the current patient's needs and preferences (Schrijvers et al. 2012).

Building the Interdisciplinary Care Team
"The aim of a care pathway is to improve the quality of care by strengthening shared decision-making, enhancing the organization of care process and

optimizing the use of resources" (Vanhaecht 2007, 138). The task of identifying and managing those resources lies mainly with primary care providers. In an attempt to distribute the responsibility, we are providing communication guidelines for all members of the integrative healthcare team—biomedical and complementary providers, including recommendations for the patient—that address the following:

- Create a framework for collaboration that facilitates clear and effective communication.

- Set treatment goals and outcome measures.

- Identify the approach(es) that best meet the treatment goals, and the patient's biopsychosocial needs.

- Select the complementary care provider(s) who best meet the treatment goals, and address the patient's biopsychosocial needs.

- Modify expectations for the team collaboratively—treatment goals and outcome measures.

- Monitor and evaluate outcomes, individually and comparatively.

Guidelines for communication
Multiple perspectives in health care offer the benefit of diverse knowledge and experience and require high-quality teamwork (Mitchell et al. 2012). Before the complementary approach(es) has been identified and a provider selected, identify guidelines for communication to ensure effective collaboration.

Collaboration depends on shared goals, clear roles, mutual trust, and measureable processes and outcomes (Mitchell et al. 2012). Clear, consistent, professional communication is the key, and requires honesty, discipline, creativity, humility, and curiosity (Launso and Haahr 2007). This requires time and commitment to the team relationship; one must become familiar with the variety of complementary approaches and language subsets and create opportunities for discussion.

Communication issues are similar regardless of the practice environment, but strategies may vary. With an emphasis on collaboration, there are a few guidelines to consider prior to building the inter-disciplinary team.

Communication guidelines for PCPs in integrative healthcare practices

- Think as a team member, avoid unilateral decision-making when possible, identify and put aside personal interests and prejudices.

- Demonstrate an openness and willingness to learn from others, cooperate, and embrace other approaches and theoretical constructs.

- Be vulnerable, humble, curious, and aware of your own strengths and weaknesses.

- Actively listen and ask clarifying questions.

- Reflect on your contributions to the team and consider how you might improve communications.

Networking guidelines for complementary providers

Massage, movement, and mindfulness (MMM) practices are full of patients in pain who found their way to complementary care without the support of bio-medical providers. Without a functional relationship with referring providers, complementary providers have become competent in working independently. With the demand for integrative health care and the exciting opportunity of working collaboratively, MMM providers need to be equipped to articulate their skills. Expect to provide this information to providers—and patients—when a complementary approach is added to the care plan. Proactively, use this information to seek out relationships with pain specialists and build your own network of providers. This will prepare you for joining an interdisciplinary team. Consider the following:

- scope of practice: what does a session entail, what are your theoretical underpinnings that inform treatment planning and clinical reasoning, how do you measure progress (this is important for collaborative treatment goal setting)?

- affiliations, including code of ethics, conduct, standards of practice

- professional experience (depth and breadth) and specific education in area of specialty, such as pain management, post-surgical work, or hospice care

- communication practices, documentation, report writing

- research, available literature supporting techniques, clinical effectiveness

- fees, availability for third party reimbursement

Guidelines for identifying massage, movement, and mindfulness approaches to pain management

Many people seek information from sources such as family, friends, and the media about pain care options, or in general about integrative health practices (Ock 2009). It is sensible for healthcare providers to become an informed resource. Providers who are perceived to be poorly informed or share negative feelings about complementary approaches induce patient anxiety and safety concerns, and may compromise the therapeutic relationship (Smithson et al. 2010). In contrast, open discussions and advice about complementary services are highly valued by patients (Smithson et al. 2010). Similar to the model of shared decision-making in chronic conditions provided by Gionfriddo and colleagues (2013), we suggest a process by which the primary care provider can be a source of information and facilitate a discussion on available care options to draw in the patient's engagement. This discussion should include: descriptions of the approaches, the evidence supporting their use (including research and clinical experience) and the PCP's evidence-informed clinical opinion, detailing which integrative health approaches might work well for the patient (Sherman 2005).

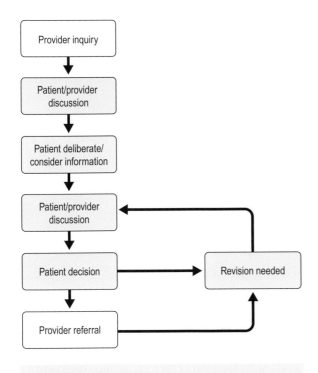

Figure 17.3
Provider/patient-facilitated discussion model:
Suggested communication for patient-centered,
shared decision-making.

Just as biomedical providers often work with patients to titrate a medication to the unique expression of a patient's biochemistry, attention and consideration should be applied when recommending an integrative health approach to a patient in pain. The approach should be available, accessible, and comfortable to the patient and their loved ones. This consideration spans geographic, economic, cultural, and social factors specific to the individual patient. In the USA, 83% of massage therapy providers are women (Young 2015); there may be cultural or religious barriers to being touched by a woman. Once the sociocultural and economic factors are understood, the provider can clarify preferences, and begin to build the interdisciplinary team.

Take into account the patient's current self-care strategies when selecting complementary approaches. Is the patient already effectively implementing daily self-care? Would a movement approach to care complement their treatment goals? Inquire if the patient would prefer active movement in a classroom setting or individual sessions of passive/interactive movement with an emphasis on developing kinesthetic awareness. Is stress all-consuming, interfering with the patient's ability to make healthy choices? Discuss if a massage is best to intercept the sympathetic overstimulation and create a parasympathetic experience, or if a home meditation practice would be easier to schedule.

Topics for discussing complementary approaches with your patient:

- access: economic, geographic, social and cultural considerations

- severity of condition: ready and able to move or needs more support or kinesthetic awareness before incorporating a movement practice

- motivation: eager to move, or fearful and unsure of balance

- commitment: willing to attend a series of weekly appointments or classes, incorporate daily self-care practice

- setting: classes, one-on-one sessions, co-located in biomedical practice or off-site

- systems: musculoskeletal, lymphatic, mind–body, structural, movement, strength, or multiple systems affected and possibly needs multiple approaches, or a provider trained in multiple modalities

Merge what you glean from the patient discussion with your clinical expertise to illuminate a care pathway and build a team that satisfies the therapeutic needs, treatment goals and personal preferences of the patient (see Figure 17.3).

Guidelines for choosing massage, movement, and mindfulness providers

The interdisciplinary team approach should encompass more than treating just illness or pain. Include team members who can improve patient sleep, increase function, alleviate stress, and improve self-image (Butts 2001; Dunigan, King, and Morse 2011). Providers should also promote self-management of pain (IOM 2011). Include team members who educate and empower patients to incorporate daily self-care tools such as discovering ways to move or positions to alleviate or manage pain, and self-massage to address the ongoing musculoskeletal pain or swelling.

Patients may have a preference regarding the location of the provider. Geography is only one issue of access, and relates to both availability of care for the patient and ease of collaboration between providers. Patients are split on their preference for co-located or parallel care models (Smithson et al. 2010). A blend of these offerings may provide greater patient choice, addressing healing environment preferences, transportation issues, and safety concerns.

Variation in professionalization puts a burden on the referring provider, and makes integration efforts challenging. As with most professions, education and regulation vary widely internationally. The complementary approaches in this book—massage, movement, and mindfulness—are no different. In Europe, for example, Germany, Austria, Finland, Hungary, Italy, and the UK provide certification or licensure for massage therapy at the medical level (De Leonardo 2012). Forty-five states in the USA, the District of Columbia, and five Canadian provinces have passed laws to regulate the massage profession—usually through licensure, certification, or registration (see Figure 17.4) (Massage Magazine 2015).

Where governmental regulations are absent, organizational structure steps in. For example, Trager, Feldenkrais, yoga, and structural integration all have strict education and advanced training requirements to maintain certification or membership. Massage therapy in Australia is not regulated through the government but has many requirements necessary for recognition by biomedical providers: diploma of remedial massage, registered with a recognized association, current first aid and indemnity insurance coverage, and therapists are held to a code of practice by the Association and Healthcare Complaints Commission.

Diversity in terminology and application of approaches exists. A patient's experience of massage therapy can vary widely, given the vast array of modalities massage therapists specialize in. Similarly, yoga can be taught as a form of stretching, a vigorous workout, therapeutic in nature, focused on rehabilitation or can be a spiritual practice. Any of the practices included in this book can be valuable contributions to general health, both physical and mental, and can be used to treat specific pain conditions.

Both the referring provider and the patient can interview prospective complementary providers to ensure the best match for the patient.

Guidelines for identifying qualified complementary care providers:

- regulation: licensed/registered/certified, and have no complaints filed

- affiliations: member of a professional association, abiding by codes of ethics and standards of practice, maintaining educational standards

- experience: years in the profession/and experience with pain

- documentation: routinely documents patient encounters/writes progress reports, and literate in biomedical terminology

- communication: agrees to share progress reports with team, and meet for patient case review (timeline determined by team)

- research: familiar with the literature and incorporates the evidence when applicable

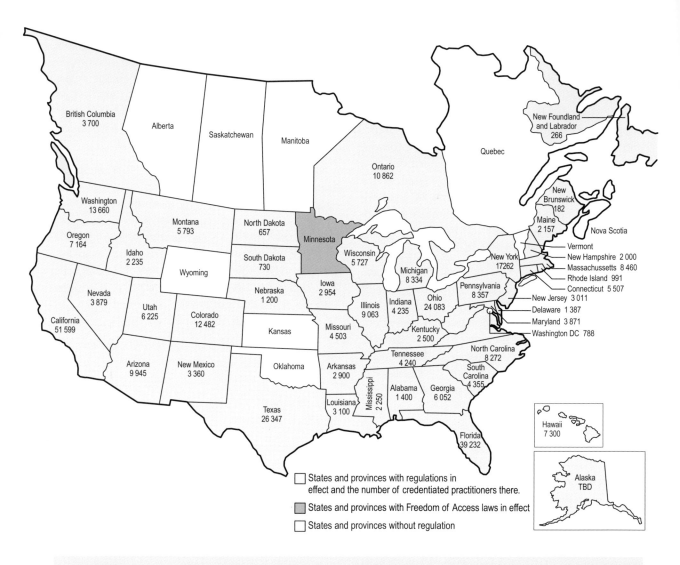

Figure 17.4

US states and Canadian provinces with massage licensure.

(Reprinted with permission *Massage Magazine*. Webpage accessed August 2, 2015.)

- insurance coverage: credentialed/accept third-party reimbursement or federally funded payment, where available and if necessary for patient access

Guidelines for team communication

The next step in creating a care pathway is to facilitate communication among team members, and with patients and loved ones.

	✓	Notes
Licensed/certified/regulated		
Professional affiliation		
Standards of practice		
Codes of ethics		
Professional experience with patients in pain		
Communication		
Familiar with biomedical language		
Willing to participate in meetings		
Documents patient encounters		
Writes progress reports		
Research literate		
Third party reimbursement provider*		

*May not be applicable

Table 17.1
Simplified checklist for choosing a complementary provider.

Interdisciplinary communication strategies

- Strive for familiarity with the language and paradigms of complementary disciplines.

- Engage team members in developing care pathways/setting treatment goals. MMM goals are often based in activities of daily living, contributing meaningful, quantifiable functional progress.

- Create opportunities to discuss clinical observations and patient experiences that aren't likely to become part of the medical record. Many MMM providers spend 30–90 minutes a session with patients, prompting deep, personal discussions.

- Include complementary providers in team meetings. Keep in mind they might not be paid for attendance, but are likely to cultivate the relationship and value inclusion.

- Schedule meetings when adding a new team member, discuss next steps, or celebrate successes of a complicated patient case.

- Facilitate access to electronic health records and the ability for complementary care to be documented within biomedical notes. Parallel care teams may not currently have access, but strive for one patient medical record as technology opportunities surface. In the meantime, communicate via progress reports.

- State communication preferences: phone, text, email, fax, etc., and respond when team members reach out. These may vary based on co-located or parallel care models.

Clarify expectations of the team

- State goals for care specific to each provider. It would be better to ask for goals from provider, and be willing to collaboratively modify if the team is not aligned.

- Identify preferred outcomes to measure, based on goals specific to the approach and provider's area of expertise (sleep measure, pain scales, functional goals, etc.).

- Request progress reports and share with other team members.

- Support the complementary provider's recommendations for patient self-care. Check in with patient regarding compliance and satisfaction.

- Request support for care plans. Know that MMM providers can easily incorporate support for your care plan, given the nature of the therapeutic relationship and the time and frequency of sessions (Hawk, Ndetan, and Evans 2012).

MMM communication guidelines for interdisciplinary care team

All of the communication strategies above apply to complementary team members. However, without diagnostic scope, and dependent upon referrals from PCPs, complementary providers are often expected to conform to the biomedical paradigm and learn the language of the primary discipline. Most complementary providers are eager to bridge the gap and to take the necessary steps to ensure a collaborative process.

Create opportunities for communication

- Maintain patient health records and chart treatment notes for every patient encounter, according to regulations or best practices. If available, document treatment sessions in electronic health records alongside the biomedical providers' notes.

- Write progress reports regularly, and with patient permission share reports with the healthcare team.

- Become familiar with biomedical language and abbreviations; avoid jargon when describing your own practice.

- Attend team meetings (when not cost prohibitive).

- Participate in developing care pathways/setting treatment goals.

- Share verifiable observations, avoiding personal opinions. You may know more about the patient's needs and desires than a PCP does, given the length and intimacy of the provider/patient relationship. Respect confidentiality. Avoid triangulating.

- State preferred communication pathways: phone, text, email, fax, etc., and return messages when team members reach out. These may vary based on co-located or parallel care models.

Consider ways of improving patient access to care

- Develop community or group classes when applicable.

- Emphasize self-care.

- Teach loved ones to provide care or maintain treatment effects between sessions.

Follow through on expectations

- Discuss and develop treatment goals, and be willing to modify collaboratively if not aligned with the team and the patient.

- Identify outcomes (sleep, pain, function, etc.) to measure, based on goals.

- Send progress reports within the agreed or expected timeframes.

- Incorporate and monitor patient self-care.

- Support the care plans of other team members. The literature suggests complementary providers are uniquely positioned to support the care plans of biomedical providers (Hawk et al. 2012).

Emerging Opportunities from Monitoring Outcomes

Much of clinical reasoning is rooted not only in scientific information, but also in clinical experience. The role of a healthcare provider, whether complementary or biomedical, doesn't end at the referral. Unique patient encounters build clinical expertise and inform future cases for care and referrals. Ongoing communication between biomedical and complementary providers—tracking outcomes and discussing patient experiences—not only helps build clinical expertise, but will also inform successful integration of complementary approaches into mainstream health care. This is an extraordinary time in health care, with many opportunities for improving the lives of patients who suffer from pain and could benefit from individualized integrative approaches to pain management.

Conclusion

The current healthcare climate is ripe with opportunity for biomedical and complementary providers to come together and take a central role in addressing the epidemic of pain. Patients are demanding access, biomedical providers are listening, insurance companies are starting to cover services, and complementary approaches are becoming more evidence-based. In this transitional time, both biomedical and complementary providers have a responsibility to improve communication and make the full scope of services available to pain patients. Once good communication—between providers, within interdisciplinary care teams and systematized into health care—is operationalized, pain patients will reap the benefits of continuity of care, assurance of safety and effectiveness, and receive the much needed support to navigate the vast range of services available that address the unique aspects of the patient's biopsychosocial needs.

This book describes the current climate of integrative health care, provides an understanding of pain anatomy and insightful theoretical perspectives on pain, and gives in-depth, evidence-informed descriptions of common approaches to managing pain: massage, movement, and mindfulness (Clarke et al. 2015). This final chapter provides the reader with guidelines for building effective interdisciplinary teams, incorporating research and clinical expertise to inform care recommendations, and much needed strategies to improve communication. *Integrative Pain Management* provides the tools necessary to integrate massage, movement, and mindfulness approaches into healthcare practice and enable patients to access effective pain care.

References

AMTA. 2014. Industry fact sheet. https://www.amtamassage.org/infocenter/economic_industry-fact-sheet.html (accessed July 31, 2015). https://www.amtamassage.org/career_guidance/detail/220?typeId=2 (accessed July 31, 2015).

Berman, B.M. 2003. Integrative approaches to pain management: how to get the best of both worlds. *BMJ*. 14; 326(7402):1320–1.

Butts, J. B. 2001. Outcomes of comfort touch in institutionalized elderly female residents. *Geriatr Nurs* Jul–Aug; 22(4):180–4.

Clarke, T. C., L. I. Black, B. J. Stussman, P. M. Barnes, and R. L. Nahin. 2015. Trends in the use of complementary health approaches among adults: United States, 2002–2012. *National Health Statistics Reports*; no 79. Hyattsville, MD: National Center for Health Statistics.

Davis, K., and J. Ballreich. 2014. Equitable access to care — how the United States ranks internationally. *New England Journal of Medicine* 371; 17.1567–70.

De Leonardo. 2012. *ECTS, ECVET, NQF and Massage Professions in Europe: State of the Art Report*. http://bbwkg.de/wp-content/uploads/2013/02/State-of-the-Art-Report-NQF-ECVET-ECTS-and-massage-professions-in-Europe.pdf (accessed July 31, 2015).

Drinka, T. J. K., and P. G. Clark. 2000. *Healthcare teamwork: Interdisciplinary practice and teaching*. Westport, CT: Auburn House.

Dubois, M. Y., R. M. Gallagher, and P. M. Lippe. 2009. Pain medicine position paper, The American Academy of Pain Medicine. *Pain Medicine* 10:6, doi: 10.1111/j1526-4637.2009.00696.x

Dunigan, B. J., T. K. King, and B. J. Morse. 2011. A preliminary examination of the effect of massage on state body image. *Body Image* Sep; 8(4):411–4. doi: 10.1016/j.bodyim.2011.06.004. Epub Jul 20, 2011.

Epstein, R. M. and R. L. Street Jr. 2011. The values and value of patient-centered care. *Ann Fam Me*. Mar–Apr; 9(2):100–3. doi: 10.1370/afm.1239.

Estrin Dashe, A. A. 2012. Integrating massage, chiropractic, and acupuncture in university clinics: a guided student observation. *Int J Ther Massage Bodywork* 5(2):3–8. Epub Jun 30, 2012.

Fulton-Kehoe, D, M. D. Sullivan, J. A. Turner, R. K. Garg, A. M. Bauer, T. M. Wickizer, and G. M. Franklin. 2015. Opioid poisonings in Washington State Medicaid. *Medical Care* 53(8):679. doi: 10.1097/MLR.0000000000000384.

Giannelli, M., M. Cuttini, M. Da Frè, and E. Buiatti. 2007. General practitioners' knowledge and practice of complementary/ alternative medicine and its relationship with life-styles: a population-based survey in Italy. *BMC Family Practice* 8:30. doi: 10.1186/1471-2296-8-30.

Gionfriddo, M. R., A. L. Leppin, J. P. Brito, A. LeBlanc, N. D. Shah, and V. M. Montori. 2013. Shared decision-making and comparative effectiveness research for patients with chronic conditions: an urgent synergy for better health. *Journal of Comparative Effectiveness Research* 2(6):595–603. doi:10.2217/cer.13.69.

Goldberg, D. S. and S. J. McGee. 2011. Pain as a global public health priority. *BMC PublicHealth* 11:770. doi: 10.1186/1471-2458-11-770 http://www.biomedcentral.com/1471-2458/11/770 (accessed July 6, 2015).

Gulliford, M., J. Figueroa-Munoz, M. Morgan, D. Hughes, B. Gibson, R. Beech, and M. Hudson. 2002. What does 'access to healthcare' mean? *J Health Serv Res Policy* Jul; 7(3):186–8.

Hawk, C., H. Ndetan, and M. W. Evans Jr. 2012. Potential role of complementary and alternative healthcare providers in chronic disease prevention and health promotion: an analysis of National Health Interview Survey data. *Prev Med* Jan; 54(1):18–22. doi: 10.1016/j.ypmed.2011.07.002. Epub Jul 13, 2011.

Integrative Healthcare Policy Consortium (IHPC). 2015. http://www.ihpc.org/section-2706/ (accessed August 3, 2015).

Institute of Medicine (IOM). 2011. *Relieving pain in America: A blueprint for transforming prevention, care, education, and research*. Washington, DC: The National Academies Press.

Kamper, S.J., A. T. Apeldoorn, A. Chiarotto, R. J. Smeets, R. W. Ostelo, J. Guzman, and M. W. van Tulder. 2014. Multidisciplinary biopsychosocial rehabilitation for chronic low back pain. Cochrane Database Syst Rev. Sept 2; 9:CD000963. doi: 10.1002/114651858.CD000963.pub3.

Launso, L., and N. Haahr. 2007. Bridge Building and Integrative Treatment of People with Multiple Sclerosis. Research-based Evaluation of a Team-building Process. *Journal of Complementary and Integrative Medicine* 4:1, Article 7.

Massage Magazine. 2015. Laws and Legislation. http://www.massagemag.com/laws/ (accessed July 31, 2015).

Menard, M., A. Nielsen, H. Tick, W. Meeker, K. Wilson, and J. Weeks. 2014. Policy brief never only opiods: the imperative for early integration of non-pharmacological approaches and practitioners in the treatment of patients with pain. *Pains Project Transforming the Way Pain is Perceived, Judged and Treated* Fall: Issue 5.

Mitchell, P. H., M. K. Wynia, R. Golden, B. McNellis, S. Okun, C. E. Webb, V. Rohrbach, and I. Von Kohorn. 2012. *Core principles & values of effective team-based healthcare*. Discussion Paper, Institute of Medicine, Washington, DC. www.iom.edu/tbc. Pain Page. National Institutes of Health. National Center for Complementary and Integrative Health. https://nccih.nih.gov/health/pain (accessed July 31, 2015).

Ock, S. M., J. Y. Choi, Y. S. Cha, J. Lee, M. S. Chun, C. H. Huh, and S. J. Lee. 2009. The use of complementary and alternative medicine in a general population in South Korea: Results from a National Survey in 2006. *Journal of Korean Medical Science* 24(1): 1–6. doi: 10.3346/jkms.2009.24.1.1.

Pain Management Taskforce. Veterans Administration. 2015. http://www.regenesisbio.com/pdfs/journal/Pain_Management_Task_Force_Report.pdf (accessed June 29, 2015).

Pain Page. 2015. National Institutes of Health. National Center for Complementary and Integrative Health. https://nccih.nih.gov/health/pain (accessed July 2, 2015).

Plastaras, C., S. Schran, N. Kim, D. Darr, and M. S. Chen. 2013. Manipulative therapy (Feldenkrais, massage, chiropractic manipulation) for neck pain. *Curr Rheumotl Rep* Jul; 15(7): 339. doi: 10.1007/s11926-013-0339-x. file:///C:/Users/Marissa/Downloads/Manipulative%20Therapy%20for%20Neck%20Pain.pdf (accessed July 8, 2015).

Schrijvers, G., A. van Hoorn, and N. Huiskes. 2012. The care pathway: concepts and theories: an introduction. *International Journal of Integrated Care* 18 September2-ISSN1568-4156URN: NBN:NL:U:I10-1-113788 Vol. 12, SpecialEditionIntegratedCarePathways.

Sherman, K. J., D. C. Cherkin, J. Erro, D. L. Miglioretti, and R. A. Deyo. 2005. Comparing yoga, exercise, and a self-care book for chronic low back pain: a randomized, controlled trial. *Ann Intern Med* 143: 849–56. doi:10.7326/0003-4819-143-12-200512200-00003.

Smith, J. M., S. J. Sullivan, and G. D. Baxter. 2011. A descriptive study of the practice patterns of massage New Zealand massage **therapists.** *Int J Ther Massage Bodywork* Mar 30; 4(1):18–27.

Smithson, J., C. Paterson, N. Britten, M. Evans, and G. Lewith. 2010. Cancer patients' experiences of using complementary therapies: polarization and integration. *Journal of Health Services Research & Policy* 15(Suppl 2):54–61.

Soklaridis, S., M. Kelner, R. L. Love, and J. D. Cassidy. 2009. Integrative healthcare in a hospital setting: Communication patterns between CAM and biomedical practitioners. *Journal of Interprofessional Care* November; 23(6):655–667.

Vanhaecht, K., K. De Witte, and W. Sermeus. 2007. *The impact of clinical pathways on the organisation of care processes.* PhD dissertation, Belgium: KU Leuven.

World Health Organization (WHO). 2004. Media release. http://www.who.int/mediacentre/news/releases/2004/pr70/en/ (accessed 7/6/15).

Young. L. 2015. re: Data from ABMP membership and Corona survey of massage therapists. email to ABMP VP leslie@abmp.com, July 31 (accessed July 31, 2015).

Additional Resources

National Institutes of Health Pain Consortium: http://painconsortium.nih.gov/index.html

INDEX

Note: Page references in *italics* refer to Figures

3B Scientific Kinesiology Tape   129

A

A-beta fibres   130
A-delta fibre   20, 130
A-delta nociceptors   20
Academic Consortium for
    Complementary and Alternative
    Health Care (ACCAHC)   6, 7
access to integrative health care   254
    components   254, *255*
    limitations to   254–255
    provider role in   255
accommodation   3–4
acetaminophen   18
activities of daily living (ADLs)   86, 122
acupressure   11, 55, 145, 148, 236
Acupressure Taping   129
acupuncture   4, 11, 82, 116, 145, 148,
    150, 153, and 154
adhesions/fixations   82–83, 84, 87
    formation, postoperative   79
adhesive capsulitis   86
afferent discharge   24
Affordable Care Act (ACA)   250–251
alcoholic polyneuropathy   24
Alexander Technique   235
allodynia   25, *26*
American Board of Integrative
    Medicine   7
American Board of Medical
    Specialties   7
amygdala   28
A Mo   147
anandamide   18
Anat Baniel Method®   162
Anatomy Trains   99, 182
ankle sprain   99–100
anterior cingulate cortex (ACC)   51
antidepressants   18
anti-inflammatories   18
Applied Kinesiology Challenge/Therapy
    Localization Test   132
Aristotle   34, 35, 36, 191
arthritis   103
asana   195–197, *196*
assimilation   4
Aston-Patterning   97
athletic taping   127–128
attention regulation   236
attentional response   236
avoidance/distraction strategies   242

Awareness Through Movement®
    159–160, 170
axillary web syndrome (AWS)   86
axon   17, 18, 19–20, 22–23
Ayurvedic constitution   193

B

back pain, low   40
beliefs   40
Bi syndrome   154
biceps tendonitis   103
biomechanical model   114
biomedical providers   249–253, 255,
    257, 258
biopsychosocial model   2, 39–40
    clinical reasoning and   40–43
biotensegrity   127
blood-letting   35, 36
body awareness   233–246
    capacity to regulate attention   236
    case study   245–246
    clinical trials   239–240
    depression   237
    developmental phenomenology
        of   234
    distraction   237–238
    emotional reaction and attentional
        response   236
    fear-avoidance   237
    history of   235–236
    ignoring pain   238
    maladaptive body perception   238
    methodology   242–245
    mind-body integration   236–237
    neurophysiology of pain and
        233–234
    noticing   236
    pain catastrophizing   237, 238
    recovery expectation   238
    relevance for body therapy approaches
        to pain management   234–235
    research   238–239
    theoretical framework   236–237
    treatment of pain   236–239
    trusting   237
body modifications   33, 34
body-self neuromatrix   38, 190
Bones For Life®   162
bone-setting therapy   145
brachial plexopathy   86
bradykinin   20
breast cancer surgery   84, 85–86

breathing exercises   58
Brief Pain Inventory   192
Buchanan, Patricia   167–168
Buddhism   220
burns   16
bursitis   103

C

C-fibers   19–20, *20*, 130
calcitonin gene-related peptide
    (CGRP)   20
cancer, massage therapy in   85–86
cancer-related fatigue   53
cannabinoid   18
carpal tunnel syndrome   24
Cartesian model of pain   36
case formulation approach   41, 42
catecholamines   28
causalgia   26
central control system   38
central sensitization (CS)   24–25
cervical plexopathy   86
cesarean section scar   79
Chartered Society of Massage and
    Gymnastics   49
Chartered Society of
    Physiotherapists   49
chemoreceptors   101
chemotherapy   24, 85
chickenpox   25
Child'Space® Chava Shelhav
    Method   162
children, pain, Qi and meridian
    systems in   150
Chinese herbal medicine   150
chronic fatigue   221
chronic low back pain (cLBP)   10
chronic pelvic pain syndrome   27
chronic regional pain syndrome
    (CRPS)   26
cicatricial scar   82
C-nociceptors   30
codeine   18
cognitive behavioral therapy (CBT)   10,
    220, 238
common compensatory pattern
    (CCP)   118
communication   249–250, *251*, 253,
    255, 256–257, 260–261
    follow through on expectation   262
    MMM guidelines for interdisciplinary
        care team   261–262

communication (*Continued*)
  networking for complementary
    providers   257
  opportunities   262
  patient access   262
  PCPs   257
  team expectations   261
compassion meditation (CM)   221
complementary and alternative medicine
    (CAM)   2, 3–5
  expenditure on   3
complex regional pain syndrome   24
conditioned learning   40
Consortium of Academic Health
    Centers for Integrative Medicine
    (CAHCIM)   6–7
contracture   82
conventional medicine   1
cortisol   51, 80
counter strain (CS)   112
Cozen's test for lateral epicondylitis   151
craniosacral therapy (CST)   122
cutaneous pain   22

D

Da Tui Na   151
decompression somatics   182
deep pain   22
deep tissue   97, 105
deep tissue massage (DTM)   50
deep vein thrombosis   87
degenerative disc disease   23
degloving injury   79
depression   84–5, 237
Dercum's disease   78
dermatomes   25, 95
Descartes, Rene   27, 36
developmental stage model of body
    awareness   239
dharana   198
dhyana   198
diabetic neuropathy   24
distraction   237–238
dopamine   80
dorsal root ganglion (DRG)   23
dukkha   189
dynamic systems theory   163

E

ectopic axonal activation   *22*
ectopic disruption   95

ectopic nociceptive pain   22, 23
edema   26, 65, 67–68, 72–73
efferent neural processes   129, 220
effleurage   49, 81
electromyography (EMG)
    biofeedback   228
emotional body language (EBL)   28
emotional pain   36
emotional reaction   236
endocannabinoid   116
endometritis   35
endorphins   18
entrapment neuropathies   24
epinephrine   28
epistemology   1, 4
evidence-based care   6, 8–9
evidence-based medicine (EBM)   9
evidence-informed care   8–9, 9–10
exercise   58
exteroception   246

F

false sciatica   95
fascia   56
fascia system   15
fascial balancing   95–108
Fascial Movement Taping   129
fascial release   80
fear-avoidance model   177, 237
Feldenkrais, Moshe   161, *161*
Feldenkrais Method®   11, 101,
    159–171, 235
  assessment   164–165
  case study   169–170
  history   161–162
  models based on teachings of   162
  monitoring outcomes   167
  overview   159
  strategy   165–167
    communication   165–166
    constraints   166–167
    creating safe and supportive learning
      environment   165
    education for self-care   167
    imagination   166
    reference postures and
      movements   166
    repetition   166
    rest   166
    reversibility   166
    small movements   166
  theoretical approaches to pain
    management   162–164
fibromyalgia   10, 27, 209, 221

fight-or-flight response   28, 165
focusing   81–82
frostbite   16
functional connectivity   164
Functional Integration® (FI)   159,
    160–161, 170
functional interdisciplinary care   250
Functional Rating Index   122
functional taping   127–41
  assessment   133–134
  case study   139–141
  history and overview   127
  kinesiology taping   127,
    128–129, 133
  McConnell taping   127, 128
  methodology   133–139
  theoretical approaches to pain
    management   129–130
    microcirculatory effects   130–131
    neurosensory effects   129, 130
    structural effects   131–132
  traditional athletic taping   127–128
functional technique (FT)   112, 121

G

Galen   34, 35
gastrointestinal lymphoid tissue
    (GALT)   114
Gate Control Theory (GCT)   36,
    37–39, 130
General System Theory   39
Guillain-Barre syndrome   24
Gun Fa, Rolling Technique   147, *148*

H

Haller, Nancy   168–169
hamstring tear   79
Hanna Somatic Education®   162
heroin   18
herpes zoster infections   25
high-velocity, low-amplitude (HVLA)
    thrust techniques   122
hippocampus   28
Hippocrates   34, 35, 66, 80
histamine   20, 67
HIV sensory neuropathy   24
hook-up   173, 175, 176, 177–178, 180,
    182, 183
hydrotherapy   82, 90
hyperalgesia   25
hyperthermia   147–148

hypertrophic scarring (HTS) 81–82
hypervigilance 233
hypochondriasis 233
hypothalamus 28
hypothalamus-pituitary-adrenal (HPA)
      axis 28
hypotonia 149
hysteralgia 35

I

ignoring pain 238
immunomodulatory effects 70
incidence of pain 249
individualized care team approach 252
inpatient integrative pain management
      (IPM) service 10–11
Integrated Healthcare Policy Consortium
      (IHPC) 6
integrative care 4
   multiple models of 7–8
integrative clinical care pathways 250,
      255–256
integrative health care 1, 249
   defining 5
   vs integrative medicine 6–7
   in the USA 1–5
integrative healthcare clinics 10
integrative medicine 1, 4
   defining 5
   vs integrative health care 6–10
integrative practice models 253
interdisciplinary care team 8,
      249, 252
interdisciplinary care team
      guidelines 256
   communication 256–257, 260–261
   follow through on expectation 262
   MMM guidelines for interdisciplinary
      care team 261–262
   networking for complementary
      providers 257
   opportunities 262
   patient access 262
   PCPs 257
   team expectations 261
   massage, movement and mindfulness
      approaches 257–258
   massage, movement and mindfulness
      providers 259–260
   monitoring outcomes 262
International Association for the Study of
      Pain 16
interoception 11, 233, 246
irritable bowel syndrome 221

J

Japanese orthopedic association
      (JOA) 154
joint pain 10
juvenile rheumatoid arthritis 10

K

keloid scar 81, 82, *87*
kidney Qi deficiency 152
Kinesio® Taping Method 129, 132, *133*,
      134, 136, 137–139, *140*
   self-care applications 139
Kinesio® Tex Tape 129, 134
kinesiology taping cuts 127, 134–135
   donut strip 137, *137*
   fan strip 136–137, *136*
   i-strip 134–135, *135*
   Y-strip 135–136, *135*

L

leprosy (Hansen's disease) 15
limbic system 28
lipomatosis doloros 78
Loesser's Onion Skin Theory of
      Pain 133
Loving kindness meditation (LKM) 221
low back pain (LBP) 10, 154
lumbosacral pain 116
lymph drainage therapy (LDT) 66
lymph system, anatomy *75*
lymphatic facilitation 81
lymphatic pump techniques (LPT) 114
lymphedema 65, 67–68, 73–75
lymphedema tardum 68
lymphology 66

M

macroneuromas 83
maladaptive body perception 238
mantra 194
manual lymph drainage (MLD) 66, 67,
      86, 122
manual therapies 29–30
marijuana 18
massage 10
massage licensure, US and Canada *260*

massage therapy 47–60
   cancer-related pain and 52
   case study 59–60
   clinical care process 56–58
   contemporary 50
   deep tissue massage (DTM) 50
   definition 47–48, 49
   effectiveness 52
   evaluation 58
   goals of 54–56
   history and development 48–51
   improved sleep cycle 51
   interventions and practice 57–58
   methodology 53–54
   patient interviews 50
   positioning and care 57
   research 50, 51
   self-management program 58–59
   social rejection and pain 51
   Swedish 49, 51, 54
   touch 51
   treatment plan 56
   see also massage therapy: lymphatic
      techniques; massage therapy:
      scars and pain
massage therapy: lymphatic
      techniques 65–78
   case study 76–77
   compression techniques and
      bandaging 66–67
   contraindications 72
   decongestive techniques 66
   edema vs. lymphedema 67–68
   history 66–67
   home care 66, 67
   interviews and assessments 71–72
   methodology 69–70
   self-care techniques 76
   theoretic approaches 67–69
   treatment in edema 72–73
   treatment in lymphedema 73–75
   treatment planning 70–71
massage therapy: scars and pain
      79–91
   assessment and interviews 87–88
   benefits 86–87
   case study 90–91
   complications of scar pain 83–84
   history 80–81
   methodology 87–90
   patient education and self-care
      89–90
   postoperative: cancer 85–86
   psychosocial trauma 84–85
   scar types 81–83
   sources of pain 83

Index

massage therapy: scars and
     pain (*Continued*)
   theoretical approaches 81–87
   trauma response *86*
   treatment outcomes 89
   treatment planning 88–89
mastectomy 84, 85
McConnell taping 127, 128
mechanoreceptors 128
Meige's syndrome/praecox 68
Mentastics® 173, 175, 177
meridians 150
metabolic-energy model 114–115
microneuromas 83
migraine headaches 27
migraines 95
Milroy's syndrome 68
mind-body divide 27–28, 36
mind-body integration 236–237
mind–body therapies 11, 236
mindful awareness 224
Mindful Awareness in Body-oriented
     Therapy (MABT) 235, 242, 244
mindful meditation 219, 221, 223,
     226, 236
Mindfulness-Based Childbirth and
     Parenting 220
Mindfulness-Based Cognitive Behavioral
     Therapy 220
Mindfulness-Based Functional
     Therapy 220
mindfulness-based interventions
     219–230
   clinical populations 221–223
   history of 220–221
   mechanisms 223–224
     attention regulation 223
     body awareness 223
     changes in perspective on the
        self 224
     emotional regulation 223–224
     extinction learning 223–224
     pain as sensation 223
     reappraisal 223
   methodology 224
   principles 224–225
     case study 229–230
     cognitive 225–226
     emotional 225
     group model 226, 227
     individual model 228–229
     physical 225
   theoretical approaches to pain
        management 221–224
Mindfulness-Based Living Well with Pain
     and Illness 221

Mindfulness-Based Relapse
     Prevention 220
Mindfulness-Based Stress Reduction
     (MBSR) 226, 235, 251
mirror therapy 38
morphine 18
moxibustion 150
mudras 195, *195*
Mueller Kinesiology Tape 129
Multidimensional Assessment of
     Interoceptive Awareness (MAIA)
     scale 11, 238, 239, *240–241*, 242
multidisciplinary teams 8
multi-microvacuolar collagenic absorbing
     system 99
muscle energy technique (MET) 112,
     118–120
myofascial dysfunction 86
Myofascial Release® (MFR) 54, 81, 89,
     97, 122
myotomes 95

N

National Center for Health Workforce
     Analysis 5
Neck Disability Index 122
nerve compression 24
nerve trunk pain 23
nervi nervorum 23, 95
neural correlates of consciousness
     (NCC) 51
neurological model 114
neuroma 23–24, 83
neuroma in continuity 23
neuromatrix model 38, 133
neuromodulation 18
neuromodules 38
neuropathic pain 24, 85
neuropathy 23, 86
neuroplasticity 25
NeuroStructural Taping 129
neurotransmitters 18, 31
neutral alignment 98
nidra 193, 198
niyama 188, 198
nociception 16, *17*
nociceptive pain 21–22, 85
nociceptor activation 20–21
nociceptors 16, 18–19, *21*, 31
   types of 19–20
non-steroidal anti-inflammatory drugs
     (NSAIDs) 50
norepinephrine 28

noticing 236
numbness 15
nutritional deficiency neuropathies 24

O

observational learning 40
Office of Alternative Medicine (OAM) 2, 4
onion ring model 40
open reduction and internal fixation
     (ORIF) 145
opening meridiens 146
opioids 18
opium 18
Ortho-Bionomy 122
osteoarthritis 10, 103, 116, 209
osteopathic manipulative treatment
     (OMT) 112
osteopathic techniques 111–123
   assessment 117–118
     evidence of acute and chronic
        changes 118
     fascial assessment 118
     osteopathic physical
        examination 117
     other examinations 118
     palpatory assessment 118
     regional range of motion
        testing 118
     segmental motion testing 118
     static postural examination 117
   case study 122–123
   classification of techniques
        118–122, *119*
   global practice 112–113
   history 111–113
   measurement tools 121
   methodology 116–117
   models of health 113–115
   origins 111–112
   theoretical approach to pain 115–116
Oswestry disability index (ODI) 154
oxycodone 18
oxytocin 51, 58

P

pain, definition 15, 16, 32–34
pain as part of sensory system 15–16
pain behavior 40
pain catastrophizing 237, 238
pain diary 58

pain filters, loss of   25–27
pain pathways   16–18
  modulation   17–18
  perception   17
  transduction   16–17
  transmission   17
pain relief   34–35
pain responses   27
palpation   50
Pancamaya model   189, *189*
paradigm appropriation   4
Parkinson's disease   28
Parkinson's mask   28
patient interview questionnaires   34
Patient Protection and Affordable Care
    Act (ACA) (2010)   5
patient-centered care   252–253
Patient-Centered Outcomes Research
    Institute (PCORI)   9
perception of pain   37
peripheral nerve damage   23–24
peripheral nervous system (PNS)   23
person-in-pain   31–32
petrissage   49, 81
phantom limb pain   24, 38
phantom pain   83, 85
Phoenix Rising Yoga Therapy   198
Physical Culture   174
plexopathy   86
pluralism   4
polio   47
polymodal nociceptor   20
polyneuropathy, alcoholic   24
polyradiculopathy, acute and chronic
    demyelinating   24
positional release techniques   120
positive nerve provocation tests   23
post-Cartesian models   36–37
postherpetic neuropathy   24, 25
post-mastectomy syndrome   86
post-radiation plexopathy   24
pranayama   194–195
pratyahara   197
presencing *see* hook-up
proprioception   233
prostaglandin   20
prostaglandin E   67
pruritis   80, 82
psychobehavioral model   115

Q

Qi   206
Qi Gong   236

quality of life   86
questionnaires   192

R

radiculopathy   24
radiotherapy   85
Raja yoga   187–188, 192
randomized, controlled clinical trial
    (RCT)   9
reaction, pain   37
receptive field   19
recovery expectation   238
referrals   251–252
reflex sympathetic dystrophy   26
reiki   55
relaxation exercises   58
relocating joint   147
respiratory-circulatory model   114
rheumatoid arthritis   10, 209, 210
Rock Tape   129
Rolfing (tissue mobilization) *see*
    Structural Integration
rotator cuff compression   86
rotator cuff tear   79

S

Samadhi   188
savasana   197
Scale of Body Connection (SBC)   239
scar types   81–84
  adhesions/fixations   79, 82–83, 84, 87
  cicatricial   82
  contracture   82
  formation, postoperative   79
  hypertrophic scarring (HTS)   81–82
  keloid scar   81, 82
  see also massage therapy: scars
    and pain
scoliosis   104, 105
sensory motor amnesia   180
serotonin   20, 58, 80, 85
shingles   25
sleep hygiene plan   58
Society of Trained Masseurs   49
soft tissue manipulation   145
Sounder Sleep System®   162
specificity theory   36
spinal manipulative therapy (SMT)   108
spiral line   *100*
spiritual pain   36

spirituality   34, 35
START acronym   118
straight leg test for sciatica   151
Strain-CounterStrain (SCS)   120–121
stress response systems
  hormonal reactions   28
  motor reactions   28–29
structural bodywork   95–108
  case study   108
  methodology   101–108
    global and local assessment
      methods   102–108
    global functional assessment   103
    introduction and session flow
      101–102
    soft tissue assessment at the
      table   103
    specialized orthopedic tests   103–104
    visual assessment   102–103
    weight-bearing palpation
      (WBP)   102, *102*
  theoretical approaches to pain
    management   97–101
    compensation, force transmission
      and biotensegrity   99–100
    fascial interfaces   99, *99*
    posture and awareness   98–99
    posture as neutral and non-neutral
      alignment   98
  treatment goals and strategies   104
  treatment methods   105–107
    client education   106
    client self-care   106–107
    clinical outcomes   107
    tissue mobilization   105–106
Structural Integration   95, 96–97,
    105, 107
structural relief therapy   122
Substance P   20
summation theory   36
Swedish massage   10, 49, 51, 54,
    66, 81
sympathetic adrenal medulla (SAM)   28

T

Tai Chi/Qi Gong   11, 203–215, 236
  accessing   213–215
  balancing yin and yang   206–207
  belief and outcome expectation   210
  case study   215
  history and overview   203–205
  home practice and self-care   212–213
  important principles   211–212

Index

Tai Chi/Qi Gong (*Continued*)
  meaning of   205–206
  meaning of Qi   206
  methodology   210
  mind-body exercise   205
  patient education   210
  patient safety   210
  theory and philosophy in treating
      pain   207–210
  treatment goals and strategy   211
  treatment methods   211–213
TART acronym   118
tattoo   33
Tellington Touch®   168
temporomandibular dysfunction   95
tendonitis   69
tensegrity   *100*
theories of pain
  Ancient Greek   35–36
  Early Egyptian   35–36
  historical   34–35
TheraBand™ Kinesiology Tape   129
thoracic outlet syndrome   24, 95
Tic douloureux (trigeminal neuralgia)   24
tissue dialogue   57
torticollis, congenital   150
touch, sense of   16, 61
toxic exposure neuropathies   24
traditional Chinese medicine
      (TCM)   145–156
Trager®   173–183
  case study   182–183
  changing the mind   177
  clients' responses and
      interactivity   179
  decompression somatics   182
  establishing trust   176
  finding resonance   176
  focusing and bodywork   181–182
  history   173–174
  indirect method   181
  interacting with client   179
  no pain   175
  pain management theoretical
      approaches   174–175
  pain vs suffering   181
  positional release and   180–181
  presence (hook-up)   173, 175, 176,
      177–178, 180, 182, 183
  self-care   175
  shared presence   179–180
  side-lying somatics   180

turning towards pain   178
traumatic scarring   84
trigeminal neuralgia   24
Tui Na   145
  blood circulation and   147–148
  case study   155–156
  children and   150
  diagnostic methods   151–154
    auscultation and olfaction
        151–152
    breathing   152
    coughing   152
    interrogation   152–153
    observation   151
    pulse taking and palpation   153
  endorphins and   148–149
  function of   145–147
  joints and   149
  medical services in China   150–151
  modern history of   147
  muscular hypotonia   149
  outcome measures   154–155
  related modalities   147
  self-care education   155
  stomach pain   149–150
trust   237

U

ujjayi breathing   194

V

Vancouver Scar Scale (VSS)   84
viscerotomes   95
visual analogue scale (VAS)   103, 154,
      167, *167*
Visual, Musculoskeletal, and Balance
      Complaints questionnaire   167

W

weight-bearing palpation (WBP)
      102, *102*
Western Ontario and McMaster
      Universities Arthritis Index
      (WOMAC)   103

wholism   53
withdrawal reflex, simple   27

X

Xiao Tui Na   151

Y

yamas   188, 198
Yang   146, 206
Yi Zhi Chan Tui Fa: One Finger Meditation
      Pushing Method   146, *146*
Yin   146, 206
yoga   10, 11, 96, 236
yoga therapy   187–200
  assessment techniques   192–193
  case study   198–200
  hands-on adjustments and physical
      treatments   197–198
  history of   187–189
  methodology   191–192
  objective assessment
      components   193
  outcome measures   198
  pain recovery mode: self-care
      complex   *191*
  subjective assessment   192
  theoretical approaches to pain
      management   189–191
  therapy techniques for pain
      192-7

Z

Snafu organs   150
zero balancing   122